MEDICAL RADIOLOGY
Radiation Oncology

Editors:
L. W. Brady, Philadelphia
H.-P. Heilmann, Hamburg
M. Molls, Munich
C. Nieder, Bodø

P. Rubin · L. S. Constine
L. B. Marks · P. Okunieff (Eds.)

CURED II · LENT
Cancer Survivorship Research and Education
Late Effects on Normal Tissues

With Contributions by

M. J. Adams · M. S. Anscher · L. Baker · M. Bishop-Jodoin · W. Bosch · J. Boyett
D. J. Brenner · M. G. Cicchetti · R. Comis · L. S. Constine · J. Deasy · A. Eisbruch
T. J. FitzGerald · D. L. Friedman · P. R. Graves · J. S. Greenberger · C. A. Hahn
D. E. Hallahan · R. Hanusik · J. L. Hubbs · G. Ibbott · S. Kessel · M. Knopp
A. Konski · L. Kun · F. Laurie · S. E. Lipshultz · B. Lu · L. B. Marks · K. McCarten
J. Matthews · R. Mikkelsen · M. T. Milano · B. Mittal · L. Moretti
K. M. Mustian · J. Nam · H. Nelson · P. Okunieff · D. Ota · M. Parliament
R. Pieters · J. Purdy · U. Ramamurthy · G. Reaman · N. Rosen · B. S. Rosenstein
P. Rubin · J. Saltz · R. Schilsky · M. Schnall · L. Schwartz · R. G. Schwartz
A. Sharma · I. Shuryak · E. Siegel · L. B. Travis · K. Ulin · M. Urie · S. Voss
Z. Vujaskovic · K. White · J. P. Williams · E. S. Yang · J. Yorty · S. Zhou

Foreword by

L. W. Brady, H.-P. Heilmann, M. Molls, and C. Nieder

With 39 Figures in 62 Separate Illustrations, 42 in Color and 25 Tables

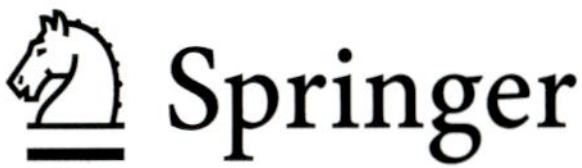

Philip Rubin, MD
Professor Emeritus
Chair Emeritus
Department of Radiation Oncology
University of Rochester
School of Medicine and Dentistry
601 Elmwood Avenue, Box 647
Rochester, NY 14642
USA

Louis S. Constine, MD
Professor of Radiation Oncology and Pediatrics
Vice Chair, Department of Radiation Oncology
James P. Wilmot Cancer Center
University of Rochester
School of Medicine and Dentistry
601 Elmwood Avenue, Box 704
Rochester, NY 14642
USA

Lawrence B. Marks, MD
Professor and Chair
Department of Radiation Oncology
University of North Carolina at Chapel Hill
Campus Box 7512
Chapel Hill, NC 27599
USA
and
Duke University Medical Center
P.O. Box 3085
Durham, NC 27710
USA

Paul Okunieff, MD
Philip Rubin Professor of Radiation Oncology
Chair, Department of Radiation Oncology
University of Rochester
School of Medicine and Dentistry
601 Elmwood Avenue, Box 647
Rochester, NY 14642
USA

Medical Radiology · Diagnostic Imaging and Radiation Oncology
Series Editors:
A. L. Baert · L. W. Brady · H.-P. Heilmann · M. Knauth · M. Molls · C. Nieder

Continuation of Handbuch der medizinischen Radiologie
Encyclopedia of Medical Radiology

ISBN 978-3-540-76270-6   e-ISBN 978-3-540-76271-3

DOI 10.1007 / 978-3-540-76271-3

Medical Radiology · Diagnostic Imaging and Radiation Oncology ISSN 0942-5373

Library of Congress Control Number: 2008920292

Cover Design and Layout: PublishingServices Teichmann, 69256 Mauer, Germany
Printed on acid-free paper
9 8 7 6 5 4 3 2 1
springer.com

Dedications

Dedication to Joel Tepper for CURED II meeting

Joel E. Tepper: Dedicated scholar, teacher, physician and leader

Joel was born in Brooklyn, soon after WWII, making him one of the earliest baby boomers. He grew up in Massachusetts and attended college at the Massachusetts Institute of Technology, where he studied electrical engineering. He went on to medical school at Washington University in St. Louis, graduating in 1972. Joel did his medical internship at Presbyterian-St. Luke's in Chicago.

He continued his training as a resident and fellow in Radiation Medicine at the Massachusetts General Hospital. There, he had the good fortune to train under many giants in our field, including Herman Suit and C.C. Wang. There, he started what would prove to be his very prolific career as an author, penning many manuscripts, including several dealing with the initial world-wide experience with proton beam radiation therapy. Following training, Joel served as the Chief of Radiation Therapy at the Malcolm Grow Air Force Medical Center. Joel then spent several years as a senior investigator at the National Cancer Institute, and had the good fortune to work with Eli Glatsein, Tim Kinsella, Allen Lichter, Steve Rosenberg, Jim Mitchell, Liz Travis, and many other talented investigators. There, he gained experience with intra-operative radiation therapy techniques, gastrointestinal cancers and soft tissue sarcomas.

Joel returned to MGH in 1981. During the subsequent six years, he further developed his expertise in several areas including intra-operative radiation therapy, soft tissue sarcoma, and most notably gastrointestinal malignancies. He rapidly became one the nation's experts in the care of patients with gastrointestinal malignancies, and in the use of combined modality therapy. He is at present Principal Investigator of the UNC GI SPORE grant, a prestigious NCI translational research award that spans many departments within the medical school.

In 1987, Joel moved to the University of North Carolina at Chapel Hill to become Professor and Chairman of the Department of Radiation Oncology. During the subsequent 20 years at UNC, Joel has proved to be a dedicated scholar, physician teacher, and leader.

As a scholar, Joel has authored over 150 publications on a wide array of topics, and has conducted numerous clinical trials. Through these efforts, Joel has helped to define the optimal treatment for most GI malignancies. His broad expertise is evident by his work as the founding editor of Seminars in Radiation Oncology, and his authorship of several books. His expertise extends well beyond radiation oncology, as he has helped to lead efforts to better define the roles of surgery, chemotherapy and radiation in GI malignancies. He is a true oncologist.

As a physician teacher, Joel has strived to provide outstanding care for many patients-both through his direct interactions with patients, and through his educational and scholarly activities. He has lectured extensively throughout the world, helping to spread knowledge to others. He has helped to organize numerous education conferences, such as being co-Director for three years of the ASCO/AACR Vail Conference on Clinical Trial Methodology, and has mentored countless residents, students and young faculty. Through these efforts, Joel has helped to train a generation of physicians and leaders in our field.

Joel's most impressive accomplishments lie in the realm of leadership where he has applied his skills in a broad array of local, national and international capacities. At UNC, in addition to serving as Chairman of the Department of Radiation Oncology, he served as an Associate Director of the Lineberger Cancer Center, and has held many leadership/administrative positions within the UNC Health System.

Nationally and internationally, Joel has served the greater oncology community on multiple levels. He served on countless ASTRO, ASCO, CALBG, AACR committees. Most notably, he is the chair of the NCI GI-Intergroup (GI Steering Committee), is on the ASCO Board of Directors, and has served as ASTRO President from 2002 – 2003, and subsequently as ASTRO Chairman of the Board. Through these many efforts, he has been a strong advocate for the fields of oncology, radiation oncology, and, most importantly, patients with cancer. His outstanding service to our field was recognized by his nomination to the first class of ASTRO Fellows in November, 2006.

Joel and his wife Laurie are active in the local Durham Chapel Hill Jewish community- serving on various committees to help the community at large. Joel is fortunate to have two daughters and three grandchildren.

Perhaps one of the most humbling aspects of reviewing Joel's outstanding career is the recognition that he has done all of this despite serious personal challenges. It is with great admiration and respect that the CURED II meeting, and this publication, is dedicated to the career and accomplishments of Dr. Joel E. Tepper.

LAWRENCE B. MARKS

Foreword

The evolution of treatment programs for cancer has been predicated on the safe intensification of radiation therapy, chemotherapy, and biologic adjuvants. The emphasis on combined integrative multimodal programs of management have led to markedly increased survivorship, which now exceeds 64% overall, and is much higher for selected malignancies, such as 87% for breast cancer and 80% for all childhood cancers combined.

Combined integrative multimodal programs of management are more aggressive in character and often miss the potential risk of normal tissue reactions or tolerance. This past emphasis has led to increased efforts to prevent or avoid normal tissue damage during combined modality treatment and to manage and rehabilitate affected patients. This requires understanding of tissue tolerances to treatment and dealing effectively with not only early but also late effects on normal tissues. Concomitant with this requirement is the need to follow the patients carefully for years after completion of treatment. Late effects may not occur early but may occur long after the cessation of treatment. This balance requires understanding of the maximum potential of benefit versus decreasing the potential for toxicity from the treatment.

The second volume on late effects in normal tissues by Rubin et al. is an important statement with regards to early and late effects from radiation therapy, as well as from combined therapy. It contributes significantly to the basic understanding of the problem, the need for long-term follow-up, and the criteria by which one would identify and treat the early and late effects of treatment. The volume represents a significant contribution in this field of endeavor.

Philadelphia   LUTHER W. BRADY
Hamburg   HANS-PETER HEILMANN
Munich   MICHAEL MOLLS
Bodø   CARSTEN NIEDER

Introduction

Multimodal treatment is the hallmark for the rising success of cancer cure rates. The more aggressive the treatment delivery in terms of dose, time and volume for radiation and chemotherapy, the more adverse effects in normal tissues can be anticipated. The major paradigm shift is to be aware of the new focus of cancer survivorship; that is to say, the promise of prolonging life means that quality of life needs to be maintained. The life worth saving must be worth living. The issues that need to be addressed can be stated succinctly. The new definition of a cancer survivor is not 5 years cancer free survival, but begins at Day 0, before treatment is initiated.

Anatomy is foremost for the radiation oncologist to focus upon with our new sophisticated techniques of intensity modulated radiation treatment (IMRT) and image-guided radiation treatment (IGRT). The ability to concentrate and increase the tumor dose is at the price of exposing surrounding normal tissues to significant radiation doses. Although such normal tissue radiation doses are well within tolerance, any radiation dose to a normal tissue is above threshold. Restated, radiation (and chemotherapy) use up the mitotic potential of a normal tissue, accelerate senescence, and cause mutations and genome instability that in time may be expressed as a second malignant tumor (SMT). Collateral unintended damage is inevitable in surrounding neighboring sites as rotational techniques focus on the tumor volume. Our highly refined computerized technology-driven radiation delivery systems concentrate high tumor doses on target; however, the anatomic sites in the immediate neighboring environment are also irradiated. Thus, the gross, clinical, and planning tumor volumes (GTV, CTV, PTV) expressed as a series of repetitive contours need to be replaced by the in situ normal tissues contents. Our physics, not our biology, has created the illusion of a selective effect in our ability to ablate cancers by heightening doses beyond 50–60 Gy to smaller tumor volumes. However, there is a parallel need to concentrate on the normal tissue volumes (NTV) being simultaneously exposed (Rubin CURED I). These fall into three categories and each deserves to be carefully assessed. They are expressed in terms of TNM cancer nomenclature:

NT are normal tissues inside the Tumor volumes GTV, CTV, PTV.

NN are normal tissues in Neighboring sites in the same transverse axial planes outside the CTV.

NM are normal tissues in more reMote systemic sites and receive scattered radiation from leakage to the whole body.

NTV: The normal tissue sites within the GTV, CTV, PTV that receive doses approaching or exceeding tolerance doses, i.e., 50–60 Gy

NNV: The neighboring normal tissue volumes surrounding the cancer that receive below tolerance doses that are well above the threshold, i.e., >10 Gy.

NMV: The more remote systemic tissues that receive minimal doses that reside in creating genomic instability and mutate chromosomal DNA, i.e., >1 Gy

Biology of the biocontinuum is essential to comprehend the complexity of molecular, subcellular mitochondrial components, nuclear DNA and cytoplasmic RNA and protein messengers triggered by all modalities, i.e., radiation, chemotherapy, and surgery. Each mode releases a microarray of molecular events resulting in a perpetual cascade of cytokines and chemokines that are the paracrine, autocrine, and endocrine messages amongst cells in normal tissues. The multimodal treatment causes normal tissues to respond both to subtolerance high doses and to above threshold lower doses beyond the range of target tumor volumes. Embedded in normal tissues that constitute organs are a large variety of cells that fall into five major categories: the parenchymal stem cell, the endothelial cell or vascular component, the fibroblast (cyte), the macrophage, lymphocyte, in the interstitium and then unique mature functioning parenchymal cells, critical to its structure and physiology. Microstructure as to tissue organization is as essential as the anatomy's macrostructure to complete the picture of events triggered by cancer treatments.

Biocontinuum refers to the sequence of ongoing events once a normal tissue or organ is perturbed by radiation chemotherapy. Rubin and Casarett's paradigm of the continuing effect in normal tissue(s) over time is built on a number of key premises:

Radiation doses that exceed the tolerance will be expressed differently over time depending on the tissue's cell kinetics, i.e., fast, slow, or no cell renewal.

There is no latent period histologically in that cellular changes always precede clinical manifestations.

There is the persistence of the memory of the radiation and compensatory mechanisms of cell regeneration or cell repopulation determining the severity of the ultimate injury expressed clinically.

There is an acceleration of the aging process expressed by the slope of cellular depletion, tissue atrophy, or the organ's senescence that is altered by radiation (dose, time, volume factors).

Another injurious event by any form of trauma (surgery) or drugs (chemotherapy) can be additive or synergistic and alter the aging slope in time uncovering radiation residual damage, i.e., recall reaction.

Co-morbidities such as infection, hypertension, diabetes, and obesity can contribute to the slope of the senescing tissues and accelerate the late effect earlier.

Common Toxicity Criteria (CTC) have been applied to assess the quality of survival as applied to cancer patient long-term survivorship. In the 1950s, the concept of late effects was considered unique to radiation. However, over the past two decades the Common Toxicity Criteria scales initially applied to chemotherapy's acute adverse events (v1.0). Since late changes due to drugs were not recognized until years later, v2.0 incorporated radiation acute toxicity, and, more recently, in v3.0 incorporated radiation's late toxicity, by recognizing that these criteria were equally applicable to chemotherapy. It is with the creation of the Office of Cancer Survivorship at NCI that long-term effects of chemotherapy were recognized as indistinguishable from late effects. It is with the publication of IOM/NRC "Cancer Survivor to Cancer Patient, Lost in Transition" that late effects are being listed and are applicable to all cancer treatment modalities.

There is a price to pay for being a cancer survivor, but one needs to be a long-term cure to have a late effect.

Rochester	PHILIP RUBIN
Rochester	LOUIS S. CONSTINE
Durham	LAWRENCE B. MARKS
Rochester	PAUL OKUNIEFF

Contents

CONCURED:

Defining the Leading Edge in Research of Adverse Effects of Treatment for Adult-Onset Cancers

LOIS B. TRAVIS

CONTENTS

1.1 Introduction

The number of cancer survivors in the United States has tripled since 1971, and is growing by 2% each year [1]. The burgeoning number of patients reflects improvements in early detection, supportive care, and therapy. In 2003, there were an estimated 10.5 million cancer survivors, representing 3.5% of the US population [2]. Among all cancer patients, the 5-year relative survival rate is now almost 66% [2]. Given the increasing survival after a cancer diagnosis, identification and quantification of the late effects of cancer and its therapy have become critical.

L. B. TRAVIS, MD, ScD
1275 East First Avenue, #159, New York, NY 10065, USA

Further, this growing and heterogeneous population provides important opportunities for clinical and epidemiologic research into cancer biology, long-term treatment effects, and prevention. In November 2004, the National Cancer Institute sponsored a workshop, whose major objective was to provide perspective on the research agenda, design considerations, and infrastructure needed to understand the underlying genetic mechanisms of late neoplastic effects in cancer survivors and thus, to facilitate the development of evidence-based long-term management and intervention strategies. Participants represented a group of experts in the fields of epidemiology, statistics, molecular genetics, clinical genetics, pharmacogenomics, informatics, radiation biology, medical oncology, pediatric oncology, and radiation oncology, and the advocacy community. Workshop proceedings were published as a Commentary in [3]. Although the focus of the workshop was second primary cancers, given the high associated mortality [4–6], participants emphasized that most of the infrastructural and design approaches that support research in this area also provide a sound basis for the study of other important physiologic late effects and psychosocial concerns in cancer survivors [7].

1.2 Research Infrastructure for Studies of Cancer Survivorship

Recommendations of the NCI-sponsored workshop are reproduced in Table 1.1. First, there was a high level of enthusiasm for the establishment of a multi-center cancer survivor cohort derived from large institutions [3]. The advantages of such a cancer survivorship coalition, as now realized by the Consortium for Cancer Research and Education

Table 1.1. Workshop recommendations for future research: genetic susceptibility and second primary cancers (modified from [3])

Develop research infrastructure for studies of cancer survivorship	**Promote the development of new technology, bioinformatics, and biomarkers**
• Institute a systematic, national approach to develop research infrastructure for studies of genetic modifiers of late effects of cancer treatment, including second malignancies • Provide for rigorous ascertainment of multiple primary cancers with clinical annotation, detailed treatment data, and biospecimen collection • Establish multicenter cohorts of cancer survivors, with recruitment of trans-disciplinary research teams dedicated to research the late effects of therapy • Expand the capacity of National Cancer Institute cooperative groups to ascertain and study long-term outcomes in clinical trial populations, in support of survivorship research	• Identify new technologies for the analysis of germline and somatic genetic alterations to determine their contributions to second cancer risk • Reduce the amount of tissue and DNA needed for various assays, with standardization of protocols for whole genome amplification • Develop molecular profiles of tumors that incorporate analyses of etiologic pathways and therapeutic targets related to second cancers and other late outcomes
Create a coordinated system for biospecimen collection	**Support the development of new epidemiologic methods**
• Standardize biospecimen collection, laboratory procedures, and documentation for blood and other DNA sources, normal tissue from target organs, and tumor tissue • Develop a centralized biospecimen repository or a tracking system ("virtual repository") to permit sample retrieval from multiple storage centers. Institute mechanisms for scientific review of specimen use and administrative procedures for specimen control • Support methodologic research to enhance the quality and lower the cost of biospecimen collection, processing, storage, and distribution	• Develop efficient epidemiologic study designs to investigate the role of genetic susceptibility to multiple primary cancers, including genetic modifiers of risk associated with treatment effects or other etiologic factors • Develop optimal approaches for selection of controls for case-control studies in which both treatment and genetic susceptibility play important roles • Include a biospecimen component in all study designs
	Develop evidence-based clinical practice guidelines
	• Implement pilot studies of interventions to prevent second cancers within genetically defined, high-risk groups of patients • Integrate smoking cessation programs into research designs • Support research to provide evidence-based follow-up care for cancer survivors

(CONCURED), are numerous. In institutions which comprise CONCURED, the status of cancer patients is usually updated routinely through hospital-based tumor registries. Detailed information with regard to cancer diagnosis and exposure data (radiation therapy and chemotherapy) is available and of high quality. Even though a number of cancer centers have independently initiated their own cancer survivorship programs, as reviewed in TRAVIS et al. [3], NCI workshop participants foresaw that only a coalition of centers would have sufficient statistical power to serve as a platform for additional research into late effects, in particular gene-environment interactions. CONCURED represents the first step in the realization of the vision published in 2006 [3]. The success of this collaborative approach is already reflected in the investigation by KLEM et al. [8] examining features of breast cancer after Hodgkin lymphoma. In this study, a total of 264 patients with second primary breast cancer was assembled from numerous, collaborating institutions across the US. In contrast, in the largest previous study to date, an international effort among population-based cancer registries, was required to assemble 105 women who developed breast cancer after being treated for HL at age 30 or less [9].

As pointed out by participants at the 2004 NCI-sponsored workshop, CONCURED can also serve as the source of patient subcohorts that are selected based on eligibility criteria that enrich populations for those at high risk of late effects. Such criteria include specific cancer treatments previously demonstrated to carry a high risk of second cancers (e.g., high-dose, extended-field radiation therapy for Hodgkin lymphoma [10]; long-term, high cumulative doses of alkylating agents [11, 12]; a specific clinical phenotype at the time of the first cancer diagnosis that might elevate the risk of treatment-related cancer (e.g., nevoid basal cell carcinoma syndrome); the presence of field effects in normal tissues that represent an increased risk; or specific genetic traits). CONCURED might serve as a study base to examine the potential risk of second cancers and other late effects associated with newer treatment modalities such as intensity-modulated radiotherapy (IMRT) [13], with the prospective identification and follow-up of patients. Importantly, CONCURED should also have sufficient statistical power to examine the under-studied area of the influence of race and ethnicity in the susceptibility to late effects of cancer treatment, as reviewed at the May 2007 meeting [14].

1.3
A Platform for Studies of Gene–Environment Interactions

Two of the five major recommendations put forth by participants in the 2004 NCI-sponsored workshop [3] were directed to the creation of a coordinated, multi-center system for biospecimen collection and the promotion of the development of new technology, bioinformatics, and biomarkers, respectively (Table 1.1). In this regard, it was noted that an infrastructure based on large cancer centers also provided the advantage that biologic specimens (peripheral blood and tumor and normal tissue from target organ) could be prospectively collected from cancer patients at presentation. This is in contrast to other cohort sources, such as population-based cancer registries, in which available specimens must be requested from constituent hospitals and laboratories, who typically store only archived paraffin-embedded tissues. The limitation of single cancer center studies to date has been the relatively small sample size; it was recognized by participants in the 2004 NCI-sponsored workshop [3] that only a multi-center effort would have sufficient statistical power to address the role of gene-environment interactions in the late effects of treatment. Thus, the vision outlined by NCI workshop participants included the establishment of programs at multiple centers using common infrastructure, common data collection instruments, and common state-of-the-art biospecimen collection, processing, storage, and distribution systems, in support of hypothesis-generating and hypothesis-testing research, with a goal of the identification of those genetic characteristics that might make cancer survivors especially susceptible to treatment-related second cancers [3]. This type of comprehensive approach to biobanking is another goal of CONCURED, and at the recent meeting, several proposals which address the issue of gene–environment interactions in the role of late effects were presented [15, 16].

1.4
Development of Epidemiologic Methods and Predictive Models

In the NCI-sponsored workshop, the use of a large survivorship network to serve as the study base for the development of new epidemiologic methods was discussed (Table 1.1) [3]. The application of traditional cohort and nested case-control designs to studies of treatment-related second primary cancers was recently reviewed [17], with both designs applicable to the study of other late effects. However, whereas standard methods have proven highly effective in defining dose–response relations between treatment and adverse outcomes, new analytic paradigms are needed to explore gene–environment and gene–gene interactions [18]. For case-control studies, these include counter-matching on therapy in studies where both treatment and genetic susceptibility may play important roles [18]. In general, new types of hypothesis-generating models and customized research methods are needed to more efficiently study the various determinants of second cancers and other late effects.

There is an increasing emphasis on the development of predictive models for the occurrence of the adverse sequelae of treatment. Travis et al. [19] recently published estimates of the cumulative absolute risk of breast cancer 10, 20, and 30 years after treatment for HL according to various dose categories of mantle radiotherapy and the administration of alkylating agents. As emphasized in an accompanying editorial by Longo [20], these types of risk estimates, which are easily communicated to patients, would be optimal for all adverse outcomes of cancer treatment. Already in CONCURED, proposals are being considered to predict the risk of second cancers comparing photon megavoltage IMRT versus conformal proton treatment [21].

1.5
Evidence-Based Clinical Practice Guidelines

The implications for research opportunities in large cohorts of cancer survivors also include the provision of definitive recommendations for evidence-based care and cost-effective strategies for patient follow-up [3] (Table 1.1). Pilot studies of interventions to prevent or ameliorate the risk of late effects can also be undertaken. Thus, as part of the CONCURED effort, NG et al. [22] present a progress report of the effectiveness of breast MRI screening in female survivors of HL. Moreover, a new proposal to examine the feasibility of using chest CT to screen for lung cancer in survivors of HL who smoke was discussed by NG, given the multiplicative interaction reported between either chest radiotherapy or alkylating agent treatment for HL and tobacco use and subsequent lung cancer risk [23, 24].

At the CONCURED meeting, a proposal to screen for second cancers of the gastrointestinal tract in survivors of HL who received pelvic and abdominal irradiation was also evaluated [25]. Based on additional analyses of the results of an international study by HODGSON et al. [26], a cumulative risk of 20% for colorectal cancer in HL patients over 50 years of age was predicted. Thus, the rationale for such a feasibility study seems well-founded.

Whether long-term cardiovascular complications in survivors of HL can be ameliorated by exercise may also be explored in other CONCURED research endeavors [27]. Already, a greater survival has been shown in physically active breast cancer survivors with high vegetable-fruit intake regardless of obesity [28]. Thus, the application of interventions such as lifestyle modifications in cancer survivors holds great promise, and deserves further study.

1.6

A Trans-disciplinary Approach

The successful establishment of effective trans-disciplinary cancer survivorship programs requires the attention of dedicated clinical and research teams [3]. For example, in the Living Well After Cancer Program (www.pennhealth.com), a multidisciplinary team of clinicians (including medical oncologists, radiation oncologists, clinical oncology nurse practitioners, nutritionists, cardiologists, cancer rehabilitation specialists, psychiatrists, and psychologists) and researchers (including those with expertise in genomics, cancer biology, biostatistics, epidemiology, and behavioral science) integrate the clinical and research arms of the program. An institutional review board-approved clinical research protocol follows data on symptoms, follow-up, and quality of life; provides feedback to health care providers regarding these problems in individual patients; and manages the recruitment of patients into studies. Participants at the 2004 NCI-sponsored workshop [3] emphasized the importance of dedicated survivorship staff and the need to budget for the costs of screening, etc. in developing these resources.

Comment

In 2005, the Institute of Medicine and the National Research Council of the National Academies issued a report, *From Cancer Patient to Cancer Survivor: Lost in Transition* [29]. Indeed, one chapter of this report was devoted to survivorship research, and emphasized the need to study large number of patients who survive their cancers for many years. The report pointed out that sample sizes should also be large enough to include individuals who will manifest unusual late sequelae. As did participants at the 2004 NCI-sponsored Workshop [3], the report stated that one mechanism to accrue large numbers of cancer survivors who represent the diversity of the US is to conduct multi-institutional collaborative research [29]. Thus, CONCURED represents in part the realization of the research component of the IOM report. Until the results of research undertaken in large survivorship programs are available, scientific progress over the last few decades has made it possible nonetheless to identify selected treatment regimens which are associated with exceptionally high risks of late effects. Although individual susceptibility factors remain largely unknown, groups of exposed patients can still be selected for close monitoring. Whenever effective screening methods (e.g., mammographic examination) are available, these should be included in patient follow-up. Preventive strategies (e.g., smoking cessation, avoidance of ultraviolet light) may also diminish the risk of selected late effects, and cancer survivors should be encouraged to adopt practices consistent with a healthy lifestyle. Even though cancer treatment represents a double-edged sword, it should be kept in mind that many treatments have been accompanied by sizable improvements in patient survival. Thus, the benefits associated with many cancer treatments greatly exceed the risk of developing adverse effects. Further, it should always be kept in mind that the late adverse effects of cancer and its treatment may not necessarily be attributable to prior therapy, but also reflect the effect of shared etiologic factors, environmental exposures, host characteristics, patient co-morbidities, underlying hepatic and renal function, lifestyle factors and combinations of influences, including gene–environment and gene–gene interactions [30]. Research undertaken in large well-constructed cohorts of survivors, such as CONCURED, should be able to clarify the roles of these various influences on the risk of late effects, identify genetically susceptible populations, and also provide the basis for evidence-based prevention and intervention efforts.

Acknowledgement

I am indebted to Ms. Janice Chau for editorial support.

References

1. Anonymous [No authors listed] (2004) Cancer survivors: living longer, and now, better [editorial]. Lancet 364:2153–2154
2. Ries L, Eisner M, Kosary C, Hankey B, Miller B, Clegg L et al (2006) SEER cancer statistics review. 1975–2003. National Cancer Institute, Bethesda
3. Travis LB, Rabkin CS, Brown LM, Allan JM, Alter BP, Ambrosone CB, Begg CB, Caporaso N, Chanock S, DeMichele A et al (2006) Cancer survivorship – genetic susceptibility and second primary cancers: research strategies and recommendations. J Natl Cancer Inst 98:15–25
4. Hoppe RT (1997) Hodgkin's disease: complications of therapy and excess mortality. Ann Oncol 8[Suppl 1]:115–118
5. Dores G, Schonfeld S, Chen J, Hodgson D, Fosså S, Gilbert E et al (2005) Long-term cause-specific mortality among 41–146 one-year survivors of Hodgkin lymphoma (HL). Proc Am Soc Clin Oncol 23:562S
6. Mauch PM, Kalish LA, Marcus KC, Shulman LN, Krill E, Tarbell NJ, Silver B, Weinstein H, Come S, Canellos GP et al (1995) Long-term survival in Hodgkin's disease. Cancer J Sci Am 1:33
7. Aziz NM (2002) Cancer survivorship research: challenge and opportunity. J Nutr 132[11 Suppl]:3494S–3503S
8. Klem ML (2008) The characteristics and management of breast cancer in Hodgkin lymphoma survivors. Personal communication at CURED III LENT meeting, Rochester, NY, in May 2008
9. Travis LB, Hill DA, Dores GM, Gospodarowicz M, Van Leeuwen FE, Holowaty E, Glimelius B, Andersson M, Wiklund T, Lynch CF et al (2003) Breast cancer following radiotherapy and chemotherapy among young women with Hodgkin disease. JAMA 290:465–475
10. Ng AK, Bernardo MV, Weller E, Backstrand K, Silver B, Marcus KC, Tarbell NJ, Stevenson MA, Friedberg JW, Mauch PM (2002) Second malignancy after Hodgkin disease treated with radiation therapy with or without chemotherapy: long-term risks and risk factors. Blood 100:1989–1996
11. Greene MH, Harris EL, Gershenson DM, Malkasian GD Jr, Melton LJ 3ʳᵈ, Dembo AJ, Bennett JM, Moloney WC, Boice JD Jr (1986) Melphalan may be a more potent leukemogen than cyclophosphamide. Ann Intern Med 105:360–367
12. Travis LB, Curtis RE, Stovall M, Holowaty EJ, Van Leeuwen FE, Glimelius B, Lynch CF, Hagenbeek A, Li CY, Banks PM et al (1994) Risk of leukemia following treatment for non-Hodgkin's lymphoma. J Natl Cancer Inst 86:1450–1457
13. Hall EJ, Wuu CS (2003) Radiation-induced second cancers: the impact of 3D-CRT and IMRT. Int J Radiat Oncol Biol Phys 56:83–88
14. Wynn RB (2008) The influence of race in the susceptibility to late effects following cancer therapy. Personal communication at CURED III LENT meeting, Rochester, NY, in May 2008
15. Rosenstein BS (2008) Association between single nucleotide polymorphisms and susceptibility for the development of adverse effects resulting from radiation therapy. In: Rubin P et al. (Eds) CURED II · LENT. Springer, Berlin Heidelberg pp 25–34
16. Friedman DL (2008) Risk factors for second malignancies following stem cell transplant. In: Rubin P et al. (Eds) CURED II · LENT. Springer, Berlin Heidelberg pp 155–162
17. Travis LB (2004) Second cancers: methods and recent results among patients with Hodgkin lymphoma. Proc Am Soc Clin Oncol pp 425–433
18. Bernstein JL, Langholz B, Haile RW, Bernstein L, Thomas DC, Stovall M, Malone KE, Lynch CF, Olsen JH, Anton-Culver H et al (2004) Study design: evaluating gene–environment interactions in the etiology of breast cancer – the WECARE study. Breast Cancer Res 6:R199–214
19. Travis LB, Hill D, Dores GM, Gospodarowicz M, van Leeuwen FE, Holowaty E, Glimelius B, Andersson M, Pukkala E, Lynch CF et al (2005) Cumulative absolute breast cancer risk for young women treated for Hodgkin lymphoma. J Natl Cancer Inst 97:1428–1437
20. Longo DL (2005) Radiation therapy in Hodgkin disease: why risk a Pyrrhic victory? J Natl Cancer Inst 97:1394–1395
21. Brenner DJ, Shuryak I (2008) Prospective second-cancer risk estimation for contemporary radiotherapeutic protocols. In: Rubin P et al. (Eds) CURED II · LENT. Springer, Berlin Heidelberg pp 33–40
22. Ng AK (2008) Breast cancer screening for second malignant tumors in Hodgkin lymphoma survivors. Personal communication at CURED III LENT meeting, Rochester, NY, in May 2008
23. Travis LB, Gospodarowicz M, Curtis RE, Clarke A, Andersson M, Glimelius B, et al (2002) Lung cancer following chemotherapy and radiotherapy for Hodgkin's disease. J Natl Cancer Inst 94:182–192
24. Gilbert ES, Stovall M, Gospodarowicz M, Van Leeuwen FE, Andersson M, Glimelius B, Joensuu T, Lynch CF, Curtis RE, Holowaty E et al (2003) Lung cancer after treatment for Hodgkin's disease: focus on radiation effects. Radiat Res 159:161–173
25. Hodgson DC (2008) Screening for second malignant tumors in the gastrointestinal tract in patients irradiated for Hodgkin lymphoma. Personal communication at CURED III LENT meeting, Rochester, NY, in May 2008
26. Hodgson DC, Gilbert ES, Dores GM, Schonfeld SJ, Lynch CF, Storm H, Hall P, Langmark F, Pukkala E, Andersson

M et al (2007) Long-term solid cancer risk among 5-year survivors of Hodgkin's lymphoma. J Clin Oncol 25:1489–1497

27. Mustian KM, Adams J, Schwartz RG, Lipshultz SE, Constine LS (2008) Cardiotoxic Effects of Radiation Therapy in Hodgkin's Lymphoma and Breast Cancer Survivors and the Potential Mitigating Effects of Exercise. In: Rubin P et al. (Eds) CURED II · LENT. Springer, Berlin Heidelberg pp 103–116

28. Pierce JP, Stefanick ML, Flatt SW, Natarajan L, Sternfeld B, Madlensky L, Al-Delaimy WK, Thomson CA, Kealey S, Hajek R (2007) Greater survival after breast cancer in physically active women with high vegetable-fruit intake regardless of obesity. J Clin Oncol 25:2345–2351

29. Hewitt M, Grenfield S, Stovall E (2005) From cancer patient to cancer survivor: lost in transition. Committee on Cancer survivorship: improving care and quality of life, IoMaNRC (ed). National Academies Press, Washington, DC, p 536

30. Travis LB (2002) Therapy-associated solid tumors. Acta Oncol 41:323-333

Bioimaging In Vivo to Discern the Evolution of Late Effects Temporally and Spatially

Jessica L. Hubbs, Jiho Nam, Sumin Zhou, Carol A. Hahn, and Lawrence B. Marks

CONTENTS

Summary

- Imaging is a powerful tool for measuring regional radiation-induced normal tissue changes, independent of radiation volumes.
- Several functional imaging tools (e.g., single photon emission computed tomography [SPECT], positron emission tomography [PET], and magnetic resonance imaging [MRI]), have been used to monitor radiation-induced injury in a variety of different tissues, including the lung, heart, brain, liver, and salivary glands.
- The degree/extent of changes in regional imaging may be associated with changes in global organ function (e.g., clinical symptoms) at various time points.

J. L. Hubbs, MS; J. Nam, MD; L. B. Marks, MD
Department of Radiation Oncology, University of North Carolina at Chapel Hill, Campus Box 7512, Chapel Hill, NC 27599, USA
S. Zhou, PhD; C. A. Hahn, MD
Department of Radiation Oncology, Duke University Medical Center, Box 3085, Durham, NC 27710, USA

Introduction

The utility of radiotherapy (RT) in cancer management is based on the premise that treatment will cause greater damage to tumor than to surrounding normal tissue. Thus, the risks of normal tissue toxicity largely determine the dose and volume used clinically.

Normal tissue injury encompasses a wide range of effects with varying clinical impact, depending on treatment site and organ of interest. Further, the acceptability of RT-induced morbidities changes over time as treatment techniques evolve. If we are successful in our goals to cure more patients of their cancers, late normal tissue effects will become of greater concern. It is critical that improvements in therapies maximize both cure and quality of life (QOL).

Normal tissue injury can be expressed in several ways (Table 2.1), and the reported frequency of "injury" depends on the endpoint chosen.

The current review addresses functional imaging as a means to assess regional RT-induced normal tissue injury. Functional imaging allows for the early detection and quantification of subclinical regional injury, and is a powerful tool in this area of study.

Table 2.1. Example of different endpoints that can be used to study RT-induced injury, organized on the basis of objective vs. subjective and regional vs. global assessments

	Objective	Subjective
Regional	Imaging (e.g., CT-defined increases in tissue density)	Pain from local ulceration
Global	Creatinine clearance, pulmonary function tests	Shortness of breath, fatigue

A variety of imaging modalities have been used, including PET, SPECT, CT, and MRI. We herein review organ sites with the most available data on functional imaging and clinical endpoints: lung, heart, liver, brain, and salivary glands.

2.2
Lung Injury

Symptomatic pulmonary injury following RT for cancers in and around the thorax is common, occurring in up to a third of patients. The early phase of RT-induced lung injury (radiation pneumonitis) usually presents within 6 months of RT, and is commonly characterized by cough and dyspnea [1]. Late fibrotic injury usually evolves and becomes clinically manifested ≥ 6 months post-RT, and is characterized by progressive dyspnea, radiologic findings, and possible mortality [1, 2]. For patients treated for lung cancer, ~ 5%–35% will develop symptomatic lung injury, and 50%–100% will develop radiologic evidence of lung injury (the majority of which are asymptomatic) [3–8]. Similarly, for patients treated for breast cancer, 0%–34% may develop symptomatic lung injury, and 0%–63% of patients may develop radiologic changes [9–14].

Review of RT-induced lung injury by several investigators using various non-invasive imaging techniques has been previously described in detail [15, 16]. In brief, nuclear medicine imaging provides a sensitive means to assess regional lung function. Investigators from the Netherlands Cancer Insti-

tute (NKI), Princess Margaret Hospital (PMH), and Duke University have related changes in regional perfusion/ventilation [via single photon emission computed tomography (SPECT)] and/or tissue density [via computed tomography (CT)] to the 3D radiation dose map. There is a clear association between regional dose and changes in regional perfusion/ventilation/density. Further, there appears to be an association, albeit weak, between the integrated response (e.g., the sum of changes in regional perfusion) and changes in whole lung function [7, 17, 18].

Recent reports have focused on radiation-induced lung injury in the context of stereotactic radiosurgery. In a study of 31 patients receiving stereotactic radiosurgery for primary or metastatic lung lesions, AOKI et al. noted asymptomatic increases in CT density 2–6 months post-RT, and later fibrotic reactions at 6–15 months post-RT [19]. While all 31 patients developed radiographic changes, no patients developed severe symptoms (e.g., Grade ≥ 2 or requiring steroids). When follow-up CTs were compared to the dose distribution on the treatment planning CT, investigators observed that the minimal dose for the development of CT-defined changes in lung tissue ranged from 16 to 36 Gy. Figure 2.1 illustrates the pre- and post-RT change in CT for a patient treated at Duke with radiosurgery for synchronous pulmonary lesions.

Contrast-enhanced magnetic resonance imaging (MRI) may also be used to describe perfusion characteristics of various phases of RT-induced lung injury [20]. Several studies from Japan suggest MRI can detect RT-induced lung injury in animal models. In the clinical setting, YANKELEVITZ et al. and OGASAWARA et al. used MRI to study perfusion characteristics of

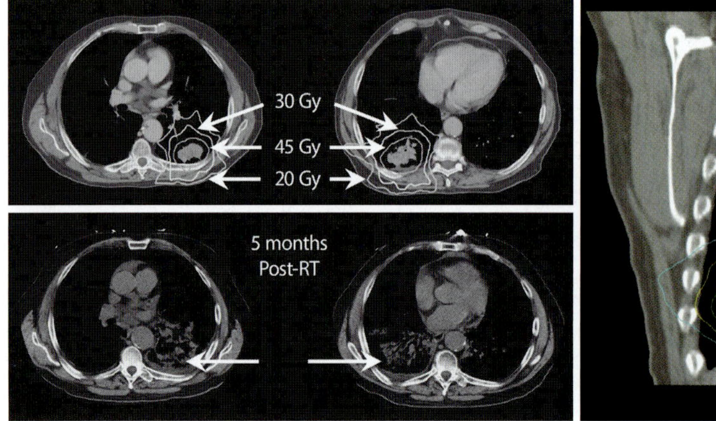

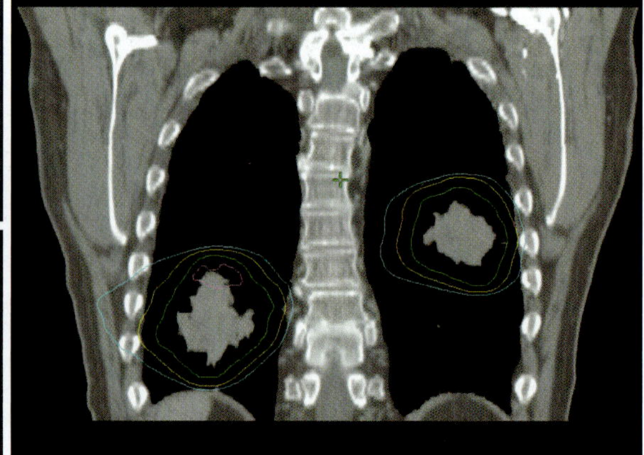

Fig. 2.1. Patient with synchronous bilateral lung lesions treated with radiosurgery at Duke University. Follow-up CTs at 5 months post-RT showed marked increases in regional tissue density in the symptomatic patient

Table 2.2. Frequency of radiographic and symptomatic changes following thoracic irradiation

Reference	No. of cases	Disease site	Radiographic follow-up	Radiologic endpoint	Rate	Clinical endpoint	Rate
CT/radiographs							
[129]	54	Lung, breast, Hodgkin's disease	6 Months	↑ Lung density	36/54 (67%)	RP	10/54 (19%)
[12]	33	Breast	9 Months	↑ Lung density	24/33 (73%)	Cough/ dyspnea	13/33 (39%)
[130]	37	Breast	0.7–10 Years	↑ Radiopacity	16/37 (43%)	–	0/37 (0%)
[131]	75	Hodgkin's disease	3–10 Years	↑ Radiopacity	12/75 (16%)	–	0/45 (0%)
[6]	184	Lung, breast, lymphoma	24 Months	↑ Lung density	162/259 (63%)	Dyspnea	34/175 (19%)
SPECT/scintigraphies							
[131]	75	Hodgkin's disease	3–10 Years	↓ Perfusion	29/45 (64%)	–	0/45 (0%)
[137]	25	Lymphoma	18 Months	Dose-dependent reductions in perfusion/ ventilation and partial recovery	25/25 (100%)	RP	4/25 (16%)
[135]	110	Breast, lymphoma	48 months	Dose-dependent reductions in perfusion/ ventilation and partial recovery	110/110 (100%)	–	–
[136]	106	Lung	3 Months	Dose-effect relation for perfusion and CT density	25/25 (100%)	–	–
[6]	184	Lung, breast, lymphoma	24 Months	↓ Perfusion	168/230 (81%)	Dyspnea	34/175 (19%)
[132]	79	Lung, lymphoma, breast, other thoracic tumors	~65 Months	Progressive dose-dependent reductions in regional perfusion	79/79 (100%)	–	–
[134]	20	Breast	1 Year	↓ Lung clearance	10/10 (100%)	Mild RP	2/20 (10%)
MRI							
[21]	10	Lung	3.5 Years	↑ Signal intensity on T1 and T2 weighted images	10/10 (100%)	–	–
[20]	9	Lung	0.5–7 Months	Asymmetric enhancement on dynamic perfusion MR	9/9 (100%)	Acute RP/ RT fibrosis	–
[133]	40	Lung, esophagus	None (pre RT image)	↑ Vascular resistance on velocity-encoded cine MR in patients with RP	–	RP	9/40 (23%)
PET							
[138]	73	Lung	38 Months	↑ FDG uptake	55/73 (75%)	–	–
[24]	36	Esophagus	1–3 Months	Linear relation between radiation dose and normalized FDG uptake	36/36 (100%)	–	–
[23]	101	Esophagus	3–12 Weeks	Linear relation between radiation dose and normalized FDG uptake	–	≥Grade 2 CTC symptoms	66/101 (66%)

RP, radiation pneumonitis; FDG, fluorodeoxyglucose
Some data estimated from published reports

RT-induced lung injury (Table 2.2) [20, 21]. In a recent study by Muryama et al., velocity-encoded cine (VEC) MRI was used to investigate whether pulmonary arterial flow as a function of time could be used to predict radiation pneumonitis (RP) [22].

A recent study from M.D. Anderson noted dose dependent changes in regional FDG-PET activity in 101 patients assessed 3–12 weeks post-RT for esophageal cancer [23]. Further, the severity of these regional inflammatory changes appeared to be significantly correlated to the probability of symptoms.

Data from several studies regarding radiographic changes in the lung following thoracic RT, seen on SPECT, CT, MRI, and PET, are summarized in Table 2.2. Figure 2.2 illustrates some of these imaging findings and correlation to dose.

2.3
Heart Injury

RT to the thorax may induce both early and late cardiac effects if portions of the heart are included in the radiation field. Patients with breast cancer

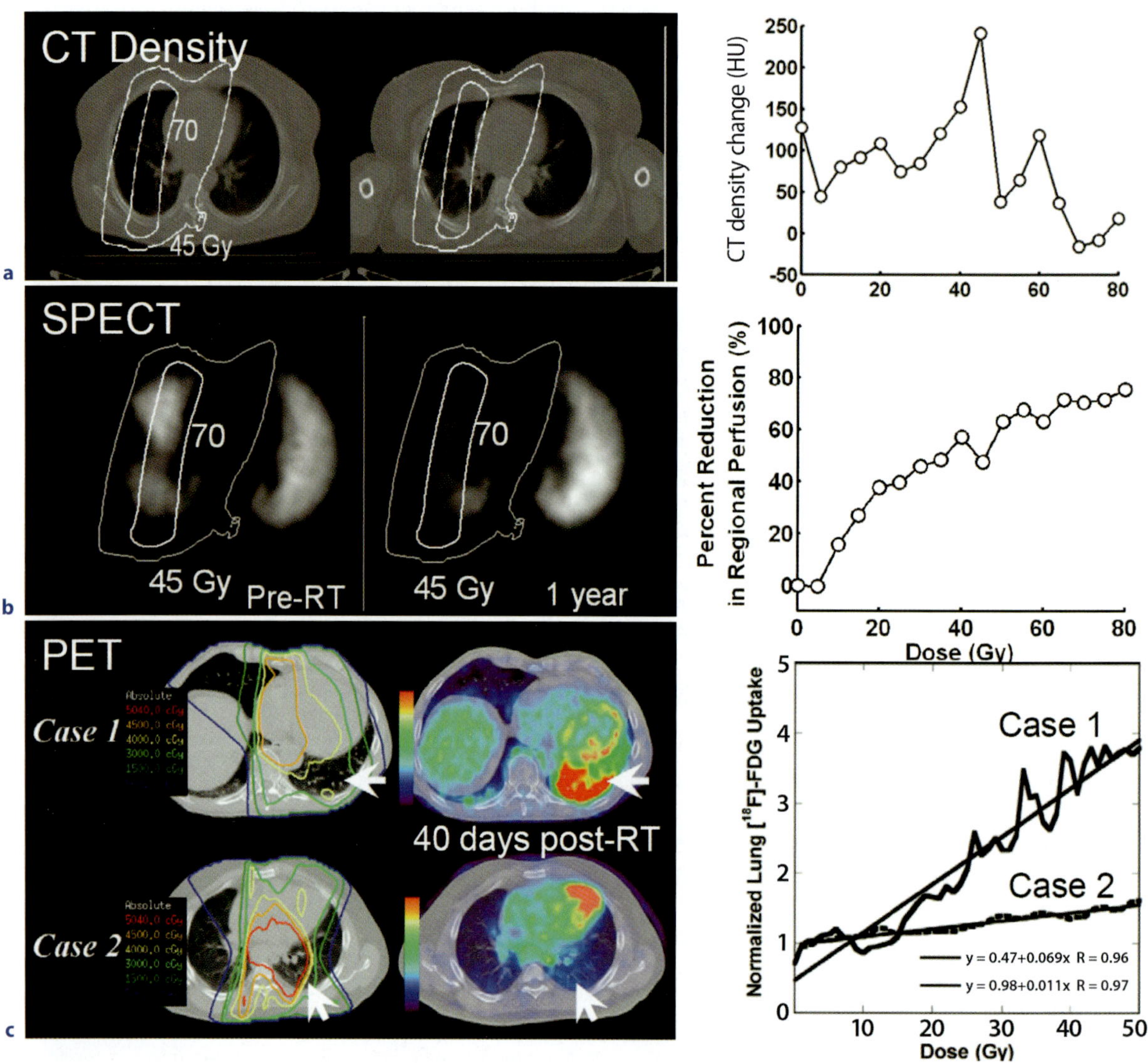

Fig. 2.2a–c. Pre- and post-RT lung CT (Panel **a**, from Duke), SPECT perfusion scans (Panel **b**, from Duke), and FTG-PET images (Panel **c** from MDAH, [24]). For each image pair, the associated isodose lines are shown. On the right side are dose response curves for changes in regional density, perfusion, and metabolic activity, respectively

and Hodgkin's disease are particularly at risk for developing late myocardial damage, due to their longevity and possibly also due to the frequent use of anthracycline-containing chemotherapy. In general, one has to wait at least 10 years post-treatment to see these effects manifest clinically [25]. The use of radiologic methods may allow for the early detection of treatment-associated dysfunction. Recent studies have investigated the incidence of cardiac effects on patients receiving RT for lung and esophageal cancer. There are some preliminary data available on newer imaging technologies such as cardiac MRI and PET to assess RT-induced cardiac injury in patients with thoracic cancers. The vast majority, however, of available data regarding the imaging of RT-induced heart injury use SPECT myocardial perfusion imaging in patients with breast cancer and Hodgkin's disease. An in-depth discussion of RT-induced cardiovascular injury in lymphoma patients is discussed elsewhere in this book (see Chap. 10).

2.3.1
SPECT

SPECT scans provide a noninvasive assessment of myocardial perfusion and function (changes in wall motion and left ventricular ejection fraction). Scans taken in early years following RT may be able to assess early the subclinical damage. The incidence of perfusion defects appears to be related to the volume of left ventricle irradiated and largely persists up to 6 years after RT in patients irradiated for breast cancer [26–28]. Perfusion defects have been associated with episodes of chest pain, and wall motion abnormalities [26, 28–30], but their clinical implications may not be well understood. Further, relatively large perfusion defects may cause reductions in ejection fraction [26, 31]. Data from several studies relating radiographic changes in the heart, as seen on SPECT, in patients treated for breast cancer and Hodgkin's disease, and preliminary data from studies in esophageal and lung cancer are shown in Table 2.3. Unlike the data for breast cancer, the results as assessed by SPECT for esophageal and lung cancer are limited and somewhat mixed. It may be more difficult to draw conclusions about the incidence of RT-induced cardiac injury in this group of patients as many may have pre-existing heart disease and associated related risks. Additional follow-up may be needed.

There is some concern that the abnormalities detected on SPECT may be due to attenuation artifacts related to RT-induced scarring of the breast/chest-wall; i.e., RT causes pericardial scarring that may lead to an "artificial" defect in the anterior myocardium. Additional study is underway to assess for this confounding issue.

2.3.2
MRI

Nuclear medicine imaging provides both qualitative and quantitative information about regional and global cardiac function [32] and has been suggested to be a sensitive means to assess myocardial injury in patients with coronary artery disease [33, 34]. MRI provides assessments of myocardial wall thickness and, with delayed hyper-enhancement, allows direct visualization of myocardial injury/fibrosis, and is more sensitive in assessing subendocardial injury. Both MRI and the nuclear medicine techniques provide information regarding wall motion and ejection fraction, but MRI has better spatial resolution and thus may be more accurate [35–37]. Conversely, quantification of myocardial perfusion is better developed with SPECT than with MRI [36, 37]. While SPECT images only the left ventricle, MRI affords the possibility to assess global cardiac function.

At this time, MRI has only been applied to the study of RT-induced cardiac disease for a small number of patients with lung cancer. In preliminary abstracts from MD Anderson and Duke University, no apparent changes on cardiac MRI have been observed in the small patient numbers evaluable [38, 139]

2.3.3
Cardiac PET

There is increased interest in the use of cardiac positron emission tomography (PET) to provide a map of regional myocardial perfusion. PET has been suggested as having improved resolution and accuracy as compared to SPECT. In addition, PET may require shorter exam times than SPECT, but is similarly limited to imaging only the left ventricle [39]. A case report noted increased FDG uptake within cardiac regions receiving ≥ 25 Gy approximately 4 years earlier [40]. The patient was asymptomatic and had a normal ECG.

Table 2.3. Summary of studies using myocardial perfusion scintigraphy/SPECT to assess for RT-induced cardiac injury in patients with thoracic malignancies. (Adapted with permission from [128])

Reference[a]	Years of RT	No. of cases	Median radiographic follow-up	Subgroup	Perfusion defects	
Breast cancer – retrospective						
[41]	1971–1976	37	18.4 Years	Left-sided photons or electrons	25%	(5/20)
			19 Years	Right-sided photons or electrons	0%	(0/17)
[42]	1978–1983	90	13 Years	Left-sided RT	12%	(4/34)
				Right-sided or no RT	4%	(2/56)
[43]	1982–1990	16	7.9 Years	Left-sided electrons	44%	(4/9)
				No RT	57%	(4/7)
[44]	1987–1993	17	8.4 Years	Left-sided photons	0%	(0/17)
[30]	1987–1995	36	6.7 Years	Left-sided photons	71%	(17/24)
			8.3 Years	Right-sided photons	17%	(2/12)
Breast cancer – prospective						
[45]	1993–1994	12	1.1 Year	Left-sided photons	100%	(4/4)
				Left-sided electrons	25%	(2/8)
[26][b]	1998–2001	114	0.5 Year	Left-sided photons	27%	(21/77)
			1 Year	Left-sided photons	29%	(16/55)
			1.5 Years	Left-sided photons	38%	(13/34)
			2 Years	Left-sided photons	42%	(11/26)
[28][b]	1998–2006	44	3 Years	Left-sided photons	38%	(3/8)
			4 Years	Left-sided photons	58%	(7/12)
			5 Years	Left-sided photons	67%	(4/6)
			6 Years	Left-sided photons	67%	(2/3)
Other disease sites						
[46]	1967–1985	16	9.3 (2.5–21.5) Years	Lymphoma	0%	(0/16)
[47]		26	15 (4–20) Years	Lymphoma	61%	(14/23)
[48]	1978–1988	31	7 (3–11) Years	Lymphoma	84%	(21/25)
[49]	1964–1992	112	11.2 (1.0–31.5) Years	Lymphoma	7%	(7/100)
[50]		49	75 (28–208) Months	Lymphoma	78%	(32/41)
[51]	1964–1994	294	6.5 (4.0–8.4) Years	Lymphoma	12%	(32/274)
[52]	2005–2006	51	3 Months	Esophageal cancer	54%	(14/26)
				No RT	16%	(4/25)
[38]		13	2 Months, 6 months	Lung cancer	–	–[a]
[139]	2006–2007	12	3, 6, 12, and 18 months	Lung cancer, Mesothelioma	50%	(6/12)

[a] At least one patient with a new perfusion abnormality. Limited data in available abstract
[b] Some patient overlap, incidence of new perfusion defects listed
Some data estimated from published reports

2.4

Liver Injury

Previous radiation therapy techniques limited the utility of radiation to the liver, due to the liver's low whole organ tolerance. Data from studies dating back to the 1960s indicated that doses to the whole liver up to 30–35 Gy using standard fractionation resulted in a 5% risk of radiation-induced liver disease (RILD), while smaller volumes of the liver could tolerate higher doses [53–56]. With the advent of 3D conformal therapy and more recently IMRT, it has become increasingly important to assess the impact RT-induced liver injury. Radiologic changes are often evident on irradiated livers prior to, or even in the absence of, clinical symptoms [54, 57]. Such imaging changes have been reported 6 months to 6 years post-RT [53, 54, 58] (Table 2.4).

2.4.1

CT Perfusion Studies

Investigators at the University of Michigan have used CT to detect RT-induced liver injury. CTs obtained 2–3 months post-RT revealed low attenuation within irradiated areas in of 74% of 31 patients studied [66]. Using CT-based perfusion imaging, Cao et al. assessed the relationship between local radiation dose and changes in regional por-

tal vein perfusion, similar to perfusion imaging studies of the lung and heart post-RT from other institutions noted above [58]. In 10 patients with unresectable primary or metastatic hepatic tumors, reductions in regional portal vein perfusion ~1.5 and 3 weeks into treatment (i.e., during RT) were related to changes in perfusion at 1 month post-RT. Conceivably, one may be able to alter therapy based on normal tissue changes noted early-on during a proposed course of therapy, thereby further individualizing therapy.

Munden et al. noted new CT liver abnormalities in 40% (8/20) of patients ≈ 8 (range 5–11) weeks post-IMRT for mesothelioma [59]. The abnormalities were in the liver periphery, corresponding to the regions receiving > 45 Gy. All patients with CT-defined abnormalities were asymptomatic and had normal liver function tests. For those patients with limited additional follow-up, the majority of the abnormalities resolved; however, additional data with longer follow-up is warranted.

2.4.2

MRI

MRI also provides a non-invasive method of imaging the RT-induced liver disease. On conventional MR images, irradiated liver tissues show T1-weighted hypointensity and T2-weighted hyperintensity, potentially due to increased water content

Table 2.4. Imaging assessment of RT-induced liver disease

Reference	No. of cases	Disease	RT technique median dose (range)	Follow-up	Radiologic changes	Clinical RT-hepatitis
CT						
[66]	31	Primary or metastatic hepatic tumors	High-dose conformal RT 59 Gy (48–73 Gy)	8- to 12 -Week intervals	74%	6%
[59]	20	Mesothelioma	IMRT in 25 fractions to 45–50 Gy	16 Weeks Range (3–116)	40%	0%
[58]	10	Primary or metastatic hepatic tumors	67.5 Gy (48–78 Gy)	1.5, 3 Weeks during RT; 1 month post-RT	↓Regional perfusion	–
MRI						
[60]	10	Hodgkin's disease	–	2, 4, 6, 12 Weeks	30%	0%

ᵃ For post-contrast T_1-weighted images
Some data estimated from published reports

[60, 61]. However, severe hepatic fibrosis can cause hypointensity on T2-weighted images that has been observed in irradiated patients with Budd-Chiari syndrome [62].

Special MR imaging techniques may provide a more precise differential diagnosis of radiation-induced hepatic injury. In gadolinium-enhanced dynamic studies, the irradiated liver parenchyma shows early hyperintensity that becomes more prominent and persists at the end of the dynamic studies [61]. Superparamagnetic iron oxide-enhanced (SPIO) MR imaging may also be a sensitive modality for early and late radiation-induced liver injury [62–65].

2.5
Brain Injury

Symptomatic brain injury from radiotherapy is common and likely underestimated due to limited lifespan of the majority of treated patients and the subtlety of findings [67–71]. Neurocognitive alterations can range from subtle cognitive dysfunction, such as mild short-term memory loss 1–6 months after treatment, to global irreversible/progressive neuropsychological deficits such as personality change and an overt decrease in IQ > 6 months post RT [72–75]. The situation is further complicated by neurotoxic effects of the tumor as well as effects of surgery and/or chemotherapy. The changes in normal brain following therapy for brain tumors is often complex; however there is an ever-increasing volume of data using imaging studies to better differentiate changes in normal brain tissue post-RT from recurrent disease. There is, however, limited data on the implications of these radiologic findings and changes in the neurocognitive function of patients receiving RT (Table 2.5).

Animal studies reveal that cranial irradiation leads to deficits in learning and memory, which may be comparable to human reports of cognitive dysfunction following RT [76]. In these animal reports, there is anatomic variability in radiosensitivity, as well as dose related deficits of learning and memory [77–81].

Post-RT, conventional CT and MRI can reveal morphologic abnormalities in the brain. However, these are non-specific and may reflect RT-induced normal tissue changes/inflammation/necrosis, tu-

mor-related changes, or surgery-induced changes (e.g., enhancement along the resection margin) [82]. Functional brain imaging (e.g., SPECT and PET) may be able to distinguish between recurrent tumor and normal tissue changes such as radiation necrosis [82–85]. The majority of studies have evaluated the response of tumor to radiotherapy rather than the effect on normal tissue.

2.5.1
SPECT

SPECT can illustrate changes in cranial blood flow following RT. A Japanese study by Araki et al. utilized Xenon 133 SPECT to evaluate changes in mean cerebral blood flow of non-tumor bearing areas in 40 patients as compared with 40 normal volunteers [86]. Mean blood flow increased during therapy in some patients, compared to normal controls. At 3 months post-RT, significant reductions in blood flow were seen in three patients.

Harila-Saari et al. studied 25 patients with acute lymphoblastic leukemia (ALL) treated with either intrathecal (IT) chemotherapy or RT. SPECT perfusion defects were noted in 11/25 (44%), eight of whom received chemotherapy alone and three who received cranial RT [87]. The degree of SPECT abnormality has not been associated with neuropsychologic changes post-RT.

2.5.2
PET

There are limited data regarding the effects of RT on glucose metabolism in the brain via FDG-PET and clinical symptoms, and the available data is contradictory. Kahkonen et al. evaluated 40 long term survivors of ALL, half of whom received methotrexate and cranial RT [88]. No major differences were found in regional glucose metabolism in various defined cortical and subcortical anatomical areas for irradiated vs. non-irradiated groups. Pre-RT imaging was not available in these patients. Munley et al. retrospectively evaluated eight patients with both pre- and post-RT FDG-PET imaging [89]. There were no changes in regional metabolic activity in areas of brain receiving doses up to 50 Gy. Above 50 Gy, the effects varied, one decreasing and others increasing to varying degrees. Both of these studies were very small.

Table 2.5. Radiographic changes to the brain after irradiation

Reference	No. of cases	Radiographic follow-up	Post-RT radiographic response/outcome
SPECT			
[86][a]	40	3 Months	• ↑ Mean blood flow during RT • ↓ In blood flow in three RT patients post-RT
[87]	25	Varied (9–13 months)[b]	• Defects in 44% (11/25) – eight chemo alone, three RT alone • Impairment in neuropsychological functioning in 19/22 (86%) • No significant difference in intelligence testing between normal vs. abnormal SPECT
Diffusion weighted (DW)-MRI			
[110]	18	1–3 Month intervals starting 4 months post-RT	• ADC ratios and means significantly ↓ for recurrent vs. non-recurrent lesions
[111]	17	–	• Marked hypointensity [67%, (8/12)], in lesions due to RT-injury vs. recurrent tumor • Maximal ADC values significantly ↓ for recurrent vs. non-recurrent lesions
^{1}HMRSI			
[97]	9	0.5–10.5 Years	• Widespread chemical changes in white matter after RT
[112]	18	Mean 4.6 years (range 3.0–9.6 years)	• ↓ NAA in RT-induced temporal lobe changes • Cr levels relatively more stable than Cho or NAA levels • Cho levels may be increased, normal, or reduced
[113] (MRS and DW-MRI)	55	2-Month intervals (1.5–12 months) 3–4 months intervals (12–36 months)	• Cho/ NAA, Cho/Cr, and ADC ratios and means significantly ↓ in regions of RT injury vs. recurrent tumor • MRS with DW MRI correctly classified 96.4% of subjects as recurrent disease or RT injury (100% correct for RT injury group)
[114] (I-IMT SPECT ^{1}HMRS)	25	9.7 Months	• I-IMT SPECT significantly ↓ for recurrent disease vs. treatment related changes • SPECT yielded more favorable results in differentiating recurrent tumor vs. post-RT changes
[115]	100	2 Years	• Oscillations in Cho/NAA and Cho/Cr ratios seen in 8 month cycles • Maxima in Cho/NAA and Cho/Cr ratios seen 2 months after RT
PET			
[91]	11	3 Weeks; 6 months	• ↓ FDG uptake, correlating with neuropsychological deficits

[a] Data extracted from abstract

[b] Radiographic follow-up not distinguished between patients with and without RT. Follow-up time measured from end of systemic therapy or RT

[1] HMRSI, proton MR spectroscopic imaging; ADC, apparent diffusion coefficient; NAA, N-acetyl-aspartate; DW, diffusion-weighted; Cr, creatine; Cho, choline; I-IMT, 123-iodine-α-methyl tyrosine

Some data estimated from published reports

Mineura et al. reported on seven patients studied with ^{15}O PET before and after RT for gliomas [90]. At 1 month post-RT, there were increases in PET-defined regional blood flow in the contralateral grey matter felt to be normal tissue by CT. At longer time points, there were significant decreases in blood flow from pre treatment compared with later studies.

Early data from a prospective Duke study of 11 patients utilizing FDG and O–15 PET revealed reductions in FDG uptake in regions of the brain receiving >40 Gy in comparison to pre-treatment scans [91]. These FDG changes were found additionally to correlate with changes on neuropsychologic testing. Additional study, however, is needed to confirm and more precisely characterize these findings.

2.5.3
MRI

In animal models, changes in brain tissue on MRI have been found to be dependent on dose and are progressive with time [92]. Diffusion-weighted MRI has been used to characterize and differentiate morphologic features including edema, necrosis, and tumor tissue. This approach is based on differences in apparent diffusion coefficient (ADC), resulting from changes in the balance between intracellular and extracellular water and changes in structure of the two compartments, with these conditions [93].

Price et al. studied four patients who received RT for low grade gliomas with MR perfusion imaging. There appeared to be RT-induced decreases in relative cerebral blood volume (rCBV) and blood flow (rCBF) within 3 months of RT in regions receiving >32 Gy [94]. In children with brain tumors, radiotherapy combined with or without chemotherapy often leads to the development of late neurocognitive sequelae. Using high-resolution MRI, Liu et al. measured the thickness of the cerebral cortex in medulloblastoma patients [95]. Cortical thickness maps showed relatively thinner cortex in multiple brain regions that were age and gender related. They reported that the areas of cortex undergoing development are more sensitive to the effects of treatment of medulloblastoma.

2.5.4
Magnetic Resonance Spectroscopy

Magnetic resonance spectroscopy (MRS) can measure aspects of brain metabolism in vivo by showing the spatial distribution and ratios of compounds that are present within the neurons, or participate in membrane or energy metabolism, e.g., N-acetyl aspartate (NAA), choline (Ch), and creatine (Cr) [96, 97]. Signals from multiple metabolites can be noninvasively measured within a single measurement period. In normal brain tissue, the largest signal arises for NAA, which serves as a marker of neuronal density and neuron functionality [98, 99]. Several studies have demonstrated decreases in NAA levels in normal brain after conventionally fractionated radiotherapy, which may occur even with low dose RT (<6 Gy) and recover within months after completing RT.

Kaminaga and Shirai serially studied 20 patients with MRS pre-RT, and ≈ 9 days and 15 months post treatment. They noted decreased NAA and increased choline at the longer follow-up time [104]. Choline was found in cellular membranes at high levels, which investigators suggested led to rapid membrane turnover or disruption. In a similar study from Zeng et al., MRS and diffusion-weighted imaging were performed 6 weeks post-RT, and serially every 2 months for the first year, then at 3- to 4-month intervals over 2 and 3 years [105]. Investigators found significantly lower levels of CH/NAA and Ch/Cr ratios ($p < 0.01$) in 55 patients assessed for radiation injury vs recurrent disease. These two variables reportedly could differentiate recurrent disease vs. normal tissue toxicity in 85.5% of the 55 subjects. With the addition of diffusion weighted imaging data [and the apparent diffusion coefficient (ADC)], authors reported a higher accuracy when differentiating radiation-induced injury vs. recurrent gliomas. Plotkin et al. compared the ability of I-IMT SPECT and H^{1}MRSI to differentiate recurrent tumor vs. radiation changes in 25 patients previously treated with RT for glioma. Using a 1.62 cutoff for I-IMT SPECT uptake, SPECT yielded a higher sensitivity, specificity, and accuracy as compared to H^{1}MRSI.

2.5.5
Functional Magnetic Resonance Imaging

Another modality being utilized increasingly to study brain plasticity in diseased patients is functional magnetic resonance imaging (fMRI) [106]. Blood-oxygen-level-dependent (BOLD)-based fMRI is based upon changes in brain oxygen content, which occur with changes in neuronal activity [107]. These changes can be induced by a number of stimuli, most commonly visual but inclusive of cognitive tasks [108]. One small study of 16 survivors of childhood cancers and 27 healthy subjects, demonstrated feasibility of using this technique to investigate brain function in survivors of childhood cancer, and found that the BOLD signal for both survivors and healthy subjects was qualitatively similar in timing and shape [109]. However, computer-aided analyses did detect significant quantitative differences in the BOLD signal of the survivors vs. healthy subjects.

2.6
Parotid Gland Injury

The parotid glands may be injured by RT during therapy for head and neck tumors, and can impact speech, chewing, and swallowing [117]. The incidence of clinical parotid dysfunction appears to be most related to the RT dose delivered, the percent of parotid volume irradiated, and the pre-RT parotid function [118].

2.6.1
SPECT and PET

^{11}C-methionine PET activity in the parotid glands is reduced following RT for head and neck cancer [119]. As has been done for the lung and heart, changes in planar salivary gland scintigraphy (SGS) and SPECT can be related to the RT dose in order to define the dose-response relationship for parotid dysfunction [118, 120]. It appears that doses as low as 10–15 Gy can result in a >50% loss of salivary gland function, measured by comparing the pre- and post-RT salivary excretion fraction (SEF) seen on SPECT. In a

study from Medical University of Lübeck (Germany), significant alterations in radiotracer uptake in irradiated salivary glands of rabbits demonstrated that functional impairment could be assessed by scintigraphy as early as 24 h post-irradiation [117].

2.6.2
MRI

MRI has been used to evaluate salivary gland diseases, due to its excellent soft tissue contrast and the visualization of characteristic changes resulting from RT [121, 122]. A reduction in MRI-defined apparent diffusion coefficients (ADC) has been noted in patients with RT-induced dysfunction as assessed by scintigraphy [122].

Data from several studies relating radiographic changes in the parotid gland using PET, SPECT, and MRI, are shown in Table 2.6.

2.7
Conclusions

Functional imaging can be used quantitatively to detect RT-induced normal tissue injury in a variety of organs. In general, these imaging abnormalities manifest soon after (or even during) RT. Hence, it may be a powerful tool for the early detection of normal tissue injury and for the study of potential mitigators of such injury in humans. Radiologically defined normal tissue injury may be related to short/long-term clinically meaningful injury (e.g., global organ function), but further study is needed to better quantify this association (Table 2.7). Additional work is needed to develop methods and standards to quantitatively score radiologic injury.

Acknowledgements

Supported in part by grants NIH R01 CA69579, Department of Defense Grants 17-98-1-8071, BC010663, and a grant from the Lance Armstrong Foundation. Thanks to the University of North Carolina at Chapel Hill for PLUNC planning software.

Portions of this document were adapted from [15].

Table 2.6. Radiographic changes in the parotid glands after irradiation of the head and neck

Reference	No. of cases	Radiographic follow-up months post-RT Median (range)	Type of radiographic study	Radiographic response/outcome
[119]	8	6 Months (minimum)	^{11}C-methionine PET	Metabolic clearance of ^{11}C-methionine in the parotid and submandibular glands decreased with increasing RT dose
[123][a]	12	21 Months (8–54)	^{11}C-methionine PET	Dose-response analysis revealed a sigmoid relationship with a threshold dose of 16 Gy, and mean TD_{50} of 30 Gy
[124]	9	1.5 and 6 months	Magnetic resonance sialography (MRS)	Comparison of pre- and post-RT images revealed RT-induced decreases in visibility of the parotid and submandibular ducts, at 1.5 months, but subsequent improvement at 6 months
[121]	52	Within 24 months post-RT	MRI	RT-induced volume reduction of parotid
[122]	21	1 Month	MRI and salivary gland scintigraphy (SGS)	• Mean apparent diffusion coefficient (ADC) of dysfunctional parotids decreased by 23% on diffusion-weighted imaging post-RT • No significant change of ADCs of functional parotids
[125]	39	1 and 4 months	Salivary gland scintigraphy (SGS)	The mean loss of SEF in the spared parotid was 67% and 19% in 1 and 4 months post-RT, respectively. Normal excretion function was regained in 75% of the spared parotids
[126]	96	1.5 and 12 months	Salivary gland scintigraphy (SGS)	Reduction in salivary excretion fractions (SEF) from 44.7% to 18.7% at 6 weeks and to 32.4% at 12 months post-RT
[127]	16	1 and 9 months	Salivary gland scintigraphy (SGS)	Maximal excretion ratio dropped from 53.5% to 10.7%, and 23.3% 1 and 9 months post-IMRT, respectively
[120]	21	1 Month	Salivary gland scintigraphy (SGS) plus SPECT	Linear correlation between RT-induced changes in SEF on SGS-SPECT and RT dose
[118]	16	7 Months (6–10)	Salivary gland scintigraphy (SGS) plus SPECT	Median reduction in salivary excretion fractions (SEF) of 100% (range 17%–100%) observed 7 months post-RT

[a] Includes four of the same patients as the other Buus study [123]
SEF, salivary excretion fraction
Some data estimated from published reports

Table 2.7. Sample attempts to relate changes in regional radiologic studies to changes in global organ function

Organ	Regional radiologic assay	Degree of regional injury associated with reported global injury?
Lung	CT, SPECT PET	Yes; PFTs (Duke, NKI), symptoms (MDAH)
Heart	SPECT, MRI, PET	Unclear; EF (Duke, NKI, MDAH)
Liver	CT perfusion, MRI	Unclear, hepatitis (University of Michigan; University Tsukuba, Japan)
Brain	MRI, PET	Yes; neuropsychological deficits (Duke)
Parotid	PET, SPECT, MRI	Mixed; SEF (University of Leuven, Beligium; Toyko Medical and Dental University, Japan)

PFT, pulmonary function test; EF, ejection fraction; SEF, salivary excretion fraction.

References

1. Theuws JCM, Kwa SLS, Wagenaar AC, Boersma LJ, Damen EMF, Muller SH, Baas P, Lebesque JV (1998) Dose-effect relations for early local pulmonary injury after irradiation for malignant lymphoma and breast cancer. Radiother Oncol 48:33–43

2. Goethals I, Dierckx R, De Meerleer G, De Sutter J, De Winter O, De Neve W, Van De Wiele C (2003) The role of nuclear medicine in the prediction and detection of radiation-associated normal pulmonary and cardiac damage. J Nucl Med 44:1531–1539

3. Anscher MS, Marks LB, Shafman TD, Clough R, Huang H, Tisch A, Munley M, Herndon JE, Garst J, Crawford J, Jirtle RL (2003) Risk of long-term complications after TGF-β 1-guided very-high-dose thoracic radiotherapy. Int J Radiat Oncol Biol Phys 56:988–995

4. Marks LB (1994) The pulmonary effects of thoracic irradiation. Oncology (Williston Park, NY) 8:89–106; discussion 100, 103

5. Graham MV, Purdy JA, Emami B, Harms W, Bosch W, Lockett MA, Perez CA (1999) Clinical dose-volume histogram analysis for pneumonitis after 3D treatment for non-small cell lung cancer (NSCLC). Int J Radiat Oncol Biol Phys 45:323–329

6. Marks LB, Fan M, Clough R, Munley M, Bentel G, Coleman RE, Jaszczak R, Hollis D, Anscher M (2000) Radiation-induced pulmonary injury: symptomatic versus subclinical endpoints. Int J Radiat Biol 76:469–475

7. Fan M, Marks LB, Hollis D, Bentel GG, Anscher MS, Sibley G, Coleman RE, Jaszczak RJ, Munley MT (2001) Can we predict radiation-induced changes in pulmonary function based on the sum of predicted regional dysfunction? J Clin Oncol 19:543–550

8. Fu XL, Huang H, Bentel G, Clough R, Jirtle RL, Kong FM, Marks LB, Anscher MS (2001) Predicting the risk of symptomatic radiation-induced lung injury using both the physical and biologic parameters V30 and transforming growth factor β Int J Radiat Oncol Biol Phys 50:899–908

9. Dorr W, Bertmann S, Herrmann T (2005) Radiation induced lung reactions in breast cancer therapy: modulating factors and consequential effects. Strahlenther Onkol 181:567–573

10. Cazzaniga LF, Bossi A, Cosentino D, Frigerio M, Martinelli A, Monti A, Morresi A, Ostinelli A, Scandolaro L, Valli MC, Besana G (1998) Radiological findings when very small lung volumes are irradiated in breast and chest wall treatment. Radiat Oncol Investig 6:58–62

11. Kuhnt T, Richter C, Enke H, Dunst J (1998) Acute radiation reaction and local control in breast cancer patients treated with postmastectomy radiotherapy. Strahlenther Onkol 174:257–261

12. Rotstein S, Lax I, Svane G (1990) Influence of radiation therapy on the lung-tissue in breast cancer patients: CT-assessed density changes and associated symptoms. Int J Radiat Oncol Biol Phys 18:173–180

13. Schratter-Sehn AU, Schurawitzki H, Zach M, Schratter M (1993) High-resolution computed tomography of the lungs in irradiated breast cancer patients. Radiother Oncol 27:198–202

14. Lind PA, Wennberg B, Gagliardi G, Rosfors S, Blom-Goldman U, Lidestähl A, Svane G (2006) ROC curves and evaluation of radiation-induced pulmonary toxicity in breast cancer. Int J Radiat Oncol Biol Phys 64:765–770

15. Evans ES, Hahn CA, Kocak Z, Zhou SM, Marks LB (2007) The role of functional imaging in the diagnosis and management of late normal tissue injury. Semin Radiat Oncol 17:72–80

16. Kocak Z SL, Sullivan DC, Marks LB (2007) The role of imaging in the study of radiation-induced normal tissue injury. In: Rubin R, Marks LB, Okunieff P (eds) Cured I – LENT. Late effects of cancer treatment on normal tissue, 1st ed. Springer-Verlag, Berlin Heidelberg New York, pp 37–45

17. Fan M, Marks LB, Lind P, Hollis D, Woel RT, Bentel GG, Anscher MS, Shafman TD, Coleman RE, Jaszczak RJ, Munley MT (2001) Relating radiation-induced regional lung injury to changes in pulmonary function tests. Int J Radiat Oncol Biol Phys 51:311–317

18. Seppenwoolde Y, De Jaeger K, Boersma LJ, Belderbos JSA, Lebesque JV (2004) Regional differences in lung radiosensitivity after radiotherapy for non-small-cell lung cancer. Int J Radiat Oncol Biol Phys 60:748–758

19. Aoki T, Nagata Y, Negoro Y, Takayama K, Mizowaki T, Kokubo M, Oya N, Mitsumori M, Hiraoka M (2004) Evaluation of lung injury after three-dimensional conformal stereotactic radiation therapy for solitary lung tumors: CT appearance. Radiology 230:101–108

20. Ogasawara N, Suga K, Karino Y, Matsunaga N (2002) Perfusion characteristics of radiation-injured lung on Gd-DTPA-enhanced dynamic magnetic resonance imaging. Invest Radiol 37:448–457

21. Yankelevitz DF, Henschke CI, Batata M, Kim YS, Chu F (1994) Lung cancer: evaluation with MR imaging during and after irradiation. J Thorac Imaging 9:41–46

22. Muryama S, Akamine T, Sakai S, Oshiro Y, Kakinohana Y, Soeda H, Toita T, Adachi G (2004) Risk factor of radiation pneumonitis: assessment with velocity-encoded cine magnetic resonance imaging of pulmonary artery. J Comput Assist Tomogr 28:204–208

23. Hart JP, McCurdy MR, Ezhil M, Wei W, Khan M, Luo D, Munden RF, Johnson VE, Guerrero TM (2008) Radiation Pneumonitis: Correlation of Toxicity With Pulmonary Metabolic Radiation Response. International Journal of Radiation Oncology Biology Physics 71(4):967–971

24. Guerrero T, Johnson V, Hart J, Pan T, Khan M, Luo D, Liao Z, Ajani J, Stevens C, Komaki R (2007) Radiation pneumonitis: local dose versus [18F]-fluorodeoxyglucose uptake response in irradiated lung. Int J Radiat Oncol Biol Phys 68:1030–1035

25. Darby SC, McGale P, Taylor CW, Peto R (2005) Long-term mortality from heart disease and lung cancer after radiotherapy for early breast cancer: prospective cohort study of about 300,000 women in US SEER cancer registries. Lancet Oncol 6:557–565

26. Marks LB, Yu X, Prosnitz RG, Zhou SM, Hardenbergh PH, Blazing M, Hollis D, Lind P, Tisch A, Wong TZ, Borges-Neto S (2005) The incidence and functional consequences of RT-associated cardiac perfusion defects. Int J Radiat Oncol Biol Phys 63:214–223

27. Marks LB, Zhou S, Yu X (2003) The impact of irradiated left ventricular volume on the incidence of radiation-induced cardiac perfusion changes. Int J Radiat Oncol Biol Phys 57[2 Suppl]:S129

28. Prosnitz RG, Hubbs JL, Evans ES, Zhou SM, Yu X, Blazing MA, Hollis DR, Tisch A, Wong TZ, Borges-Neto S, Hardenbergh PH, Marks LB (2007) Prospective assessment of radiotherapy-associated cardiac toxicity in breast cancer patients: analysis of data 3 to 6 years after treatment. Cancer 110:1840–1850

29. Yu X, Prosnitz RR, Zhou S, Hardenbergh PH, Tisch A, Blazing MA, Borges-Neto S, Hollis D, Wong T, Marks LB (2003) Symptomatic cardiac events following radiation therapy for left-sided breast cancer: possible association with radiation therapy-induced changes in regional perfusion. Clin Breast Cancer 4:193–197

30. Seddon B, Cook A, Gothard L, Salmon E, Latus K, Underwood SR, Yarnold J (2002) Detection of defects in myocardial perfusion imaging in patients with early breast cancer treated with radiotherapy. Radiother Oncol 64:53–63

31. Marks LB, Prosnitz RG, Hardenbergh PH (2002) Functional consequences of radiation (RT)-induced perfusion changes in patients with left-sided breast cancer. Int J Radiat Oncol Biol Phys 54[2 Suppl]:3–4

32. Hardenbergh PH, Munley MT, Bentel GC, Kedem R, Borges-Neto S, Hollis D, Prosnitz LR, Marks LB (2001) Cardiac perfusion changes in patients treated for breast cancer with radiation therapy and doxorubicin: preliminary results. Int J Radiat Oncol Biol Phys 49:1023–1028

33. Li D, Deshpande V (2001) Magnetic resonance imaging of coronary arteries. Top Magn Reson Imaging 12:337–348

34. Hundley WG, Hamilton CA, Rerkpattanapipat P (2003) Magnetic resonance imaging assessment of cardiac function. Curr Cardiol Rep 5:69–74

35. Wagner A, Mahrholdt H, Kim RJ, Judd RM (2005) Use of cardiac magnetic resonance to assess viability. Curr Cardiol Rep 7:59–64

36. Cuocolo A, Acampa W, Imbriaco M, De Luca N, Iovino GL, Salvatore M (2005) The many ways to myocardial perfusion imaging. Q J Nucl Med Mol Imaging 49:4–18

37. Schaefer WM, Lipke CSA, Nowak B, Kaiser H-J, Reinartz P, Buecker A, Krombach GA, Buell U, Kuhl HP (2004) Validation of QGS and 4D-MSPECT for quantification of left ventricular volumes and ejection fraction from gated 18F-FDG PET: comparison with cardiac MRI. J Nucl Med 45:74–79

38. Lind PA, Larsson T, Lidestahl A, Agren-Cronqvist A, Nygren A, Brodin O (2006) 2497: heart changes on MRI and SPECT after definitive radiation therapy in patients with lung cancer. Int J Radiat Oncol Biol Phys 66[3, Suppl 1]:S487

39. Chua SC, Ganatra RH, Green DJ, Groves AM (2006) Nuclear cardiology: myocardial perfusion imaging with SPECT and PET. Imaging 18:166–177

40. Zophel K, Holzel C, Dawel M, Holscher T, Evers C, Kotzerke J (2007) PET/CT demonstrates increased myocardial FDG uptake following irradiation therapy. Eur J Nucl Med Mol Imaging 34:1322–1323

41. Gyenes G, Fornander T, Carlens P, Rutqvist LE (1994) Morbidity of ischemic heart disease in early breast cancer 15–20 years after adjuvant radiotherapy. Int J Radiat Oncol Biol Phys 28:1235–1241

42. Gustavsson A, Bendahl PO, Cwikiel M, Eskilsson J, Thapper KL, Pahlm O (1999) No serious late cardiac effects after adjuvant radiotherapy following mastectomy in premenopausal women with early breast cancer. Int J Radiat Oncol Biol Phys 43:745–754

43. Hojris I, Sand NP, Andersen J, Rehling M, Overgaard M (2000) Myocardial perfusion imaging in breast cancer patients treated with or without post-mastectomy radiotherapy. Radiother Oncol 55:163–172

44. Cowen D, Gonzague-Casabianca L, Brenot-Rossi I, Viens P, Mace L, Hannoun-Levi JM, Alzieu C, Resbeut M (1998) Thallium-201 perfusion scintigraphy in the evaluation of late myocardial damage in left-side breast cancer treated with adjuvant radiotherapy. Int J Radiat Oncol Biol Phys 41:809–815

45. Gyenes G, Fornander T, Carlens P, Glas U, Rutqvist LE (1996) Myocardial damage in breast cancer patients treated with adjuvant radiotherapy: a prospective study. Int J Radiat Oncol Biol Phys 36:899–905

46. Savage DE, Constine LS, Schwartz RG, Rubin P (1990) Radiation effects on left ventricular function and myocardial perfusion in long term survivors of Hodgkin's disease. Int J Radiat Oncol Biol Phys 19:721–727

47. Gustavsson A, Eskilsson J, Landberg T, Svahn-Tapper G, White T, Wollmer P, Akerman M (1990) Late cardiac effects after mantle radiotherapy in patients with Hodgkin's disease. Ann Oncol 1:355–363

48. Maunoury C, Pierga JY, Valette H, Tchernia G, Cosset JM, Desgrez A (1992) Myocardial perfusion damage after mediastinal irradiation for Hodgkin's disease: a thallium-201 single photon emission tomography study. Eur J Nucl Med 19:871–873

49. Glanzmann C, Kaufmann P, Jenni R, Hess OM, Huguenin P (1998) Cardiac risk after mediastinal irradiation for Hodgkin's disease. Radiother Oncol 46:51–62

50. Girinsky T, Cordova A, Rey A, Cosset JM, Tertian G, Pierga JY (2000) Thallium-201 scintigraphy is not predictive of late cardiac complications in patients with Hodgkin's disease treated with mediastinal radiation. Int J Radiat Oncol Biol Phys 48:1503–1506

51. Heidenreich PA, Schnittger I, Strauss HW, Vagelos RH, Lee BK, Mariscal CS, Tate DJ, Horning SJ, Hoppe RT, Hancock SL (2007) Screening for coronary artery disease after mediastinal irradiation for Hodgkin's disease. J Clin Oncol 25:43–49

52. Gayed IW, Liu HH, Yusuf SW, Komaki R, Wei X, Wang X, Chang JY, Swafford J, Broemeling L, Liao Z (2006) The prevalence of myocardial ischemia after concurrent chemoradiation therapy as detected by gated myocardial perfusion imaging in patients with esophageal cancer. J Nucl Med 47:1756–1762

53. Dawson LA, Ten Haken RK (2005) Partial volume tolerance of the liver to radiation. Semin Radiat Oncol 15:279–283

54. Lawrence TS, Robertson JM, Anscher MS, Jirtle RL, Ensminger WD, Fajardo LF (1995) Hepatic toxicity resulting from cancer treatment. Int J Radiat Oncol Biol Phys 31:1237–1248

55. Ingold JA, Reed GB, Kaplan HS, Bagshaw MA (1965) Radiation hepatitis. Am J Roentgenol Radium Ther Nucl Med 93:200–208

56. Reed GB Jr, Cox AJ Jr (1966) The human liver after radiation injury. A form of veno-occlusive disease. Am J Pathol 48:597–611

57. Kwek JW, Iyer RB, Dunnington J, Faria S, Silverman PM (2006) Spectrum of imaging findings in the abdomen after radiotherapy. AJR Am J Roentgenol 187:1204–1211

58. Cao Y, Platt JF, Francis IR, Balter JM, Pan C, Normolle D, Ben-Josef E, Haken RK, Lawrence TS (2007) The prediction of radiation-induced liver dysfunction using a local dose and regional venous perfusion model. Med Phys 34:604–612

59. Munden RF, Erasmus JJ, Smythe WR, Madewell JE, Forster KM, Stevens CW (2005) Radiation injury to the liver after intensity-modulated radiation therapy in patients with mesothelioma: an unusual CT appearance. AJR Am J Roentgenol 184:1091–1095

60. Yankelevitz DF, Knapp PH, Henschke CI, Nisce L, Yi Y, Cahill P (1992) MR appearance of radiation hepatitis. Clin Imaging 16:89–92

61. Onaya H, Itai Y, Ahmadi T, Yoshioka H, Okumura T, Akine Y, Tsuji H, Tsujii H (2001) Recurrent hepatocellular carcinoma versus radiation-induced hepatic injury: differential diagnosis with MR imaging. Magn Reson Imaging 19:41–46

62. Mori H, Yoshioka H, Mori K, Ahmadi T, Okumura T, Saida Y, Itai Y (2002) Radiation-induced liver injury showing low intensity on T2-weighted images noted in Budd-Chiari syndrome. Radiat Med 20:69–76

63. Mori H, Yoshioka H, Ahmadi T, Saida Y, Ohara K, Itai Y (2000) Early radiation effects on the liver demonstrated on superparamegnetic iron oxide-enhanced T1-weighted MRI. J Comput Assist Tomogr 24:648–651

64. Nohara C, Matsumine H, Suzuki K, Saito A, Ohtaka M, Mori H, Suda K, Kondo T, Hayakawa M, Kanai J, Mizuno Y (1997) [(Neurological CPC-59). A 65-year-old man with a history of gastric cancer who presented progressive loss of vision, memory loss and consciousness disturbance]. No To Shinkei 49:1041–1051

65. Yoshiokaa H, Itai Y, Saida Y, Mori K, Mori H, Okumura T (2000) Superparamagnetic iron oxide-enhanced MR imaging for early and late radiation-induced hepatic injuries. Magn Reson Imaging 18:1079–1088

66. Yamasaki SA, Marn CS, Francis IR, Robertson JM, Lawrence TS (1995) High-dose localized radiation therapy for treatment of hepatic malignant tumors: CT findings and their relation to radiation hepatitis. AJR Am J Roentgenol 165:79–84

67. Armstrong C, Mollman J, Corn BW, Alavi J, Grossman M (1993) Effects of radiation therapy on adult brain behavior: evidence for a rebound phenomenon in a phase 1 trial. Neurology 43:1961–1965

68. Meyers CA, Weitzner MA (1995) Neurobehavioral functioning and quality of life in patients treated for cancer of the central nervous system. Curr Opin Oncol 7:197–200

69. Weitzner MA, Meyers CA (1997) Cognitive functioning and quality of life in malignant glioma patients: a review of the literature. Psychooncology 6:169–177

70. Giovagnoli AR, Boiardi A (1994) Cognitive impairment and quality of life in long-term survivors of malignant brain tumors. Ital J Neurol Sci 15:481–488

71. Archibald YM, Lunn D, Ruttan LA, Macdonald DR, Del Maestro RF, Barr HW, Pexman JH, Fisher BJ, Gaspar LE, Cairncross JG (1994) Cognitive functioning in long-term survivors of high-grade glioma. J Neurosurg 80:247–253

72. Hoppe-Hirsch E, Brunet L, Laroussinie F, Cinalli G, Pierre-Kahn A, Renier D, Sainte-Rose C, Hirsch JF (1995) Intellectual outcome in children with malignant tumors of the posterior fossa: influence of the field of irradiation and quality of surgery. Childs Nerv Syst 11:340–345; discussion 345–346

73. Merchant TE, Kiehna EN, Li C, Xiong X, Mulhern RK (2005) Radiation dosimetry predicts IQ after conformal radiation therapy in pediatric patients with localized ependymoma. Int J Radiat Oncol Biol Phys 63:1546–1554

74. Crossen JR, Garwood D, Glatstein E, Neuwelt EA (1994) Neurobehavioral sequelae of cranial irradiation in adults: a review of radiation-induced encephalopathy. J Clin Oncol 12:627–642

75. Taphoorn MJ, Klein M (2004) Cognitive deficits in adult patients with brain tumours. Lancet Neurol 3:159–168

76. Armstrong C, Ruffer J, Corn B, DeVries K, Mollman J (1995) Biphasic patterns of memory deficits following moderate-dose partial-brain irradiation: neuropsychologic outcome and proposed mechanisms. J Clin Oncol 13:2263–2271

77. Calvo W, Hopewell JW, Reinhold HS, Yeung TK (1986) Radiation induced damage in the choroid plexus of the rat brain: a histological evaluation. Neuropathol Appl Neurobiol 12:47–61

78. Calvo W, Hopewell JW, Reinhold HS, Yeung TK (1988) Time- and dose-related changes in the white matter of the rat brain after single doses of X rays. Br J Radiol 61:1043–1052

79. Devi PU, Hossain M, Bisht KS (1999) Effect of late fetal irradiation on adult behavior of mouse: Dose-response relationship. Neurotoxicol Teratol 21:193–198

80. Sienkiewicz ZJ, Haylock RG, Saunders RD (1994) Prenatal irradiation and spatial memory in mice: investigation of dose-response relationship. Int J Radiat Biol 65:611–618

81. Sienkiewicz ZJ, Saunders RD, Butland BK (1992) Prenatal irradiation and spatial memory in mice: investigation of critical period. Int J Radiat Biol 62:211–219

82. Vos MJ, Hoekstra OS, Barkhof F, Berkhof J, Heimans JJ, Van Groeningen CJ, Vandertop WP, Slotman BJ, Postma TJ (2003) Thallium-201 single-photon emission computed tomography as an early predictor of outcome in recurrent glioma. J Clin Oncol 21:3559–3565

83. Spaeth N, Wyss MT, Weber B, Scheidegger S, Lutz A, Verwey J, Radovanovic I, Pahnke J, Wild D, Westera G, Weishaupt D, Hermann DM, Kaser-Hotz B, Aguzzi A, Buck A (2004) Uptake of 18F-fluorocholine, 18F-fluoroethyl-L-tyrosine, and 18F-FDG in acute cerebral radiation injury in the rat: implications for separation of radiation necrosis from tumor recurrence. J Nucl Med 45:1931–1938

84. Henze M, Mohammed A, Schlemmer HP, Herfarth KK, Hoffner S, Haufe S, Mier W, Eisenhut M, Debus J, Haberkorn U (2004) PET and SPECT for detection of tumor progression in irradiated low-grade astrocytoma: a receiver-operating-characteristic analysis. J Nucl Med 45:579–586

85. Ross DA, Sandler HM, Balter JM, Hayman JA, Archer PG, Auer DL (2005) Imaging changes after stereotactic radiosurgery of primary and secondary malignant brain tumors. J Neurooncol 56:175–181

86. Araki Y, Imao Y, Hirata T, Ando T, Sakai N, Yamada H (1990) [Cerebral blood flow of the non-affected brain in patients with malignant brain tumors as studied by SPECT; with special reference to adverse effects of radiochemotherapy]. No Shinkei Geka 18:601–608

87. Harila-Saari AH, Ahonen AK, Vainionpaa LK, Paakko EL, Pyhtinen J, Himanen AS, Torniainen PJ, Lanning BM (1997) Brain perfusion after treatment of childhood acute lymphoblastic leukemia. J Nucl Med 38:82–88

88. Kahkonen M, Metsahonkala L, Minn H, Utriainen T, Korhonen T, Norvasuo-Heila MK, Harila-Saari A, Aarimaa T, Suhonen-Polvi H, Ruotsalainen U, Solin O, Salmi TT (2000) Cerebral glucose metabolism in survivors of childhood acute lymphoblastic leukemia. Cancer 88:693–700

89. Munley MT, Marks LB, Strickland JL, Turkington TG, Wong TZ, Coleman RE, Halperin EC (1999) The effect of radiotherapy on brain metabolism using F-18 FDG PET imaging. Int J Radiat Biol 45:330–331

90. Mineura K, Suda Y, Yasuda T, Kowada M, Ogawa T, Shishido F, Uemura K (1988) Early and late stage positron emission tomography (PET) studies on the haemocirculation and metabolism of seemingly normal brain tissue in patients with gliomas following radiochemotherapy. Acta Neurochir (Wien) 93:110–115

91. Hahn CA, Zhou S, Raynor R, Tisch, A, Light K, Shafman T, Wong T, Kirkpatrick J, Turkington T, Hollis D, Marks LB (2008) Dose-dependent effects of radiation therapy on cerebral blood flow, metabolism and neurocognitive dysfunction. Int J Rad Onc Biol Phys (in press)

92. Karger CP, Munter MW, Heiland S, Peschke P, Debus J, Hartmann GH (2002) Dose-response curves and tolerance doses for late functional changes in the normal rat brain after stereotactic radiosurgery evaluated by magnetic resonance imaging: influence of end points and follow-up time. Radiat Res 157:617–625

93. Hein PA, Eskey CJ, Dunn JF, Hug EB (2004) Diffusion-weighted imaging in the follow-up of treated high-grade gliomas: tumor recurrence versus radiation injury. AJNR Am J Neuroradiol 25:201–209

94. Price SJ, Jena R, Green HA, Kirkby NF, Lynch AG, Coles CE, Pickard JD, Gillard JH, Burnet NG (2007) Early radiotherapy dose response and lack of hypersensitivity effect in normal brain tissue: a sequential dynamic susceptibility imaging study of cerebral perfusion. Clin Oncol (R Coll Radiol) 19:577–587

95. Liu AK, Marcus KJ, Fischl B, Grant PE, Young Poussaint T, Rivkin MJ, Davis P, Tarbell NJ, Yock TI (2007) Changes in cerebral cortex of children treated for medulloblastoma. Int J Radiat Oncol Biol Phys 68:992–998

96. Davidson A, Tait DM, Payne GS, Hopewell JW, Leach MO, Watson M, MacVicar AD, Britton JA, Ashley S (2000) Magnetic resonance spectroscopy in the evaluation of neurotoxicity following cranial irradiation for childhood cancer. Br J Radiol 73:421–424

97. Virta A, Patronas N, Raman R, Dwyer A, Barnett A, Bonavita S, Tedeschi G, Lundbom N (2000) Spectroscopic imaging of radiation-induced effects in the white matter of glioma patients. Magn Reson Imaging 18:851–857

98. Rango M, Spagnoli D, Tomei G, Bamonti F, Scarlato G, Zetta L (1995) Central nervous system trans-synaptic effects of acute axonal injury: a 1H magnetic resonance spectroscopy study. Magn Reson Med 33:595–600

99. Simmons ML, Frondoza CG, Coyle JT (1991) Immunocytochemical localization of N-acetyl-aspartate with monoclonal antibodies. Neuroscience 45:37–45

100. Rutkowski T, Tarnawski R, Sokol M, Maciejewski B (2003) 1H-MR spectroscopy of normal brain tissue before and after postoperative radiotherapy because of primary brain tumors. Int J Radiat Oncol Biol Phys 56:1381–1389

101. Usenius T, Usenius JP, Tenhunen M, Vainio P, Johansson R, Soimakallio S, Kauppinen R (1995) Radiation-induced changes in human brain metabolites as studied by 1H nuclear magnetic resonance spectroscopy in vivo. Int J Radiat Oncol Biol Phys 33:719–724

102. Waldrop SM, Davis PC, Padgett CA, Shapiro MB, Morris R (1998) Treatment of brain tumors in children is associated with abnormal MR spectroscopic ratios in brain tissue remote from the tumor site. AJNR Am J Neuroradiol 19:963–970

103. Esteve F, Rubin C, Grand S, Kolodie H, Le Bas JF (1998) Transient metabolic changes observed with proton MR spectroscopy in normal human brain after radiation therapy. Int J Radiat Oncol Biol Phys 40:279–286

104. Kaminaga T, Shirai K (2005) Radiation-induced brain metabolic changes in the acute and early delayed phase detected with quantitative proton magnetic resonance spectroscopy. J Comput Assist Tomogr 29:293–297

105. Zeng Q-S, Li C-F, Liu H, Zhen J-H, Feng D-C (2007) Distinction between recurrent glioma and radiation injury using magnetic resonance spectroscopy in combination with diffusion-weighted imaging. Int J Radiat Oncol Biol Phys 68:151–158

106. Rocca MA, Filippi M (2006) Functional MRI to study brain plasticity in clinical neurology. Neurol Sci 27[Suppl 1]:S24–26

107. Di Salle F, Formisano E, Linden DE, Goebel R, Bonavita S, Pepino A, Smaltino F, Tedeschi G (1999) Exploring brain function with magnetic resonance imaging. Eur J Radiol 30:84–94

108. Moritz C, Haughton V (2003) Functional MR imaging: paradigms for clinical preoperative mapping. Magn Reson Imaging Clin N Am 11:529–542

109. Zou P, Mulhern RK, Butler RW, Li CS, Langston JW, Ogg RJ (2005) BOLD responses to visual stimulation in survivors of childhood cancer. Neuroimage 24:61–69

110. Hein PA, Eskey CJ, Dunn JF, Hug EB (2004) Diffusion-weighted imaging in the follow-up of treated high-grade gliomas: tumor recurrence versus radiation injury. AJNR Am J Neuroradiol 25:201–209

111. Asao C, Korogi Y, Kitajima M, Hirai T, Baba Y, Makino K, Kochi M, Morishita S, Yamashita Y (2005) Diffusion-weighted imaging of radiation-induced brain injury for differentiation from tumor recurrence. AJNR Am J Neuroradiol 26:1455–1460

112. Chong VF, Rumpel H, Fan YF, Mukherji SK (2001) Temporal lobe changes following radiation therapy: imaging and proton MR spectroscopic findings. Eur Radiol 11:317–324

113. Zeng QS, Li CF, Liu H, Zhen JH, Feng DC (2007) Distinction between recurrent glioma and radiation injury using magnetic resonance spectroscopy in combination with diffusion-weighted imaging. Int J Radiat Oncol Biol Phys 68:151–158

114. Plotkin M, Eisenacher J, Bruhn H, Wurm R, Michel R, Stockhammer F, Feussner A, Dudeck O, Wust P, Felix R, Amthauer H (2004) 123I-IMT SPECT and 1H MR-spectroscopy at 3.0 T in the differential diagnosis of recurrent or residual gliomas: a comparative study. J Neurooncol 70:49–58

115. Matulewicz L, Sokol M, Michnik A, Wydmanski J (2006) Long-term normal-appearing brain tissue monitoring after irradiation using proton magnetic resonance spectroscopy in vivo: statistical analysis of a large group of patients. Int J Radiat Oncol Biol Phys 66:825–832

116. Hahn CA ZS, Dunn RH (2005) Dose-dependent effects of radiation therapy on cerebral blood flow, metabolism and neurocognitive dysfunction. Int J Radiat Oncol Biol Phys 62:S67

117. Hakim SG, Jacobsen H, Hermes D, Kosmehl H, Lauer I, Nadrowitz R, Sieg P (2004) Early immunohistochemical and functional markers indicating radiation damage of the parotid gland. Clin Oral Investig 8:30–35

118. Bussels B, Maes A, Flamen P, Lambin P, Erven K, Hermans R, Nuyts S, Weltens C, Cecere S, Lesaffre E, Van den Bogaert W (2004) Dose-response relationships within the parotid gland after radiotherapy for head and neck cancer. Radiother Oncol 73:297–306

119. Buus S, Grau C, Munk OL, Bender D, Jensen K, Keiding S (2004) 11C-methionine PET, a novel method for measuring regional salivary gland function after radiotherapy of head and neck cancer. Radiother Oncol 73:289–296

120. van Acker F, Flamen P, Lambin P, Maes A, Kutcher GJ, Weltens C, Hermans R, Baetens J, Dupont P, Rijnders A, Maes A, van den Bogaert W, Mortelmans L (2001) The utility of SPECT in determining the relationship between radiation dose and salivary gland dysfunction after radiotherapy. Nucl Med Commun 22:225–231

121. Nomayr A, Lell M, Sweeney R, Bautz W, Lukas P (2001) MRI appearance of radiation-induced changes of normal cervical tissues. Eur Radiol 11:1807–1817

122. Zhang L, Murata Y, Ishida R, Ohashi I, Yoshimura R, Shibuya H (2001) Functional evaluation with intravoxel incoherent motion echo-planar MRI in irradiated salivary glands: a correlative study with salivary gland scintigraphy. J Magn Reson Imaging 14:223–229

123. Buus S, Grau C, Munk OL, Rodell A, Jensen K, Mouridsen K, Keiding S (2006) Individual radiation response of parotid glands investigated by dynamic 11C-methionine PET. Radiother Oncol 78:262–269

124. Astreinidou E, Roesink JM, Raaijmakers CP, Bartels LW, Witkamp TD, Lagendijk JJ, Terhaard CH (2007) 3D MR sialography as a tool to investigate radiation-induced xerostomia: feasibility study. Int J Radiat Oncol Biol Phys 68:1310–1319

125. Maes A, Weltens C, Flamen P, Lambin P, Bogaerts R, Liu X, Baetens J, Hermans R, Van den Bogaert W (2002) Preservation of parotid function with uncomplicated conformal radiotherapy. Radiother Oncol 63:203–211

126. Roesink JM, Moerland MA, Hoekstra A, Van Rijk PP, Terhaard CH (2004) Scintigraphic assessment of early and late parotid gland function after radiotherapy for head-and-neck cancer: a prospective study of dose-volume response relationships. Int J Radiat Oncol Biol Phys 58:1451–1460

127. Hsiung CY, Ting HM, Huang HY, Lee CH, Huang EY, Hsu HC (2006) Parotid-sparing intensity-modulated radiotherapy (IMRT) for nasopharyngeal carcinoma: preserved parotid function after IMRT on quantitative salivary scintigraphy, and comparison with historical data after conventional radiotherapy. Int J Radiat Oncol Biol Phys 66:454–461

128. Prosnitz RG, Hubbs JL, Evans ES et al (2007) Prospective assessment of radiotherapy-associated cardiac toxicity in breast cancer patients: analysis of data 3 to 6 years after treatment. Cancer 110:1840–1850

129. Mah K, Van Dyk J, Keane T et al (1987) Acute radiation-induced pulmonary damage: a clinical study on the response to fractionated radiation therapy. Int J Radiat Oncol Biol Phys 13:179–188

130. Polansky SM, Ravin CE, Prosnitz LR (1980) Pulmonary changes after primary irradiationfor early breast carcinoma. AJR Am J Roentgenol 134:101–105

131. Allavena C, Conroy T, Aletti P et al (1992) Late cardiopulmonary toxicity after treatment for Hodgkin's disease. Br J Cancer 65:908–912

132. Woel RT, Munley MT, Hollis D et al (2002) The time course of radiation therapy-induced reductions in regional perfusion: a prospective study with >5 years of follow-up. Int J Radiat Oncol Biol Phys 52:58–67

133. Muryama S, Akamine T, Sakai S et al (2004) Risk factor of radiation pneumonitis: assessment with velocity-encoded cine magnetic resonance imaging of pulmonary artery. J Comput Assist Tomogr 28:204–208

134. Tokatli F, Kaya M, Kocak Z et al (2005) Sequential pulmonary effects of radiotherapy detected by functional and radiological end points in women with breast cancer. Clin Oncol (R Coll Radiol) 17:39–46

135. Theuws JC, Seppenwoolde Y, Kwa SL et al (2000) Changes in local pulmonary injury up to 48 months after irradiation for lymphoma and breast cancer. Int J Radiat Oncol Biol Phys 47:1201–1208

136. Seppenwoolde Y, Muller SH, Theuws JC et al (2000) Radiation dose-effect relations and local recovery in perfusion for patients with non-small-cell lung cancer. Int J Radiat Oncol Biol Phys 47:681–690

137. Boersma LJ, Damen EM, de Boer RW et al (1996) Recovery of overall and local lung function loss 18 months after irradiation for malignant lymphoma. J Clin Oncol 14:1431–1441

138. Hicks RJ, Mac Manus MP, Matthews JP et al (2004) Early FDG-PET imaging after radical radiotherapy for non-small-cell lung cancer: inflammatory changes in normal tissues correlate with tumor response and do not confound therapeutic response evaluation. Int J Radiat Oncol Biol Phys 60:412–418

139. Hubbs JL, Zhou SM, Ma JL et al (2008) The Prospective Assessment of RT-Associated Changes in Myocardial Perfusion and Function in Patients Irradiated for Thoracic Malignancies. Int J Radiat Oncol Biol Phys Suppl (Abstract; in press)

Association Between Single Nucleotide Polymorphisms and Susceptibility for the Development of Adverse Effects Resulting from Radiation Therapy

Barry S. Rosenstein

CONTENTS

3.1 Summary

A small, but significant number of radiotherapy patients develop adverse responses to treatment, manifested as either normal tissue/organ damage or the development of a radiation-induced cancer. The ability to predict which patients are at greatest risk for radiation toxicity would be of great benefit in optimizing treatment decisions. One promising approach for the development of a predictive assay is through the use of genetic information. The main source of genetic variation among individuals is single nucleotide polymorphisms. Much of the early work to identify single nucleotide polymorphisms (SNPs) associated with the development of

B. S. Rosenstein, PhD
Departments of Radiation Oncology, Community and Preventive Medicine and Dermatology, Mount Sinai School of Medicine, Box 1236, One Gustave Levy Place, New York, NY 10029, USA
and
Department of Radiation Oncology, New York University School of Medicine, 550 First Avenue, New York, NY 10016, USA

radiation injury focused on candidate genes. These studies have provided results indicative of a genetic basis for radiosensitivity, but it is clear that this approach is too limited in its scope to identify the SNPs that could serve as the basis for a predictive assay with clinical applicability. However, with completion of HapMap II and the development of high density SNP microarrays, it is now feasible to conduct genome wide studies which promise to lead to the identification of SNPs that will serve as the basis of an assay with sufficient sensitivity and specificity to be useful in the routine screening of cancer patients to identify those individuals at greatest risk for the development of adverse effects resulting from radiotherapy.

3.2 Introduction

The widespread recognition that modern radiation therapy can provide a sustainable cure for many people diagnosed with cancer, or at least delay disease progression, has led to its acceptance as a standard treatment option. However, as is true with all forms of cancer therapy, some patients experience morbidity resulting from their treatment. Although there are well-documented dosimetric explanations or underlying medical conditions responsible for the injury experienced by some patients who received radiotherapy, this explanation is not appropriate for many people. Often, the adverse response is simply ascribed to unknown individual variations. Important evidence in support of genetic factors being responsible for the differences in radiosensitivity between patients was obtained through an examination of radiation-induced telangiectasia in breast cancer patients [1]. It was observed in this study that the variation in the progression rate to the development of telangiectasia was relatively large for the same radiation treatment. A determination was reached that 80%–90% of the disparity was due to deterministic effects related to the existence of possibly genetic differences between individuals, whereas only 10%–20% of the variation could be explained through stochastic events arising from the random nature of radiation-induced cell killing and random variations in dosimetry and dose delivery. In addition to normal tissue injury, it must be recognized that radiation is a carcinogen. As a result, radiotherapy may increase the risk for the development of a new cancer. Extensive epidemiologic evidence has been obtained consistent with the conclusion that radiotherapy may cause many of the second malignancies observed in long-term cancer survivors for whom radiation successfully controlled their initial tumor [2–12].

3.3
Predictive Assays

The development of an assay capable of predicting which radiotherapy patients are most likely to manifest adverse radiation effects represents a long sought after goal [13]. Despite modest success, the effort to achieve this aim continues since an assay capable of predicting clinical radiosensitivity would allow customization of radiotherapy protocols. It has been estimated that a significant improvement in the therapeutic index could be achieved using this approach [14, 15]. These efforts are also reflective of the new era of "personalized" medicine [16–18], which recognizes the increasing importance of cancer survivorship for the roughly 10 million Americans who have survived a cancer diagnosis [19]. For these individuals, there is an increased focus on the quality of life 5, 10 or 20 years following treatment. The goal for this field of research is therefore to develop a robust, specific assay for cancer patients who are eligible for radiotherapy to enable individual dose adjustment based upon the response of each patient to this test [14, 15, 20, 21]. It is suggested that the area of research utilizing assays to predict the response of radiotherapy patients based upon genetic profiles be termed "radiogenomics". Hence, radiogenomics is a new manifestation of the developing field of personalized medicine, which uses detailed information about a patient's genotype in order to select a medication, therapy or preventative measure that is particularly suited specifically to that patient.

There have been numerous efforts to identify predictors of clinical radiosensitivity. However, none of these assays has been implemented in the routine practice of radiotherapy as these efforts have failed to yield biomarkers that could serve as the basis for an assay which would possess the level of level of sensitivity and specificity necessary for a clinically useful predictive test [22]. In recent years, attention has focused upon the identification of genetic factors as the basis for an assay to predict which patients are at increased risk for complications secondary to radiation treatment. With the recognition that large and well-characterized patient populations are essential for the performance of these genetic studies, several broad international efforts have begun whose aim is the creation of biorepositories and databanks of radiotherapy patients. Major biorepositories have been established under the auspices of the Gene-PARE (genetic predictors of adverse radiotherapy effects) project [22], GENEPI [23] which was initiated by ESTRO and RadGenomics [24] which is comprised of Japanese patients.

Although the emphasis for much of the research performed has focused upon susceptibility to tissue and organ damage from radiation, there is increasing recognition that the development of second malignancies, particularly in children, is of great concern. Due to the success of radiotherapy and other forms of cancer treatment, many young people are being cured of their cancers only to develop a new radiation-induced cancer some years later. It would therefore also be advantageous if a predictive assay could be advanced that would help to identify which of these patients are most likely to develop a second malignancy from the radiation used to treat their first cancer.

Hence, the overall goal of this area of research is to identify those individuals from the general patient population who are most likely to suffer pronounced radiation-induced normal tissue damage and/or a radiation-induced malignancy. Although these radiosensitive patients may be better suited to a surgical treatment approach, paradoxically, these people could alternatively represent a subset of patients who are optimal candidates for radiotherapy, given that their cancers presumably harbor the identical sequence alterations associated with normal tissue toxicity. This highlights the potential for radiotherapy dose modification as radiosensitive tumors theoretically could require lower total treatment doses than their genetically non-variant counterparts. Conversely, for the vast majority of patients who do not possess genetic variants associated with radiosensitivity, it may be possible to dose escalate and potentially achieve a larger number of cancer cures.

It should also be noted that through this research, genetic markers may be identified that are associated with radioresistance. For these patients, it may be possible, and even necessary if the possession of the SNP confers radioresistance to their cancer, to treat them with a greater dose of radiation.

3.4
Candidate Gene Studies

The sequence of the genetic material between all people is roughly 99.9% identical. However, approximately once every 1,000 nucleotides, a person may have a alternate nucleotide in the DNA sequence, which is referred to as a single nucleotide polymorphism (SNP). Many of the estimated 10 million SNPs that are thought to be present in the human genome can lead to a substitution of one amino acid for a different one in a protein, or could occur in an important functional region of a gene that can cause a person to be more likely to develop a certain disease, affect drug metabolism, or possibly render that individual more susceptible to the development of complications resulting from a radiation treatment [25].

A great deal of work has been performed in recent years in an effort to identify the candidate genes and SNPs in these genes that are associated with clinical radiosensitivity. This work is summarized in Table 3.1. Although candidate gene studies have provided critical evidence supportive of a genetic basis for clinical radiosensitivity, this approach has reached an impasse in terms of its ability to provide findings that will translate into a useful predictive assay for the following reasons: (1) Although a number of studies have detected correlations between possession of a minor SNP allele with an increased incidence of either radiation injury or second malignancy, the results of early studies have not been routinely validated in subsequent work (Table 3.1); (2) There is relative ignorance of the full spectrum of

genes and proteins that are associated with the development of radiation injury and/or radiation-induced cancers; (3) Even if all of the important genes that encode the essential protein products associated with radiation toxicity were included in candidate gene studies, it is not certain whether any of these genes would possess SNPs that would both alter protein function and be present at a high enough frequency in the population to be of importance; (4) Critical SNPs associated with radiosensitivity may not be located within genes, but in regulatory portions of the DNA.

3.5
Genome Wide SNP Association Studies

It has become now clear that candidate gene studies are far too limited in scope to enable identification of SNPs to meet two criteria for useful biomarkers to form the basis of a predictive assay. These two essential characteristics are that the SNP must be present in at least a few per cent of the overall population and that possession of the SNP confers a significant elevation in the relative risk for the development of radiation toxicity. Therefore, it is now recognized that only through the performance of genome wide association studies will it be possible to identify SNPs that could form the basis of a predictive assay. This approach has just become feasible within the past few years due to two important scientific advances that have provided the ability to screen the entire human complement of genetic material to identify SNPs associated with clinical radiation responses. The first is the HapMap Project that has identified a substantial portion of the SNPs present in the human genome [26]. The second critical advance is the development of high density SNP microarrays which has enabled genotyping for less than $0.001 per SNP [27, 28]. Hence, it is likely that the path leading to the identification of SNPs that will form the basis of a predictive assy for clinical radiosensitivity will involve the performance of genome wide association studies. This approach has achieved a great deal of success in other areas of biomedical research which is reflected in the marked increase in the number of genome wide association studies being reported in which SNPs associated with a series of diseases and treatment reactions have been discovered [29].

Table 3.1. Candidate gene studies

Reference	First author	Irradiated site	Gene(s) screened	Number of subjects [a]	Result
[24]	SUGA	Breast	999 SNPs in 137 candidate genes	399	Association between haplotype GGTT in CD44 with an increased incidence of early skin reactions. Association between haplotypes CG in MAD2L2, GTTG in PTTG1, TCC and CCG in RAD9A and GCT in LIG3 with a reduced risk for early skin reactions
[30]	HALL	Prostate	ATM	17	[b] Association between "significant mutations" with proctitis and cystitis
[31]	DUELL	[c] Self reported	XRCC1	1286	No association between the codon 399 SNP with an increased incidence of breast cancer
[32]	SEVERIN	[d] Multiple sites	RAD21	19	Association between the nucleotide 1440 SNP with adverse radiation effects
[33]	IANNUZZI	Breast	ATM	46	Association between "significant" SNPs with subcutaneous fibrosis and telangiectasia
[34]	OFFIT	Hodgkin's disease	ATM	64	No association between protein truncation mutations with the development of breast cancer
[35]	ANDREASSEN	Breast	[e] TGFB1, SOD2, XRCC3, XRCC1, APEX	41	Association between the SNPs in TGFB1 codon 10 and nucleotide -509, SOD2 codon 16, XRCC3 codon 241 and XRCC1 codon 399, with an increased risk for subcutaneous fibrosis
[36]	ANGELE	Breast	ATM	566	Association between the codon 1853 SNP with an increased risk for adverse effects. Association between the SNPs at nucleotides IVS22-77 and IVS48 + 238 with a decreased risk for adverse radiation responses
[37]	BREMER	Breast	ATM	1100	No association between protein truncation mutations with either acute or late radiation effects
[38]	MOULLAN	Breast	XRCC1	566	Association between codons 194 and 399 SNPs with adverse radiation effects
[39]	QUARMBY	Breast	TGFB1	103	Association between the nucleotide -509 and 869 SNPs with subcutaneous fibrosis
[40]	ANDREASSEN	Breast	TGFB1, SOD2, XRCC1, XRCC3, APEX and ATM	52	Association between the TGFB1 codon 10 and nucleotide -509 SNPs with an increased risk of altered breast appearance
[41]	DERUYCK	Cervix / endometrium	XRCC1, XRCC3 and OGG1	62	Association between the XRCC3 nucleotide IVS5-14 SNP with an increased risk of late radiation effects and the XRCC1 codon 194 SNP with a reduced incidence of late effects
[42]	MILLIKAN	[c] Self reported	XRCC3, NBS1, XRCC2 and BRCH2	4333	Association between possession of the minor allele for 2-4 SNPs in the screened genes with an increased risk for breast cancer and number of lifetime mammograms
[43]	ANDREASSEN	Breast	ATM	41	Association between the codon 1853 SNP with subcutaneous fibrosis

Table 3.1. Continued

Reference	First author	Irradiated site	Gene(s) screened	Number of subjects [a]	Result
[44]	ANDREASSEN	Breast	TGFB1, XRCC1, XRCC3, SOD2 and ATM	120	No association for any of the screened SNPs with risk for subcutaneous fibrosis
[45]	CESARETTI	Prostate	ATM	37	Association between missense SNPs (cause substitution of the encoded amino acid) with rectal bleeding and erectile dysfunction
[46]	DAMARAJU	Prostate	[f] Multiple genes		Association between the LIG4 codon 568 and ERCC2 codon 711 SNPs and the CYP2D6*4 splicing defect, with bladder and rectal toxicity
[47]	DERUCK	Cervix / endometrium	TGFB1	218	Association between the SNPs at nucleotides -1.552delAGG, -509 and in codon 10 were associated with development of late radiotherapy effects
[48]	CESARETTI	Prostate	ATM	108	Association between multiple SNPs with proctitis when the radiation dose to rectal tissue was quantified
[49]	EDVARDSEN	Breast	ATM	462	Association between the rs1801516 SNP with a reduced frequency of telangiectasia and the rs1800058 SNP with a reduced risk for pleural thickening and lung fibrosis
[50]	GIOTOPULOS	Breast	TGFB1 and XRCC1	167	Association between the TGFB1 -509 SNP with an increased risk of fibrosis and an association between the XRCC1 codon 399 SNP with an increased risk of telangiectasia
[51]	Ho	Breast	ATM	131	Association between the codon 1853 SNP with the development of fibrosis and telangiectasia
[52]	MEYER	Prostate	ATM	721	No association between the codon 1054 SNP with either urinary morbidity or erectile dysfunction
[53]	PETERS	Prostate	TGFB1	141	Association between SNPs at either nucleotide -509, codon 10 or in codon 25 with a decline in erectile function. Association between the SNP at nucleotide -509 with an increased risk of late rectal bleeding
[54]	EDVARDSEN	Breast	GSTM1, GSTP1, and GSTT1	542	Association between the GSTP1 codon 105 SNP with pleural thickening

[a] Includes cases and controls.

[b] Use of the term "association" indicates that a statistically significant association was reported (generally based upon use of a p-value of 0.05). It should be noted that most studies did not correct the p-value for multiple testing.

[c] Self-reported occupational and medical irradiations.

[d] Breast, tonsillar fossa, cervix, anus, vagina, testis, thymoma, and lymphoma.

[e] When multiple genes and SNPs were screened, a note was indicated only for significant associations that were detected.

[f] BRCA1, BRCA2, ESR1, XRCC1, XRCC2, XRCC3, NBN, RAD51, RAD52, LIG4, ATM, BCL2, TGFB1, MSH6, ERCC2, XPF, NR3C1, CYP1A1, CYP2C9, CYP2C19, CYP3A5, CYP2D6, CYP11B2, and CYP17A1.

Identification of the genetic factors associated with clinical radiosensitivity will have important and direct implications upon patient care as this will provide a basis to predict which patients diagnosed with cancer are at greatest risk for radiation toxicity resulting from radiotherapy. Upon detection of one or several SNPs associated with normal tissue injury or a heightened risk for a second malignancy in a particular patient, either a surgical approach to treatment can be considered, or recommendations may be made that can reduce the risk of morbidity resulting from radiotherapy. An added benefit of genetic testing is that once a potentially radiosensitive population is identified, then the vast majority of cancer patients who prove negative for possession of the SNPs associated with susceptibility to the harmful effects of radiation can consider radiotherapy with less concern regarding complications. In fact, it is possible that traditional treatment doses have been limited by the subset of radiosensitive patients as radiation oncologists generally treat to normal tissue tolerance, the dose at which complications that cause significant morbidity begin to appear in the patient population. It may therefore be feasible as a result of genetic testing to increase the standard treatment dose and possibly achieve more cancer cures among the population of people who do not harbor the genetic alterations associated with adverse radiotherapy responses.

3.6

Conclusion

The performance of genome wide studies to identify SNPs associated with a susceptibility for the development of either radiation injury or a second malignancy from radiotherapy will be of great value as this will permit the creation of a predictive assay that will help patients and their doctors to decide upon an optimal treatment plan for each individual.

Acknowledgements

This research was supported by Department of the Army grants DAMD 17-02-1-0502, DAMD 17-02-1-0503 and American Cancer Society Research Scholar Grant RSGT-05-200-01-CCE.

References

1. Safwat A, Bentzen SM, Turesson I, Hendry JH (2002) Deterministic rather than stochastic factors explain most of the variation in the expression of skin telangiectasia after radiotherapy. Int J Radiat Oncol Biol Phys 52:198–204
2. Brenner DJ, Curtis RE, Hall EJ, Ron E (2000) Second malignancies in prostate carcinoma patients after radiotherapy compared with surgery. Cancer 88:398–406
3. Boice JD Jr, Engholm G, Kleinerman R et al (1988) Radiation dose and second cancer risk in patients treated for cancer of the cervix. Radiat Res 116:3–55
4. Horwich A, Swerdlow AJ (2004) Second primary breast cancer after Hodgkin's disease. Br J Cancer 90:294–298
5. Kenney LB, Yasui Y, Inskip PD et al (2004) Breast cancer after childhood cancer: a report from the Childhood Cancer Survivor Study. Ann Intern Med 141:590–597
6. Perkins JL, Liu Y, Mitby PA et al (2005) Nonmelanoma skin cancer in survivors of childhood and adolescent cancer: a report from the childhood cancer survivor study. J Clin Oncol 23:3733–3741
7. Sigurdson AJ, Ronckers CM, Mertens AC et al (2005) Primary thyroid cancer after a first tumour in childhood (the Childhood Cancer Survivor Study): a nested case-control study. Lancet 365:2014–2023
8. Bassal M, Mertens AC, Taylor L et al (2006) Risk of selected subsequent carcinomas in survivors of childhood cancer: a report from the Childhood Cancer Survivor Study. J Clin Oncol 24:476–483
9. Ronckers CM, Sigurdson AJ, Stovall M et al (2006) Thyroid cancer in childhood cancer survivors: a detailed evaluation of radiation dose response and its modifiers. Radiat Res 166:618–628
10. Neglia JP, Robison LL, Stovall M et al (2006) New primary neoplasms of the central nervous system in survivors of childhood cancer: a report from the Childhood Cancer Survivor Study. J Natl Cancer Inst 98:1528–1537
11. Henderson TO, Whitton J, Stovall M et al (2007) Secondary sarcomas in childhood cancer survivors: a report from the Childhood Cancer Survivor Study. J Natl Cancer Inst 99:300–308
12. Dinu I, Liu Y, Leisenring W et al (2007) Prediction of second malignant neoplasm incidence in a large cohort of long-term survivors of childhood cancers. Pediatr Blood Cancer
13. Fletcher GH (1988) Regaud lecture perspectives on the history of radiotherapy. Radiother Oncol 12:iii–v, 253–271
14. Tucker SL, Geara FB, Peters LJ, Brock WA (1996) How much could the radiotherapy dose be altered for individual patients based on a predictive assay of normal-tissue radiosensitivity? Radiother Oncol 38:103–113
15. Mackay RI, Hendry JH (1999) The modelled benefits of individualizing radiotherapy patients' dose using cellular radiosensitivity assays with inherent variability. Radiother Oncol 50:67–75
16. Evans WE, Relling MV (2004) Moving towards individualized medicine with pharmacogenomics. Nature 429:464–468
17. Fierz W (2004) Challenge of personalized health care: to what extent is medicine already individualized and what are the future trends? Med Sci Monit 10:RA111–123
18. Gurwitz D, Livshits G (2006) Personalized medicine Europe: health, genes and society: Tel-Aviv University,

Tel-Aviv, Israel, June 19–21, 2005. Eur J Hum Genet 14:376–380

19. Aziz NM (2007) Cancer survivorship research: state of knowledge, challenges and opportunities. Acta Oncol 46:417–432

20. Agren A, Brahme A, Turesson I (1990) Optimization of uncomplicated control for head and neck tumors. Int J Radiat Oncol Biol Phys 19:1077–1085

21. MacKay RI, Niemierko A, Goitein M, Hendry JH (1998) Potential clinical impact of normal-tissue intrinsic radiosensitivity testing. Radiother Oncol 46:215–216

22. Ho AY, Atencio DP, Peters S et al (2006) Genetic predictors of adverse radiotherapy effects: the Gene-PARE project. Int J Radiat Oncol Biol Phys 65:646–655

23. Baumann M, Holscher T, Begg AC (2003) Towards genetic prediction of radiation responses: ESTRO's GENEPI project. Radiother Oncol 69:121–125

24. Suga T, Ishikawa A, Kohda M et al (2007) Haplotype-based analysis of genes associated with risk of adverse skin reactions after radiotherapy in breast cancer patients. Int J Radiat Oncol Biol Phys 69:685–693

25. Christensen K, Murray JC (2007) What genome-wide association studies can do for medicine. N Engl J Med 356:1094–1097

26. Frazer KA, Ballinger DG, Cox DR et al (2007) A second generation human haplotype map of over 3.1 million SNPs. Nature 449:851–861

27. Fan JB, Gunderson KL, Bibikova M et al (2006) Illumina universal bead arrays. Methods Enzymol 410:57–73

28. Ragoussis J, Elvidge G (2006) Affymetrix GeneChip system: moving from research to the clinic. Expert Rev Mol Diagn 6:145–152

29. Lango H, Weedon MN (2008) What will whole genome searches for susceptibility genes for common complex disease offer to clinical practice? J Intern Med 263:16–27

30. Hall EJ, Schiff PB, Hanks GE et al (1998) A preliminary report: frequency of A-T heterozygotes among prostate cancer patients with severe late responses to radiation therapy. Cancer J Sci Am 4:385–389

31. Duell EJ, Millikan RC, Pittman GS et al (2001) Polymorphisms in the DNA repair gene XRCC1 and breast cancer. Cancer Epidemiol Biomarkers Prev 10:217–222

32. Severin DM, Leong T, Cassidy B et al (2001) Novel DNA sequence variants in the hHR21 DNA repair gene in radiosensitive cancer patients. Int J Radiat Oncol Biol Phys 50:1323–1331

33. Iannuzzi CM, Atencio DP, Green S, Stock RG, Rosenstein BS (2002) ATM mutations in female breast cancer patients predict for an increase in radiation-induced late effects. Int J Radiat Oncol Biol Phys 52:606–613

34. Offit K, Gilad S, Paglin S et al (2002) Rare variants of ATM and risk for Hodgkin's disease and radiation-associated breast cancers. Clin Cancer Res 8:3813–3819

35. Andreassen CN, Alsner J, Overgaard M, Overgaard J (2003) Prediction of normal tissue radiosensitivity from polymorphisms in candidate genes. Radiother Oncol 69:127–135

36. Angele S, Romestaing P, Moullan N et al (2003) ATM haplotypes and cellular response to DNA damage: association with breast cancer risk and clinical radiosensitivity. Cancer Res 63:8717–8725

37. Bremer M, Klopper K, Yamini P, Bendix-Waltes R, Dork T, Karstens JH (2003) Clinical radiosensitivity in breast cancer patients carrying pathogenic ATM gene mutations: no observation of increased radiation-induced acute or late effects. Radiother Oncol 69:155–160

38. Moullan N, Cox DG, Angele S, Romestaing P, Gerard JP, Hall J (2003) Polymorphisms in the DNA repair gene XRCC1, breast cancer risk, and response to radiotherapy. Cancer Epidemiol Biomarkers Prev 12(11 Pt 1): 1168–1174

39. Quarmby S, Fakhoury H, Levine E et al (2003) Association of transforming growth factor beta-1 single nucleotide polymorphisms with radiation-induced damage to normal tissues in breast cancer patients. Int J Radiat Biol 79:137–143

40. Andreassen CN, Alsner J, Overgaard J et al (2005) TGFB1 polymorphisms are associated with risk of late normal tissue complications in the breast after radiotherapy for early breast cancer. Radiother Oncol 75:18–21

41. De Ruyck K, Van Eijkeren M, Claes K et al (2005) Radiation-induced damage to normal tissues after radiotherapy in patients treated for gynecologic tumors: association with single nucleotide polymorphisms in XRCC1, XRCC3, and OGG1 genes and in vitro chromosomal radiosensitivity in lymphocytes. Int J Radiat Oncol Biol Phys 62:1140–1149

42. Millikan RC, Player JS, Decotret AR, Tse CK, Keku T (2005) Polymorphisms in DNA repair genes, medical exposure to ionizing radiation, and breast cancer risk. Cancer Epidemiol Biomarkers Prev 14:2326–2334

43. Andreassen CN, Overgaard J, Alsner J et al (2006) ATM sequence variants and risk of radiation-induced subcutaneous fibrosis after postmastectomy radiotherapy. Int J Radiat Oncol Biol Phys 64:776–783

44. Andreassen CN, Alsner J, Overgaard M, Sorensen FB, Overgaard J (2006) Risk of radiation-induced subcutaneous fibrosis in relation to single nucleotide polymorphisms in TGFB1, SOD2, XRCC1, XRCC3, APEX and ATM – a study based on DNA from formalin fixed paraffin embedded tissue samples. Int J Radiat Biol 82:577–586

45. Cesaretti J, Stock R, Atencio D et al (2006) A genetically determined dose volume histogram predicts for rectal bleeding among patients treated with prostate brachytherapy. Int J Radiat Oncol Biol Phys 66:S37–S37

46. Damaraju S, Murray D, Dufour J et al (2006) Association of DNA repair and steroid metabolism gene polymorphisms with clinical late toxicity in patients treated with conformal radiotherapy for prostate cancer. Clin Cancer Res 12:2545–2554

47. De Ruyck K, Van Eijkeren M, Claes K et al (2006) TGF-beta1 polymorphisms and late clinical radiosensitivity in patients treated for gynecologic tumors. Int J Radiat Oncol Biol Phys 65:1240–1248

48. Cesaretti JA, Stock RG, Atencio DP et al (2007) A genetically determined dose-volume histogram predicts for rectal bleeding among patients treated with prostate brachytherapy. Int J Radiat Oncol Biol Phys 66:S37–S37

49. Edvardsen H, Tefre T, Jansen L et al (2007) Linkage disequilibrium pattern of the ATM gene in breast cancer patients and controls; association of SNPs and haplotypes to radio-sensitivity and post-lumpectomy local recurrence. Radiat Oncol 2:25

50. Giotopoulos G, Symonds RP, Foweraker K et al (2007) The late radiotherapy normal tissue injury phenotypes of telangiectasia, fibrosis and atrophy in breast cancer

patients have distinct genotype-dependent causes. Br J Cancer 96:1001–1007

51. Ho AY, Fan G, Atencio DP et al (2007) Possession of ATM sequence variants as predictor for late normal tissue responses in breast cancer patients treated with radiotherapy. Int J Radiat Oncol Biol Phys 69:677–684

52. Meyer A, Wilhelm B, Dork T et al (2007) ATM missense variant P1054R predisposes to prostate cancer. Radiother Oncol 83:283–288

53. Peters CA, Stock RG, Cesaretti JA et al (2007) TGFB1 single nucleotide polymorphisms are associated with adverse quality of life in prostate cancer patients treated with radiotherapy. Int J Radiat Oncol Biol Phys 70:752–759

54. Edvardsen H, Kristensen VN, Grenaker Alnaes GI et al (2007) Germline glutathione S-transferase variants in breast cancer: relation to diagnosis and cutaneous long-term adverse effects after two fractionation patterns of radiotherapy. Int J Radiat Oncol Biol Phys 67:1163–1171

4

Prospective Second-Cancer Risk Estimation for Contemporary Radiotherapeutic Protocols

DAVID J. BRENNER and IGOR SHURYAK

CONTENTS

Introduction: Radiotherapy-Related Second-Cancer Risks

The ability to predict radiation-induced cancer risks associated with modern radiation therapy protocols should allow the risks of second cancers to be included, and potentially minimized, in radiation therapy treatment plan optimization. This consideration is of increasing importance in light of the increasing number of younger patients undergoing radiation therapy, and with increasing survival times. As screening programs lead to earlier treatment and at younger ages, and as improvements

D. J. BRENNER, PhD, DSc
I. SHURYAK, MD
Center for Radiological Research, Columbia University Medical Center, 630 West – 168th Street, New York, NY 10032, USA

in radiotherapy result in longer survival times, the issue of radiation-induced second cancers is becoming increasingly important [1, 2]. The 5-year relative survival rate for prostate cancer in the US has increased from about 67% in the mid 1970s to about 98% in the 1990s [3], while the mean age at diagnosis decreased from 72 to 69 [4]. The corresponding 10-year relative survival rates are now 76% for both prostate and breast.

Of particular importance in this regard are radiation-induced second cancers in childhood radiotherapy survivors [5–7], who: (a) are probably inherently more sensitive to radiation-induced carcinogenesis than adults, and (b) hopefully have more years of life remaining.

An example of the magnitude of the risks of concern can be seen from the results of a retrospective tumor-registry-based study [8] which compared second cancers in prostate cancer survivors who had radiotherapy, vs. those who had surgery: Here, the risks of developing a radiation-associated second malignancy after prostate cancer radiotherapy were estimated as 1 in 290 (all years), 1 in 125 for 5+ year survivors, and 1 in 70 for 10+ year survivors. As expected, second-cancer risks are much higher in long-term survivors of pediatric radiotherapy, approaching 25% at 30 years [6].

Using retrospective techniques, many such studies of second cancer risks after radiation therapy have been reported [2, 8–19]. However, radiotherapy treatment techniques are constantly changing, particularly in terms of escalating treatment dose [20–22], altered dose fractionation/protraction [23–26], and, as discussed in the next section, differing normal-tissue dose distributions, such as from intensity-modulated radiation therapy (IMRT) [27, 28]. Consequently, results from second-cancer studies which are typically the results of treatments that took place several decades ago, cannot generally be directly applied to modern-day protocols. This issue can be addressed, as is described in this chapter, by developing models that prospectively predict, through use of organ doses or dose distributions, second cancers associated with current radiation therapeutic treatments. Such models also provide insight into the basic mechanisms of radiation carcinogenesis [29] and, as we argue, are an essential first step towards systematic reduction of long-term radiotherapy-induced second-cancer risks.

4.2
The Potential Significance of Altered Normal-Tissue Dose Distributions: Intensity-Modulated Radiation Therapy and Second-Cancer Risks

There are two potential reasons why the change from 3D conformal radiotherapy (3D-CRT) to IMRT might result in a change in radiation-induced second malignancies risks [27, 30–35]. First, compared to 3D-CRT IMRT involves smaller volumes of normal tissues receiving higher doses, but larger volumes of tissues receiving smaller doses. Clearly the significance of this in terms of radiation-induced malignancies will depend will depend on the shape of the dose-risk relationship. Second, delivery of a specified dose to the isocenter from a modulated field requires the accelerator to be energized for longer, and so more monitor units are needed, typically increases being factors of about 3, but with a range of from about 2–8 [35–37], compared with delivering the same prescribed dose from an unmodulated field. It follows that patient dose due to leakage radiation may be increased, although its spatial distribution and magnitude will depend on many interrelated factors, including the head shielding design, design and operation of the multileaf collimator, beam energy, and the details of the IMRT modulation.

To date, there have only been fairly crude estimates of second cancer risks after IMRT compared with 3D-CRT. FOLLOWILL et al. [34] estimated a fatal cancer risk after pelvic IMRT of 1.0%, compared with 0.4%–0.6% for the corresponding 3D-CRT treatment. HALL and WUU's cancer mortality estimates [27] were 1.8% (IMRT) vs. 1.0% (3D-CRT), and the fatal cancer risk estimates by KRY et al. [35] were 2.9%–3.7% (IMRT) vs. 1.7% (3D-CRT). So each of these estimates concluded that IMRT would roughly

double the second-cancer risk, compared with 3D conformal radiotherapy.

These estimates are, however, all very crude [38]. In particular they are based on linear extrapolations of low dose (≤ 2 Gy) cancer risks that were generated for radiation-protection purposes from A-bomb survivors, to high, fractionated, radiotherapeutic doses. There has been a considerable literature suggesting that this is not a reasonable approach [11, 39], though to date alternatives have not been available. Here we describe some new approaches towards understanding and predicting dose-effect relations for radiation-induced cancer at radiotherapeutic doses.

4.3
Mechanisms of Radiation-Induced Cancer at Radiotherapeutic Doses

4.3.1
The Standard Model

Radiation therapy can deliver very high doses of radiation to regions in organs that are in or close to the target volume [40]. In earlier approaches to high-dose risk estimation, radiation-induced carcinogenesis at high doses was assumed to be governed primarily by two competing cellular processes [41], "initiation" and "inactivation". Initiation is the production of changes that make a stem cell premalignant; examples are chromosomal translocations, such as the Philadelphia chromosome [42], or other cytogenetic abnormalities such as inversions, small-scale mutations, deletions, duplications, or aneuploidy [43–45]. Inactivation prevents a stem cell from having viable progeny, examples being mitotic death or apoptosis.

The assumption that radiation carcinogenesis is primarily governed by initiation and inactivation has generally been quantified using the standard linear–quadratic–exponential (LQE) equation [41]; for reviews, see [29, 46, 47]. The LQE equation describes the excess relative cancer risk (ERR) after a single acute dose of radiation (D) as

$$\text{ERR} = (aD + bD^2)\exp(-\alpha D - \beta D^2) \qquad (4.1)$$

where a and b are linear and quadratic coefficients for initiation, and α and β are linear and quadratic coefficients for inactivation. The LQE equation uses the classic linear-quadratic (LQ) form both for radiation-induced initiation $(aD + bD^2)$ and for radiation-induced inactivation $\exp(-\alpha D - \beta D^2)$.

For small and intermediate radiation doses, Equation 4.1 predicts that ERR is an increasing function of dose, as is seen epidemiologically [11, 12, 48, 49]. At high doses, however, the exponential cellular inactivation term, $\exp(-\alpha D - \beta D^2)$, in this LQE equation leads to very small predicted ERRs; that is, essentially all radiation-initiated premalignant stem cells would be inactivated by the radiation. As shown in Figure 4.1 [29], this prediction of the LQE equation is inconsistent with recent estimates of radiation-induced solid cancer risks, in that a rapid decrease in the ERR at high doses is not observed.

4.3.2
A More Realistic Model

Consequently, the standard LQE initiation–inactivation model has been extended [29] to include a third mechanism, in addition to initiation and inactivation, of radiation-induced carcinogenesis at high doses. Specifically, symmetric stem-cell proliferation (i.e., a stem cell dividing into two daughter stem cells) occurs in response to radiation-induced cell killing [55–58], and replenishes the number of stem cells in that organ. Because repopulating cells can only travel very small distances, at least for solid organs, they will have been near the treatment field at the time of irradiation, so will have received significant doses, and so will contain a significant fraction of stem cells with pre-malignant damage. Symmetric proliferation, which takes place both during and after radiation therapy, and will thus increase the high-dose cancer risk, as any proliferating stem cell that has pre-malignant damage can pass that damage on to its progeny.

In fact there is a great deal of quantitative biology in the literature about repopulation kinetics [55–58], which can be reasonably grafted on to the standard initiation/inactivation model, resulting in a quantitative initiation/inactivation/proliferation model, as discussed in the next section.

Figure 4.2 schematizes the three mechanisms which appear to dominate radiation-induced carcinogenesis at radiotherapeutic doses. The standard model incorporates only the first two mechanisms, namely initiation and inactivation.

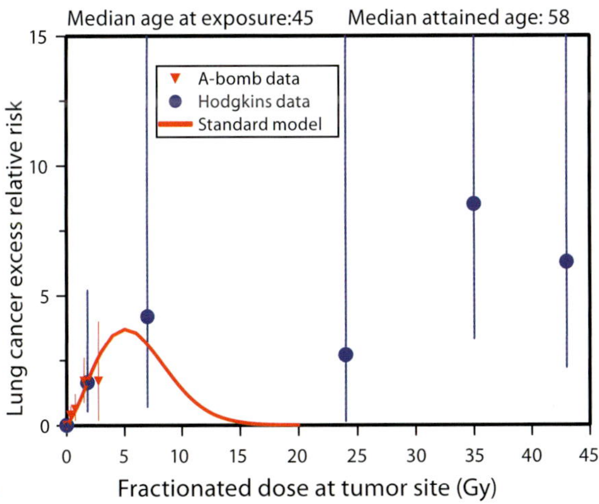

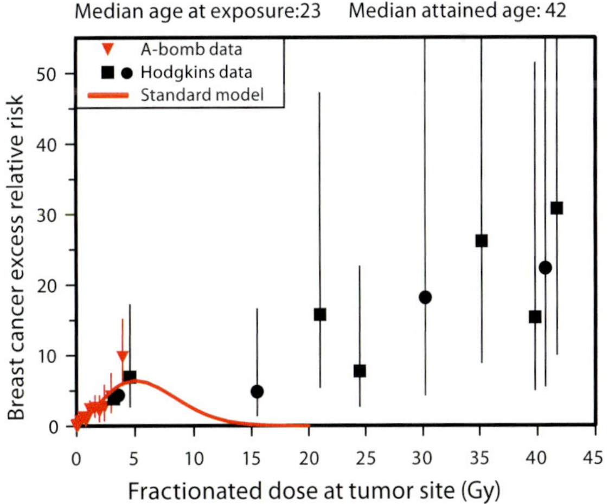

Fig. 4.1a,b. Excess relative risks for radiation-induced lung cancer (**a**) and breast cancer (**b**). The lower-dose data points from A-bomb survivors [50, 51], and the data points at high doses are from studies of lung cancer [52] and breast cancer [53, 54] after radiotherapy of Hodgkin's disease patients. The *solid curves* in each panel represent fits to the A-bomb data using the standard "initiation + killing" LQE model [41], which involves a balance solely between induction of pre-malignant cells and cell killing, without considering cellular repopulation. It is clear that the predictions of this standard LQE model are inconsistent with the high-dose data

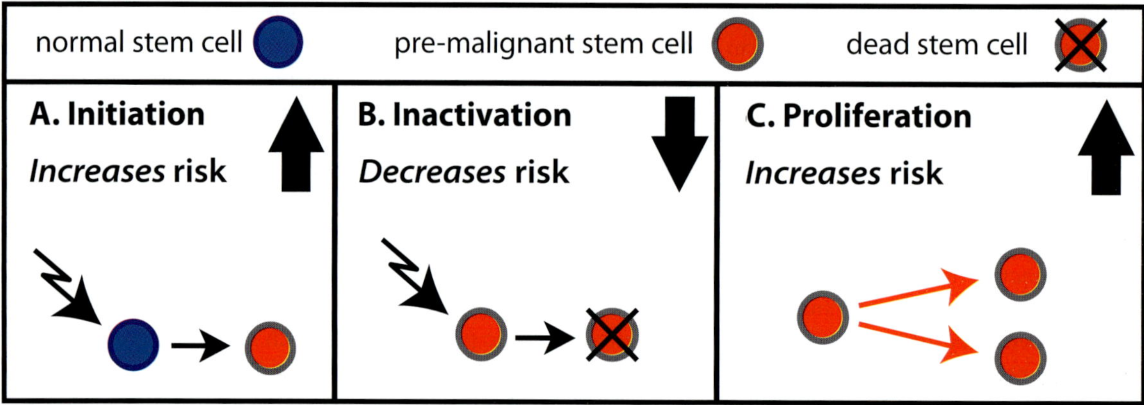

Fig. 4.2. The three dominant processes affecting the probability of radiation-induced cancer at radiotherapeutic doses. The standard model incorporates only the first two of these mechanisms

4.4

An Application: Prospective Estimation of Radiotherapy-Induced Second-Cancer Risks

The stem cell initiation/inactivation/proliferation model [29, 59, 60] outlined here provides a practical approach [61] for predicting organ-specific high-dose cancer risks based on: (a) cancer risk data from A-bomb survivors (who were exposed to lower doses), (b) the demographic variables (age, time since exposure, gender, ethnicity) of the population/individual of interest, and (c) an organ-specific parameter describing radiation-induced cellular repopulation, which has previously been estimated both for breast and lung [29]. First, ERRs are directly estimated for single radiation exposures at moderate doses, based on cancer incidence data among A-bomb survivors [50, 62]. Second, a well established methodology described by LAND and colleagues [63] (and almost identically in the recent BEIR-VII report [64]) is used to adjust the dose-dependent ERRs from the A-bomb survivors to apply to the demographics (age, time since exposure, gender, ethnicity) of the individual or group under study. These two steps are implemented through publicly available on-line software (Interactive RadioEpidemiological Program, IREP version 5.3 [65]). Finally, these moderate-dose ERR estimates for single exposures are adjusted to fractionated high-dose radiation exposure, using the initiation/inactivation/proliferation model [29] outlined above.

This augmented cancer risk model is able to well describe demographics-specific epidemiological data for radiotherapy-induced carcinogenesis [29, 59]; examples are shown in Figure 4.3.

The approach can, in principle, generate organ-specific ERR estimates for any given radiotherapeutic dose and fractionation scheme, for any given set of demographics (in particular age at exposure, and time post exposure). Essentially all that is needed are dose-volume histogram (DVH) data for the organ or organs of interest. In this "dosimetric + risk-modeling" method, each incremental small volume in the DVH, ΔV_j, is associated with a total dose $D_j = j\Delta D$. Given the associated $ERR(D_j)$, estimated as described above, the overall predicted ERR is the volume-average of these local ERRs, i.e., $ERR = (1/V) \sum_j ERR(D_j) \Delta V_j$, where V is the organ volume. An example is given in Figure 4.4, based on results reported by KOH et al. [61].

4.5

Future Directions

Understanding and quantifying second cancer risks is, we believe, the first step towards being able to reduce them, through hardware and software optimization – conceptually in the same way as classic early and late sequelae have been reduced by advances in hardware and by treatment planning. Having said

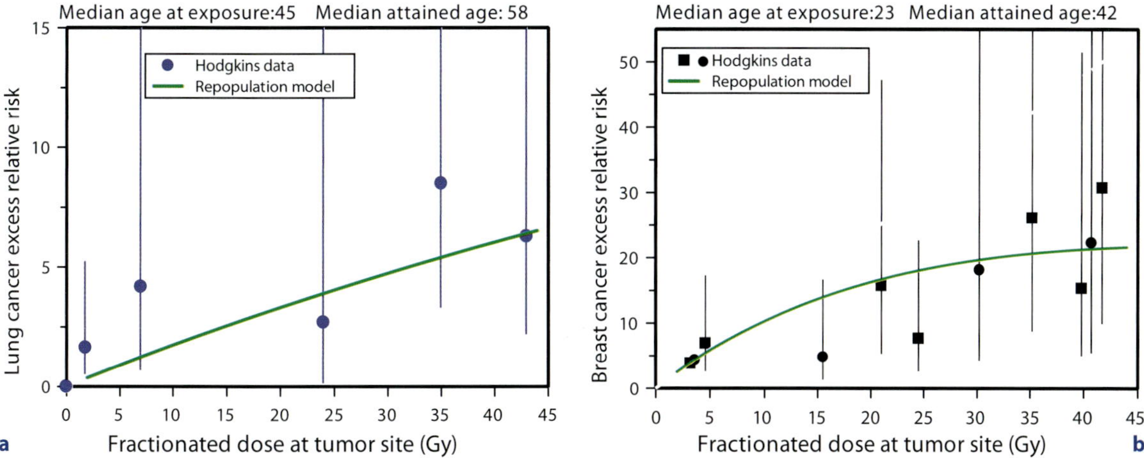

Fig. 4.3a,b. Measured and predicted excess relative risks for lung cancer (**a**) and breast cancer (**b**) induced by high doses of fractionated ionizing radiation. The data points are from studies of second cancers after radiotherapy of Hodgkin's disease patients, as in Figure 4.1, and the curves are estimates using the methodology [29] outlined here

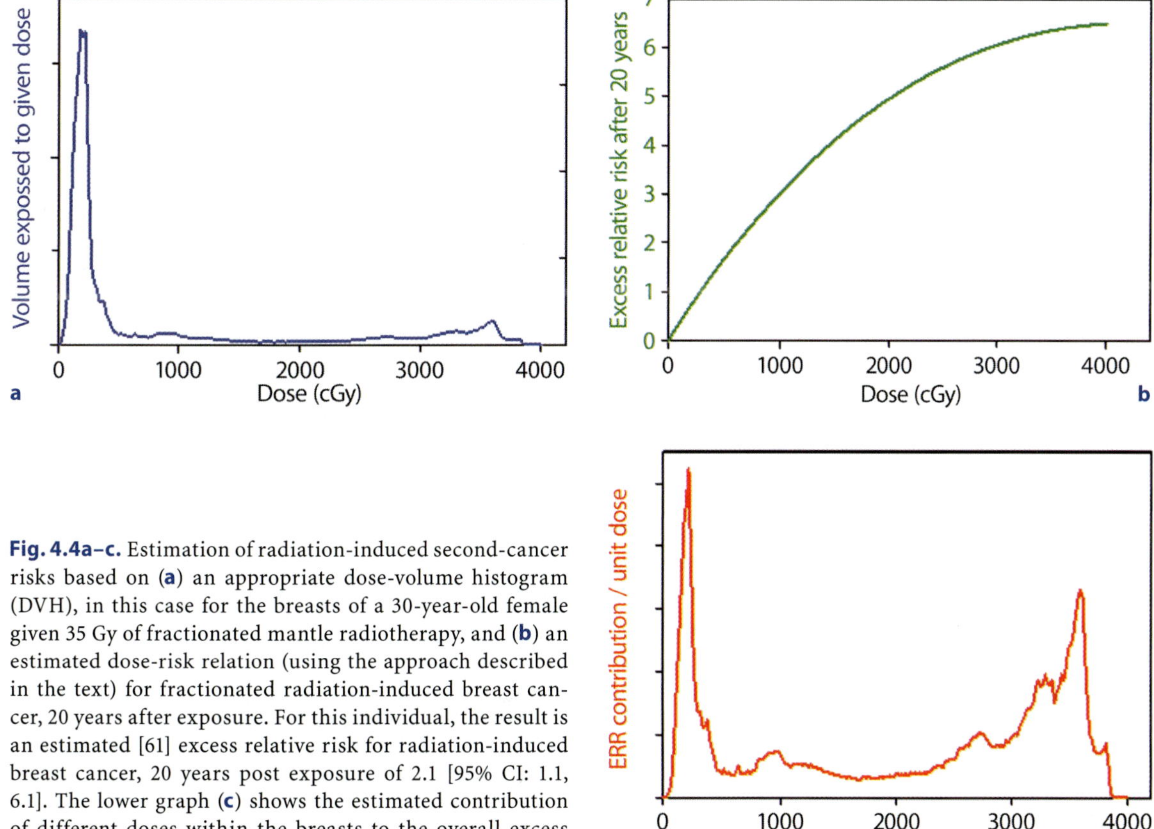

Fig. 4.4a–c. Estimation of radiation-induced second-cancer risks based on (**a**) an appropriate dose-volume histogram (DVH), in this case for the breasts of a 30-year-old female given 35 Gy of fractionated mantle radiotherapy, and (**b**) an estimated dose-risk relation (using the approach described in the text) for fractionated radiation-induced breast cancer, 20 years after exposure. For this individual, the result is an estimated [61] excess relative risk for radiation-induced breast cancer, 20 years post exposure of 2.1 [95% CI: 1.1, 6.1]. The lower graph (**c**) shows the estimated contribution of different doses within the breasts to the overall excess relative risk

this, it is crucial to ensure that any changes in treatment technique designed to decrease second-cancer risks do not impact negatively on primary tumor control.

We are a long way from being able to estimate radiation-induced cancer risks *ab initio*, i.e., solely based on biologically-based models. The approach described here, which appears to be reasonably promising, is to use cancer risks originally estimated in A-bomb survivors, modify them for the demographic cohort or individual of interest, and then extrapolate these risks to higher doses using the quantitative biological models described here. Finally, combining the results using organ-specific dose volume histograms allows realistic prospective estimates of radiotherapy-related second cancer risks.

Of course, there remain considerable uncertainties in these modeling approaches. For example, it remains unclear to what extent radiation-induced second cancer risks depend on the primary cancer, over and above the different dose distributions. A recent study of CNS tumors in survivors of childhood cancers concluded that "after adjustment for radiation dose, neither original cancer diagnosis nor chemotherapy was associated with risk" [5], but the question is still open and important.

DONALDSON and BOYER, commenting on IMRT, suggested [66] that *"the impact of multi-field, low-dose radiation exposure, and higher total body doses from leakage radiation associated with longer "beam-on" times and leaf transmission, carry risks of radiation carcinogenesis that cannot be accurately addressed"*. In this regard, we have reported here some advances towards quantitative prospective estimation of radiotherapy-induced second-cancer risks.

Acknowledgments

The advice and support of our friend and collaborator, Rainer Sachs, is gratefully acknowledged. We also thank Drs Lawrence Marks, Louis Constine and Philip Rubin for insightful comments. This work was supported with grants from the National Institutes of Health (U19 AI-67773, P41-EB-002033, and P01 CA-49062).

References

1. Travis LB (2002) Therapy-associated solid tumors. Acta Oncol 41:323–333
2. Curtis RE, Freedman DM, Ron E et al (eds) (2006) New malignancies among cancer survivors: SEER Cancer Registries, 1973–2000. National Cancer Institute, Bethesda, NIH Publication No. 05-5302, 2006
3. Jemal A, Tiwari RC, Murray T et al (2004) Cancer statistics, 2004. CA Cancer J Clin 2004:54:8–29
4. Farkas A, Schneider D, Perrotti M, Cummings KB, Ward WS (1998) National trends in the epidemiology of prostate cancer, 1973 to 1994: evidence for the effectiveness of prostate-specific antigen screening. Urology 52:444–448
5. Neglia JP, Robison LL, Stovall M et al (2006) New primary neoplasms of the central nervous system in survivors of childhood cancer: a report from the Childhood Cancer Survivor Study. J Natl Cancer Inst 98:1528–1537
6. Bhatia S, Yasui Y, Robison LL et al (2003) High risk of subsequent neoplasms continues with extended follow-up of childhood Hodgkin's disease: report from the Late Effects Study Group. J Clin Oncol 21:4386–4394
7. Gold DG, Neglia JP, Dusenbery KE (2003) Second neoplasms after megavoltage radiation for pediatric tumors. Cancer 97:2588–2596
8. Brenner DJ, Curtis RE, Hall EJ, Ron E (2000) Second malignancies in prostate carcinoma patients after radiotherapy compared with surgery. Cancer 88:398–406
9. van Leeuwen FE, Travis LB (2004) Second cancers. In: Devita VT, Hellman S, Rosenberg SA (eds) Cancer: principles and practice of oncology, 7th ed. Lippincott, Williams & Wilkins, Philadelphia
10. Ron E (2003) Cancer risks from medical radiation. Health Phys 85:47–59
11. Little MP (2001) Comparison of the risks of cancer incidence and mortality following radiation therapy for benign and malignant disease with the cancer risks observed in the Japanese A-bomb survivors. Int J Radiat Biol 77:431–464
12. Travis LB, Andersson M, Gospodarowicz M et al (2000) Treatment-associated leukemia following testicular cancer. J Natl Cancer Inst 92:1165–1171
13. Weiss HA, Darby SC, Fearn T, Doll R (1995) Leukemia mortality after X-ray treatment for ankylosing spondylitis. Radiat Res 142:1–11
14. Curtis RE, Boice JD Jr, Stovall M et al (1994) Relationship of leukemia risk to radiation dose following cancer of the uterine corpus. J Natl Cancer Inst 86:1315–1324
15. Boice JD Jr, Engholm G, Kleinerman RA et al (1988) Radiation dose and second cancer risk in patients treated for cancer of the cervix. Radiat Res 116:3–55
16. Inskip PD, Kleinerman RA, Stovall M et al (1993) Leukemia, lymphoma, and multiple myeloma after pelvic radiotherapy for benign disease. Radiat Res 135:108–124
17. Boice JD Jr, Blettner M, Kleinerman RA et al (1987) Radiation dose and leukemia risk in patients treated for cancer of the cervix. J Natl Cancer Inst 79:1295–1311
18. Little MP, Weiss HA, Boice JD Jr, Darby SC, Day NE, Muirhead CR (1999) Risks of leukemia in Japanese atomic bomb survivors, in women treated for cervical cancer, and in patients treated for ankylosing spondylitis. Radiat Res 152:280–292

19. Thomas DC, Blettner M, Day NE (1992) Case-control study of acute and nonlymphocytic leukemia. J Natl Cancer Inst 84:1600–1601

20. Zelefsky MJ, Fuks Z, Hunt M et al (2002) High-dose intensity modulated radiation therapy for prostate cancer: early toxicity and biochemical outcome in 772 patients. Int J Radiat Oncol Biol Phys 53:1111–1116

21. Arriagada R, Komaki R, Cox JD (2004) Radiation dose escalation in non-small cell carcinoma of the lung. Semin Radiat Oncol 14:287–291

22. Mangar SA, Huddart RA, Parker CC, Dearnaley DP, Khoo VS, Horwich A (2005) Technological advances in radiotherapy for the treatment of localised prostate cancer. Eur J Cancer 41:908–921

23. Stitt JA (1999) High dose rate brachytherapy in the treatment of cervical carcinoma. Hematol Oncol Clin North Am 13:585–593, vii–viii

24. Nguyen LN, Ang KK (2002) Radiotherapy for cancer of the head and neck: altered fractionation regimens. Lancet Oncol 3:693–701

25. Vicini FA, Vargas C, Edmundson G, Kestin L, Martinez A (2003) The role of high-dose rate brachytherapy in locally advanced prostate cancer. Semin Radiat Oncol 13:98–108

26. Pollack A, Hanlon AL, Horwitz EM et al (2006) Dosimetry and preliminary acute toxicity in the first 100 men treated for prostate cancer on a randomized hypofractionation dose escalation trial. Int J Radiat Oncol Biol Phys 64:518–526

27. Hall EJ, Wuu CS (2003) Radiation-induced second cancers: the impact of 3D-CRT and IMRT. Int J Radiat Oncol Biol Phys 56:83–88

28. Bucci MK, Bevan A, Roach M, 3rd (2005) Advances in radiation therapy: conventional to 3D, to IMRT, to 4D, and beyond. CA Cancer J Clin 55:117–134

29. Sachs RK, Brenner DJ (2005) Solid tumor risks after high doses of ionizing radiation. Proc Natl Acad Sci U S A 102:13040–13045

30. Williams PO, Hounsell AR (2001) X-ray leakage considerations for IMRT. Br J Radiol 74:98–100

31. Glatstein E (2002) Intensity-modulated radiation therapy: the inverse, the converse, and the perverse. Semin Radiat Oncol 12:272–281

32. Lillicrap SC, Morgan HM, Shakeshaft JT (2000) X-ray leakage during radiotherapy. Br J Radiol 73:793–794

33. Verellen D, Vanhavere F (1999) Risk assessment of radiation-induced malignancies based on whole-body equivalent dose estimates for IMRT treatment in the head and neck region. Radiother Oncol 53:199–203

34. Followill D, Geis P, Boyer A (1997) Estimates of whole-body dose equivalent produced by beam intensity modulated conformal therapy. Int J Radiat Oncol Biol Phys 38:667–672

35. Kry SF, Salehpour M, Followill DS et al (2005) The calculated risk of fatal secondary malignancies from intensity-modulated radiation therapy. Int J Radiat Oncol Biol Phys 62:1195–1203

36. Mansur DB, Klein EE, Maserang BP (2007) Measured peripheral dose in pediatric radiation therapy: a comparison of intensity-modulated and conformal techniques. Radiother Oncol 82:179–184

37. Pirzkall A, Carol M, Lohr F, Hoss A, Wannenmacher M, Debus J (2000) Comparison of intensity-modulated radiotherapy with conventional conformal radiotherapy for complex-shaped tumors. Int J Radiat Oncol Biol Phys 48:1371–1380

38. Kry SF, Followill D, White RA, Stovall M, Kuban DA, Salehpour M (2007) Uncertainty of calculated risk estimates for secondary malignancies after radiotherapy. Int J Radiat Oncol Biol Phys 68:1265–1271

39. Rubino C, de Vathaire F, Shamsaldin A, Labbe M, Le MG (2003) Radiation dose, chemotherapy, hormonal treatment and risk of second cancer after breast cancer treatment. Br J Cancer 89:840–846

40. Stovall M, Smith SA, Rosenstein M (1989) Tissue doses from radiotherapy of cancer of the uterine cervix. Med Phys 16:726–733

41. Gray LH (1965) Radiation biology and cancer. In: Cellular radiation biology; a symposium considering radiation effects in the cell and possible implications for cancer therapy, a collection of papers. William and Wilkins Co., Baltimore, pp 8–25

42. Radivoyevitch T, Hoel DG (1999) Modeling the low-LET dose-response of BCR-ABL formation: predicting stem cell numbers from A-bomb data. Math Biosci 162:85–101

43. Whang-Peng J, Young RC, Lee EC, Longo DL, Schechter GP, DeVita VT, Jr. (1988) Cytogenetic studies in patients with secondary leukemia/dysmyelopoietic syndrome after different treatment modalities. Blood 71:403–414

44. Christiansen DH, Andersen MK, Desta F, Pedersen-Bjergaard J (2005) Mutations of genes in the receptor tyrosine kinase (RTK)/RAS-BRAF signal transduction pathway in therapy-related myelodysplasia and acute myeloid leukemia. Leukemia 19:2232–2240

45. Duesberg P, Rasnick D, Li R, Winters L, Rausch C, Hehlmann R (1999) How aneuploidy may cause cancer and genetic instability. Anticancer Res 19:4887–4906

46. Bennett J, Little MP, Richardson S (2004) Flexible dose-response models for Japanese atomic bomb survivor data: Bayesian estimation and prediction of cancer risk. Radiat Environ Biophys 43:233–245

47. Dasu A, Toma-Dasu I, Olofsson J, Karlsson M (2005) The use of risk estimation models for the induction of secondary cancers following radiotherapy. Acta Oncol 44:339–347

48. Little MP (2003) Risks associated with ionizing radiation. Br Med Bull 68:259–275

49. Preston DL, Kusumi S, Tomonaga M et al (1994) Cancer incidence in atomic bomb survivors. Part III. Leukemia, lymphoma and multiple myeloma, 1950–1987. Radiat Res 137:S68–97

50. Thompson DE, Mabuchi K, Ron E et al (1994) Cancer incidence in atomic bomb survivors. Part II: Solid tumors, 1958–1987. Radiat Res 137:S17–67

51. Land CE, Tokunaga M, Koyama K et al (2003) Incidence of female breast cancer among atomic bomb survivors, Hiroshima and Nagasaki, 1950–1990. Radiat Res 160:707–717

52. Gilbert ES, Stovall M, Gospodarowicz M et al (2003) Lung cancer after treatment for Hodgkin's disease: focus on radiation effects. Radiat Res 159:161–173

53. Travis LB, Hill DA, Dores GM et al (2003) Breast cancer following radiotherapy and chemotherapy among young women with Hodgkin disease. JAMA 290:465–475

54. van Leeuwen FE, Klokman WJ, Stovall M et al (2003) Roles of radiation dose, chemotherapy, and hormonal factors in

breast cancer following Hodgkin's disease. J Natl Cancer Inst 95:971–980

55. Sacher GA, Trucco E (1966) Theory of radiation injury and recovery in self-renewing cell populations. Radiat Res 29:236–256

56. Brown JM (1970) The effect of acute x-irradiation on the cell proliferation kinetics of induced carcinomas and their normal counterpart. Radiat Res 43:627–653

57. von Wangenheim KH, Siegers MP, Feinendegen LE (1980) Repopulation ability and proliferation stimulus in the hematopoietic system of mice following gamma-irradiation. Exp Hematol 8:694–701

58. Cheshier SH, Morrison SJ, Liao X, Weissman IL (1999) In vivo proliferation and cell cycle kinetics of long-term self-renewing hematopoietic stem cells. Proc Natl Acad Sci U S A 96:3120–3125

59. Shuryak I, Sachs RK, Hlatky L, Little MP, Hahnfeldt P, Brenner DJ (2006) Radiation-induced leukemia at doses relevant to radiation therapy: modeling mechanisms and estimating risks. J Natl Cancer Inst 98:1794–1806

60. Sachs RK, Shuryak I, Brenner D, Fakir H, Hlatky L, Hahnfeldt P (2007) Second cancers after fractionated radiotherapy: stochastic population dynamics effects. J Theor Biol 249:518–531

61. Koh ES, Tran TH, Heydarian M et al (2007) A comparison of mantle versus involved-field radiotherapy for Hodgkin's lymphoma: reduction in normal tissue dose and second cancer risk. Radiat Oncol 2:13

62. Preston DL, Ron E, Tokuoka S et al (2007) Solid cancer incidence in Atomic Bomb survivors: 1958–1998. Radiat Res 168:1–64

63. Land C, Gilbert E, Smith JM, Hoffman FO, Apostoiae I, Thomas B, Kocher D (2003) Report of the NCI-CDC Working Group to Revise the 1985 NIH Radioepidemiological Tables. DHHS Publication No. 03-5387 NIH Bethesda, MD

64. NRC (2006) Health risks from exposure to low levels of ionizing radiation – BEIR VII. The National Academies Press, Washington, DC

65. Interactive RadioEpidemiological Program, IREP version 5.3. (2005)

66. Donaldson SS, Boyer AL (2000) New methods for precision radiation therapy exceed biological and clinical knowledge and institutional resources needed for implementation. Med Phys 27:2477–2479

Bioengineering in the Repair of Irradiated Normal Tissue by Bone Marrow Derived Stem Cell Populations

Joel S. Greenberger

CONTENTS

5.1
Introduction

5.1.1
The New Paradigm for Understanding Ionizing Irradiation Tissue Damage

While the basic principles of radiation chemistry and radiation molecular biology have not changed, there has been significant modification in our understanding of cellular interactions involved in ir-

J. S. Greenberger, MD
Professor and Chairman, Department of Radiation Oncology, University of Pittsburgh School of Medicine, 200 Lothrop Street, Pittsburgh, PA 15213, USA

radiation tissue damage [1–5]. Ionizing irradiation induces radiation chemical changes in cells, principally targeting oxygen and water molecules which results in formation of superoxide, hydroxyl, and other free radical moieties, within fractions of a second after radiation exposure [2]. Formation of nitric oxide, and its combination with superoxide leads to formation of peroxynitrite, a potent pro-oxidant [6, 7], which in combination with the other radical oxygen species leads to significant lipid peroxidation as well as direct binding to nuclear DNA that results in single and double strand breaks [8–11]. In the last decade, it has become clear that DNA strand breaks are repaired rapidly, certainly within 15 min after irradiation of cells in culture [4, 5], and that this repair involves a complex interaction of multiple rapid response genes, which initiate by site specific phosphorylation of the ataxia telangiectasia protein (ATM) on a specific phosphorylation site [12]. Concatenation of multiple proteins at the site of DNA strand break leads to induction of pathways for homologous recombination or homologous end joining in the case of double strand break repair [11, 12]. Deletion or inactivation or one or more components of the complex protein concatenation at DNA strand break sites leads to a reduced kinetics of DNA repair, radiosensitivity of cells in culture, and increased irradiation damage to tissues or organs in vivo [12].

While our understanding of the initial events involved in DNA strand breaks and repair, remain basically the same, there has been new appreciation for the distal steps in the pathway of ionizing irradiation response that follow rapid repair of DNA strand breaks.

Nuclear to cytoplasmic, and specifically mitochondrial communication of signals from DNA strand breaks has become the focus of intense investigation in basic radiation biology [4, 5, 13–17]. Translocation of multiple proteins from the nucleus to the mitochondria has been described following irradiation of cells in culture, including movement of p53, activation of p21, and the stress activated protein (SAP) kinases including BAX [4, 5, 18–20]. Localization of these nuclear proteins to the mitochondria after irradiation has been associated with profound biochemical and physiological changes in the mitochondrial membrane. Increased calcium transport across the mitochondrial membrane, is associated with activation of mitochondrial (neuronal) nitric oxide synthase, resulting in mitochondrial production of nitric oxide [6, 19]. Mitochondrial membrane changes associated with SAP kinase concentration include increased production of superoxide which in combination with nitric oxide leads to peroxynitrite formation and lipid peroxidation [6–9, 15]. A potentially critical element in the mitochondrial changes that are associated with irradiation induced apoptosis (programmed cell death) is the step involving interaction of Cytochrome C with cardiolipin [14]. Recent evidence has indicated that Cytochrome C, a natural component of the electron transport cascade which normally functions to stabilize mitochondrial generation of ATP during respiratory metabolism, has been shown to be associated 70% in binding to the mitochondrial phospholipid cardiolipin [14]. Only around 30% of cytochrome c is free within the inter-cisternae space between the outer and inner mitochondrial membranes [14]. Lipid peroxidation associated with ionizing irradiation induced changes in the mitochondria results in release of cardiolipin from Cytochrome C [14]. Furthermore, changes in Cytochrome C induced by ROS convert Cytochrome C into a peroxidase which can further denigrate cardiolipin and other mitochondrial lipids [14, 15]. Shunting of one of the breakdown products of cardiolipin, phosphatidyl-serine from the mitochondrial to the cell membrane is associated with annexin 5 expression, leading to one of the signals for apoptosis and/or signal for phagocytosis by inflammatory cells in the microenvironment [14, 15]. Cytochrome C leakage from the mitochondria, follows the release of Cytochrome C from cardiolipin, and represents a "point of no return" [14] in the apoptotic pathway since free Cytochrome C in the cytoplasm has been associated with activation of caspase-3, leading to PARP (poly-ADP-ribosylpolymerase) and the formation of DNA strand breaks in the nucleus that are observed in the apoptosis [4, 5].

Thus, the "new paradigm" for irradiation induced cellular injury involves initial DNA damage which is rapidly repaired, but results in a signal through the cytoplasm to the mitochondria which results in lipid peroxidative changes in the mitochondrial membrane [4, 5, 14], and release of Cytochrome C that then induces a secondary damage effect called apoptosis. There follows a delayed series of DNA strand breaks which are detected in the apotag or Olive-tail assay in vitro or identification of apoptotic bodies in vivo [4, 5, 21]. Studies from the 1960s and 1970s with alkaline sucrose gradient analysis of DNA fragmentation of the nucleus, following increasing doses of irradiation, may actually have been measuring those strand breaks induced by secondary apoptosis, rather than the initial DNA strand breaks [1].

5.1.2
General Concepts of Bioengineering for Tissue Repair

There is great enthusiasm for combining biological materials with chemically synthesized scaffolds in tissue repair. Synthetic polymer, and micro-porous materials have been utilized in maxillofacial surgery and in the therapy of non-union of bone fractures [74–81]. Combining tissue culture grown bone marrow stromal cells (progenitors of osteoblasts and chondrocytes) with scaffolding has led to novel approaches for experimental bone reconstruction [78, 81]. Biological engineering has also incorporated techniques utilizing keratinocytes, or bone marrow stromal cells, genetically engineered to express increased levels of humoral factors, including colony stimulating factors, and cytokines, involved in tissue repair [82]. Such approaches have been used to modify skin grafts for burn therapy, and also in the repair of vascular grafts including coronary microvasculature. Transplantation of embryonic stem cells, tissue derived stem cells, or bone marrow stem cells into stereotactically defined regions of the brain has been utilized in experimental approaches to treat Parkinson's Disease, stroke, and damaged tissues following brain or spinal cord injury [79, 80]. Biologically engineered cells secreting neurotrophic growth factors have also been applied in these approaches [79].

In all the above examples, the role of the tissue microenvironment into which complex organic and in-organic repair modules are inserted, has been described as of critical importance.

Ionizing irradiation damaged tissue poses a unique challenge for the use of stem cell therapies in tissue repair. Unlike burn, or traumatic tissue injury, ionizing irradiation damaged tissue may show only microscopic histopathology [2]. In the case of the oral cavity mucosa, esophagus, and lung, microvascular edema, inflammatory cell infiltrates, and then delayed apoptotic body formation may be the only indications of early irradiation damage. Circulatory elaboration of cytokines may rapidly cause systemic symptoms, but the sites of major irradiation injury may reveal damage days to weeks after injury [2]. Furthermore, the kinetics of induction of the late effects (fibrosis, vascular telangiectasias) may vary dependent upon dose, fraction size, and volume irradiated as well as sources of co-morbidity including prior surgery.

While ionizing irradiation damage poses unique challenges to tissue engineering, there are common factors which link many forms of tissue injury and can guide strategies for using stem cell transplantation in tissue repair. A common challenge in the development of stem cell therapies for bioengineering of irradiated tissue repair, is focused on the pathophysiology of the irradiated microenvironment. Irradiated tissues demonstrate many common associations with premature aging, including graying of hair, loss of elasticity of skin, and delayed healing of wounding [3]. At the biochemical level, reduction in antioxidant pools is associated with increased cumulative injury from radical oxygen species production [83–86]. Transplanting unirradiated stem cell populations into an irradiated tissue results in oxidative stress induced damage to the donor cells. In vitro systems [84] document cell contact and humoral mechanisms of induction in non-irradiated cells of molecular biologic changes and biochemical changes induced by the irradiated cells of the microenvironment [85, 86].

While recent work in experimental model systems suggests that administration of antioxidant transgenes such as MnSOD-plasmid liposomes locally to the target irradiated organ, can facilitate improved engraftment [47], it remains to be demonstrated whether sustained engraftment and robust tissue repair will follow. It may be that transient reduction in ROS by MnSOD-PL gene therapy facilitates engraftment of cell populations that can help in the initial repair of tissue integrity, but that surviving recipient stem cells provide the repopulation necessary for sustained organ function [21]. Furthermore, tissue repair of epithelial organs by bone marrow derived stem cell transplantation, may not obviate other life shortening effects of irradiation which may be a consequence of irradiation damage to the microenvironment [48, 83].

5.2
Bone Marrow Origin of Stem Cells for Epithelial Tissues

The bone marrow origin of hematopoietic progenitor cells was first demonstrated in the mouse by Till and McCullough who also established a quantitative approach toward calculation of the frequency and density of multilineage stem cells in the marrow [22]. In vitro colony assays for committed stromal or hematopoietic progenitors were next described [23, 24]. Since these pioneering studies in mouse models of marrow transplantation and correlation to human marrow, mobilized peripheral blood, and cord blood stem cell populations; the concept of a limited and quantifiable number of multilineage progenitor cells from the marrow, capable of reconstituting hematopoietic tissues has been established [25]. The entire field of bone marrow transplantation developed from these pioneering studies. Preparation of the host for accepting bone marrow stem cell engraftment by total body irradiation [23, 25] defined the role for both cells of the hematopoietic microenvironment (bone marrow stromal cells) and humoral cytokines produced by irradiated tissues, in the process [23, 24].

The bone marrow origin of cells of other than the hematopoietic lineage has remained a subject of intense investigation and continues to be controversial. Bone marrow stromal cells, recently renamed mesenchymal stem cells, were demonstrated originally by Friedenstein et al. [92] to have a quantifiable and limited number [27], and were shown to be transplantable in vivo [23]. Werts et al. [28] first demonstrated the capacity of bone marrow stromal cells to migrate from one non-irradiated site into a heavily irradiated site in the mouse marrow. Anklesaria et al. [29, 30] showed that cell lines derived from bone marrow as well as uncloned populations of marrow stromal cell lines could repopulate serial niches of irradiated target tissue by intravenous injection.

The capacity of bone marrow stromal cells to differentiate to osteoblasts, chondrocytes, adipocytes, as well as supportive tissues of the hematopoietic microenvironment is well established [31, 32]. There is controversy over the subdivisions of marrow stromal cells, and whether there is a true subpopulation that is capable of multilineage differentiation. Alternatively, all bone marrow stromal cells have been suggested to retain a multilineage differentiation capacity and the term "transdifferentiation" of the marrow stromal cell suggests that these cells have a different capacity for a lateral transfer from one epithelial lineage to another (osteoblast to chondrocyte) [111].

A very important experiment by TERRY and TRAVIS [33], first demonstrated that abdominal irradiation of mice could be rendered sublethal by bone marrow transplantation. Among the potential explanations discussed, include the possibility that bone marrow contained cells capable of reconstituting gastrointestinal stem cells. KARUS et al. [34] identified epithelial marked cells of donor origin, in mice reconstituted with a single hematopoietic stem cell. In the last 8 years, numerous publications have suggested the possibility that a subset of bone marrow stem cells is capable of reconstituting epithelial organs including liver, GI tract, esophagus, skin, glandular tissues including the pancreas, beta-islet cells of the pancreas, central nervous system, striated muscle, cardiac muscle, lung, and other tissues [35–42]. These studies can be characterized by several degrees of rigorousness: most studies demonstrate histochemical or immunohistochemical markers of epithelial tissue, in the same cells with donor chromosome or histo compatibility markers [34, 35]. A second level of rigorousness involves the serial transfer assay of sorted cells from a first generation recipient to a second generation recipient, documenting the self-renewal capacity of such cells of bone marrow origin [49]. The most rigorous assay for demonstrating bone marrow origin of epithelial tissues, is the use of a functional assay in which biochemical or immune or structural deficiencies in a recipient animal, are corrected by transplantation of bone marrow derived cells [50]. In this latter and most rigorous category of proof of bone marrow origin of epithelial tissues, partial reconstitution of the recipient organ should be demonstrated. An example of rigorous proof is the MDX mouse model of Duchenne muscular dystrophy in which striated muscle cells are deficient in components of contractile proteins and render muscles in a mouse incapable of significant functional activity [51–58]. Transplantation of subsets of muscle derived stem cells from normal donor mice into these animals has shown partial correction of the functional defect [58]. Utilizing bone marrow stem cells in this assay has also shown some positive results; however, even these studies fall short of significant correction of the defect [51–53].

Recent studies have attempted to prove that bone marrow derived cells can either replace defective lung function in (CFTR) cystic fibrosis transmembrane receptor mutant mice [59]; replace defective liver protein synthesis in mouse models of liver protein deficiency [42], or correct cardiac functional defects in mouse models of myocardial damage [53].

The present state of research in this area has gained some support from studies utilizing embryonic stem cell lines. Embryonic stem cell lines, have been demonstrated to differentiate to specific tissue elements in vitro, and subsets of ESCs can be transplanted in vivo forming organ specific tissue foci [60–62]. For applications to tissue engineering, and bioengineering, either embryonic stem cell lines or sorted subpopulations of bone marrow stem cell lines provide an attractive potential resource for repairing tissue. The challenge remains one in which absolute proof of the concept can be demonstrated, and then more importantly that subpopulation of the cells can provide reconstitution of a significant relative volume of the target organ to provide for a functional and quantifiable repair.

A compelling reason to continue research in the area of marrow stem cell reconstitution of irradiation damaged tissue is the observation that cells of bone marrow origin naturally repair radiation damaged tissues in vivo. Bone marrow origin cells have been demonstrated to reconstitute the liver of bone marrow transplant recipients [35]. Allogeneic bone marrow transplant recipients have been shown to have significant replacement of lung tissue by donor derived cell populations [63–69]. Finally, there is evidence that stem cell populations sorted from epithelial organs using the same cell separation techniques, can be transplanted into recipient animals and will reconstitute the same organ, or in some cases the bone marrow itself suggesting that there is a reversed epithelial to bone marrow reconstitution capacity [54–57]. Thus, these data suggest that multilineage epithelial stem cell populations can exist not only in the bone marrow, but in the target organ itself. It remains a major challenge of cell biology to define the parameters of isolation of bone marrow progenitors for epithelial organs, to develop ways of amplifying such cells for transplantation, and then most importantly to demonstrate reproducible engraftment of target organs with bone marrow derived cells leading to functional reconstitution in the recipient.

5.2.1
Repopulation of Recipient Target Organs with Bone Marrow Derived Stem Cell Progenitors: A Double Edged Sword

Since the first demonstration of the use of total body irradiation to prepare recipient animals for bone marrow transplantation, there has been controversy over the role of irradiation in the process [70–73]. Clinical bone marrow transplantation has gone through cycles of evolution of either utilizing total body irradiation, either single fraction or fractionated, for nearly all patients with hematopoietic malignancies, or going to protocols in which irradiation is removed and substituted with use of Busulfan and Cytoxan to reduce the pulmonary toxicity of irradiation. Over the last 30 years, marrow transplant centers have fluctuated back and forth between using total body irradiation as desirable in the preparatory method, or as undesirable because of toxicity. The most recent evolutionary step in this process has been to design a "non-myeloablative" total body irradiation dose [70–73], designed to be low enough to prevent pulmonary toxicity, but high enough to produce microenvironmental changes including upregulation of cytokines and depopulating hematopoietic stem cell niches in the recipient. The cellular and molecular mechanisms of the effect of total body irradiation are still unknown. Table 5.1 demonstrates the hypothesized positive and negative effects of total body irradiation preparing a host for bone marrow transplant.

The irradiation dose dependent "clearance" or "preparation" of a marrow site for transplantation has been demonstrated [29, 30].

5.2.2
Bone Marrow Derived Stem Cells in Bioengineering Repair of Irradiated Oral Cavity and Oropharyngeal Mucosa

Animal models of irradiation damage to the oral cavity and mucosa have been published [87, 89]. In these models, single fraction and fractionated irradiation is associated with induction of apoptotic bodies, micro-ulceration, and then sloughing of mucosal tissue. This apoptosis leads to secondary infection, severe damage to the mucosa also leads to severe dysphagia, dehydration, and weight loss. A common acute side effect of radiotherapy of head and neck cancer is mucositis. Salivary gland dam-

Table 5.1. The role of total body irradiation (TBI) in preparing the host for bone marrow transplantation

Putative positive effects of TBI
1. Removal of malignant cells from the marrow
2. Clearing "space" in bone marrow stem cell niches, removing recipient cells and providing for homing of donor cells
3. Inducing stimulatory cytokines from the marrow microenvironment which facilitate engraftment
4. Removing immuno-competent cells from the recipient to prevent graft rejection
Putative negative effects of TBI
1. Damage to the hematopoietic microenvironment, vascular and stromal cells and production of toxic cytokines and ROS
2. By removing differentiated cells stimulation of repopulation by surviving recipient stem cells which compete with donor stem cells
3. Co-morbidity of lung toxicity, GI stem cell toxicity, and toxicity to mucosal stem cells

age from irradiation has also been well documented [87]. In studies with epitope-tag, hemagglutinin-tagged MnSOD transgene, intraoral administration in the mouse model have been demonstrated to result in transgene penetration to cells in the basal layer of the epithelium, at sites where cycling stem cells are known to reside [89]. Quiescent stem cells in the mucosal basal layer are induced to cycle as part of the repopulation response of irradiated tissue. An hypothesis tested in recent experiments was that MnSOD-PL treatment of the oral mucosa could result in stabilization of the mucosal cells such that post-irradiation cell cycling would be decreased [89]. This would presumably lead to decreased destruction of stem cell populations during the fractionated irradiation program and better healing.

The question of whether bone marrow derived stem cell populations can reconstitute the oral cavity and oral mucosa has recently begun to be addressed. A recent report [90] demonstrated that mouse salivary glands are repopulated with cells coming from the bone marrow. With three-dimensional culture in vitro and in vivo explants, ductal epithelium and branching microscopic ducts were demonstrated to be of bone marrow origin. In one experiment cells were removed from the first generation recipients of bone marrow transplant, stem cell populations isolated and transplanted into a second generation of irradiated mice in which the glandular epithelium was shown to be replaced by cells originally of bone marrow origin [90]. The question of how much bone marrow derived stem cells contributes to repair of the irradiation damaged oral cavity and oral mucosa is not known. Stem cell repopulation in both salivary gland and oral cavity/oropharynx are known to occur and are part of the response to fractionated irradiation, but the question of whether circulating stem cells mobilized from the bone marrow can compete for the repopulation with the in situ epithelial stem cells is not yet known.

Other experiments in radiation protection of the oral cavity using MnSOD-plasmid liposomes in both single fraction and fractionation models have shown significant stabilization of the oral mucosa, and parotid glands [87]. In these experiments, decreased micro-ulceration, decreased weight loss, and improved survival were noted. In addition, increased saliva production by the irradiated oral cavity was demonstrated. Several experimental paradigms have been derived to determine whether bone marrow stem cell populations can replace irradiation damaged oral cavity tissues.

Fibrotic areas in the high dose irradiated sites, that receive in excess of 70 Gy, have been limited to high dose boost areas in programs of IMRT or brachytherapy. The question of whether fibroblasts forming the fibrosis come in part from marrow stromal cells (mesenchymal stem cells) that are mobilized from the bone marrow has not been conclusively demonstrated with the oral cavity or oropharynx, but since similar studies have been carried out in lung [48] and esophagus, it is possible that secondary immobilization of cells involved in oral cavity fibrosis may involve progenitors of bone marrow origin.

5.2.3
Bioengineering for Repair of Irradiation Damage in the Esophagus Using Bone Marrow Derived Stem Cell Progenitors

Recent studies in an experimental model of murine irradiation esophagitis have demonstrated significant preservation of the esophageal lining by MnSOD-plasmid liposome administration [21, 47, 91, 93–98]. Mice receiving either MnSOD-PL prior to single fraction irradiation or every third day during six- or eight-fraction radiotherapy [94] showed

improved survival, which was directly related to MnSOD biochemical levels in the irradiated tissue [96]. In the esophagus model, a stem cell population has been isolated from the basal layer of the esophageal mucosa [95]. Using techniques originally designed to isolate stem cell populations from bone marrow, and striated muscle, single cell suspensions of esophagus were sorted for Hoscht/Prodium Iodide or side population cells [95]. These side population cells have been shown to contain quiescent stem cell populations from bone marrow or from smooth muscle [95]. In a second technique a serial preplate method was utilized whereby single cell suspensions of esophagus were plated in tissue culture medium on plastic plates, and then daily for 7 days non-adherent cells removed and placed into a second cell culture [95]. By serial removal of adherent cell populations over 7 days, those cells found to be non-adherent and still in suspension on day 7 had properties of stem cells [95]. In both model systems (side populations and serial preplate) cells were isolated which when injected intravenously into esophagus irradiated mice, homed to the esophagus and formed donor origin foci. Furthermore, in mice which were chimeric for sex mismatched GFP+ bone marrow, esophagus irradiation resulted in migration to the irradiated esophagus of cells of bone marrow origin which produced GFP+ foci in the esophagus [47]. The esophageal stem cells from either primary or secondary recipients in serial transfer demonstrated properties of multilineage differentiation in vitro [98]. Cells formed multilineage colonies containing cells with myeloepithelial morphology, fibroblast morphology, and endothelial morphology [95, 98]. Histochemical staining showed that single cell derived colonies contained cells positive for vimentin, endothelin, and F480 (which was originally used as a macrophage specific marker, but has now been found in peripheral blood multilineage progenitor cells) [95, 98].

The question of whether bone marrow derived stem cell populations can reconstitute and facilitate repair of radiation damaged esophagus has recently been tested. In these experiments (Fig. 5.1) donor male mice containing ROSA marked bone marrow, Y-probe+, G418 resistance marker, and LAC-Z marker were engrafted into female C57BL/6J mice that had received 31 Gy to the esophagus 5 days previously. Unlike bone marrow, esophageal cells undergo apoptosis at 5 days after irradiation suggesting a delayed turnover of irradiation damaged cells in this squamous mucosal organ compared to

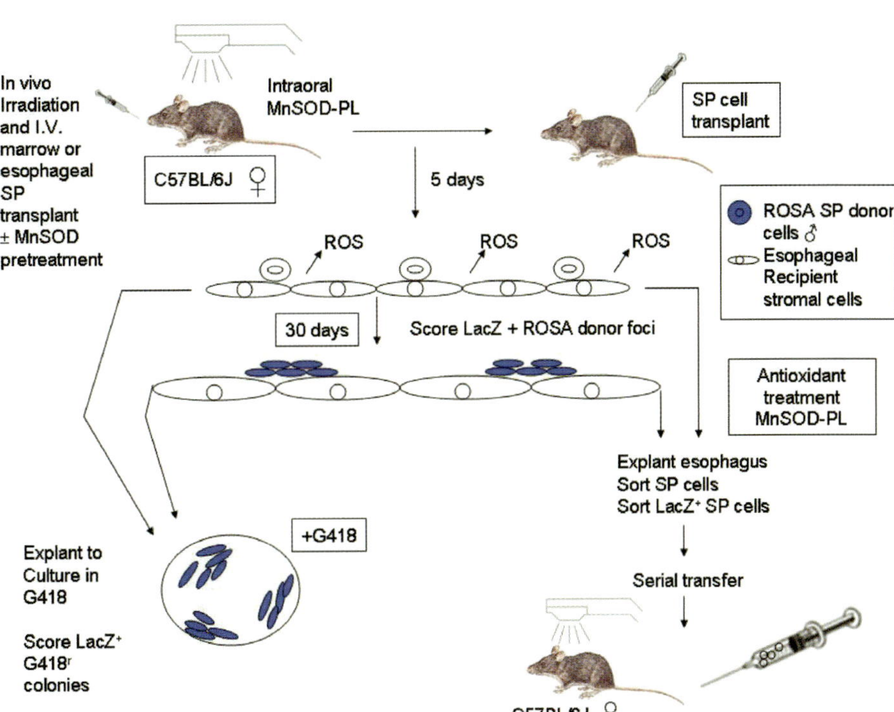

Fig. 5.1. Experimental model system to show donor marrow stem cell origin of esophageal stem cells. ROSA male donor mice have three markers (Y chromosome, G418 resistance, LAC-Z production). Recipient esophagus is irradiated 24 h after intraoral administration of MnSOD-PL, then donor marrow is given intravenously. Esophagus is removed. Cells shown to be donor origin in vivo and in vitro, and donor esophageal side population (stem cells) show self renewal by serial transfer to recipient second generation irradiated esophagus (With permission from Greenberger JS (2008) Gene Therapy Approaches for Stem Cell Protection. Gene Therapy 15:100–108)

the more rapidly proliferating hematopoietic cells in the bone marrow [97].

Removing the esophagus from marrow transplanted mice at serial time points after transplant and out to 21 days demonstrated that a significant contribution to the esophageal repair was attributable to cells that had been injected intravenously and had markers for LAC-Z, Y-probe in vivo, and following explant in culture in the presence of 50 µg/ml G418, demonstrated G418 resistance. Colonies growing in G418 also contained Y-probe and had multilineage differentiation markers [98].

Serial transfer or self-renewal of esophageal progenitor cells that were derived of bone marrow has recently been carried out. SP cells removed from the esophagus of first generation recipient mice at 14 days after marrow injection, were sorted for SP cells, and then either SP or non-SP cells injected intravenously into a second generation of C57BL/6J female mice that receive 31 Gy to the esophagus. The esophagus from the second generation mice demonstrated significant LAC-Z positive foci in situ, which were also Y-probe+, and explant of these cells to culture revealed multilineage G418 resistant esophageal colony forming cells [98].

Whether cells of bone marrow origin which provided esophageal repair, and were capable of serial transfer, are in fact multilineage stem cells remains to be rigorously tested. However, there is striking evidence that in both the first and second generation recipients, administration of MnSOD-PL intraesophageally prior to irradiation, and intravenous injection of bone marrow cells enhanced bone marrow engraftment into the esophagus [98]. These data suggest that irradiation may remove a population of esophageal progenitor or stem cells, eliciting a cell cycling response in the esophageal basal layer, recruiting quiescent stem cells into cycling for the repair process. However, the persistence of irradiation damage effects in the microenvironment may in fact work against the repopulation response [98]. The irradiation induced changes in the esophagus microenvironment have been shown to include continuous production of radical oxygen species (ROS) and inflammatory cytokines [93, 96]. Administration of MnSOD-PL prior to irradiation (and stem cell transplant) has been shown to reduce both ROS production and inflammatory cytokine production [93, 96]. Since bone marrow derived cells engrafted more efficiently into the irradiated esophagus that had been treated with MnSOD-PL, we hypothesized that irradiation cleared the space but that MnSOD-PL "cleans" the space and facilitated engraftment (Fig. 5.2). Another phenomenon associated with bone marrow derived cell migration and engraftment of the esophagus is the phenomenon of cell fusion. Bone marrow derived cells fused to esophageal as well as lung cells providing heterokaryon formation [99].

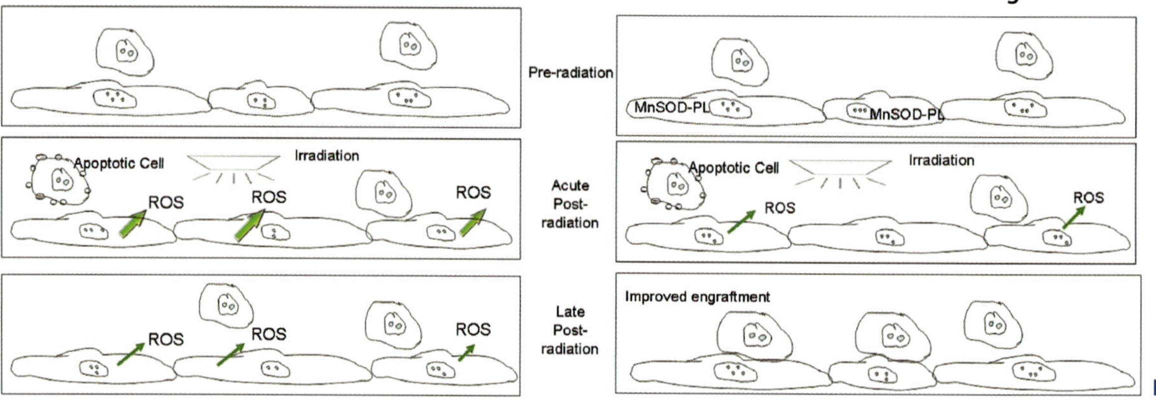

Fig. 5.2a,b. Hypothesis: MnSOD-PL administered to target organ before irradiation reduces both acute and late effects of ionizing irradiation by reducing oxygen species production. Untreated microenvironment (**a**), MnSOD-PL treated microenvironment (**b**)

The repair of mucosal surfaces including those in the oral cavity and esophagus is a complex phenomenon, but appears to involve a repopulation response which can be enhanced by providing additional cells from the circulation [100].

5.2.4
Bioengineering of Irradiation Damaged Lung Through Use of Bone Marrow Derived Stem Cell Progenitors

Radiation protection of the lung by antioxidant gene therapy has been described [101–108]. There has been much work describing the complex biology of the pulmonary stem cell [59, 63–69, 109, 110]. Work of Barry Stripp and Susan Reynolds [109, 110] demonstrated two populations of Clara cell secretory protein positive cells (CCSP) in the mouse bronchioles, one quiescent, and the other cycling. Both these cell populations appear capable of restoring the integrity of chemically damaged bronchial tissue. A cycling CCSP cell subset was removed by Naphthalene treatment and serial histopathologic examination studies of the drug treated bronchioles demonstrated repopulation by a CCSP population that was resistant to Naphthalene [109, 110]. The CCSP+ quiescent cells which resisted Naphthalene treatment, were, however, removed in another transgenic mouse strain (HSV-TK-CCSP), when the mice were treated with Gangcyclovir. This interesting mouse strain has been genetically engineered to have the Herpes virus thymidine kinase gene attached to the CCSP promoter such that its induction by Gangcyclovir results in production of toxic free radical species in both the cycling and quiescent CCSP populations [110]. Recent studies suggested that ionizing irradiation damage to the lung, either single fraction or fractionated, does destroy lung stem cells although rigorous dose response curves have not yet been carried out.

The question of whether bone marrow derived progenitors can reconstitute the irradiation damaged lung is a subject of intense investigation. Recent data [63] indicate that mouse lung when irradiated, can be reconstituted by bone marrow derived cells if animals are supplemented with G-CSF (granulocyte colony stimulating factor) mediated mobilization of bone marrow into the circulation. Confocal microscopic studies of lung sections revealed bone marrow origin cells with lung specific markers including TTF1 in experiments carried out in sex mismatched marrow chimeric mice [63]. However, in these experiments relative numbers of cells of bone marrow origin were very small, less than 5%. Similarly, small numbers of bone marrow derived progenitors were detected in the lungs of cystic fibrosis transmembrane receptor (CFTR) knockout mice, the animal model system for cystic fibrosis [59].

Under baseline conditions irradiated lung may not elicit a significant repopulation or repair response from bone marrow derived cells. However, in recent experiments, delivering by inhalation technique [104]. MnSOD-Plasmid Liposome antioxidant gene therapy (as was described above for intraesophageal administration of MnSOD to enhance bone marrow derived stem cell repair of the esophagus) increased numbers of bone marrow origin cells were found homing to and proliferating in the irradiated lung. When MnSOD-PL inhalation gene therapy was supplemented by G-CSF administration after radiation, further numbers of bone marrow derived cells were detected in the lungs. G-CSF alone may not be the optimal way to mobilize bone marrow cells into an epithelial organ for purposes of post-irradiation repair. Use of FLK-3 ligand, and VEGF supplementing G-CSF may be a more appropriate way to optimally mobilize stem cell populations from the marrow into the lung. The question of whether significant volumes of lung tissue can be replaced by bone marrow origin stem cells is still unanswered, but techniques are available to facilitate such experiments in several animal model systems.

Less controversial is the clear involvement of bone marrow derived marrow stromal cells (mesenchymal stem cells) in irradiation pulmonary fibrosis as well as the fibrosis associated with bleomycin injury to the lung [48]. Several experimental model systems have shown using intravenous bone marrow injection, or in sex mismatched chimeric mice with mismatched bone marrow, that bone marrow derived cells contribute to the fibrotic response in the irradiated lung. An attractive hypothesis is the possibility that MnSOD-PL antioxidant inhalation gene therapy can ameliorate both the acute and chronic effects of lung irradiation damage through mobilization of repairing stem cells in their early phase and inhibition of mobilization of deleterious fibrotic cells in the late time frame (Fig. 5.3). The ease of administration of inhalation MnSOD-Plasmid Liposomes, which has been carried out in fractionation irradiation experiments [1, 4]. indicates that mice in these chimera experiments could be treated with inhalation MnSOD-PL weekly, during the period of latency between the acute response and late radiation fibrosis response [48].

If bone marrow derived stem cell populations are naturally involved in repairing irradiation damaged epithelial organs perhaps at low levels, then acceleration and enhancement of this response during tissue injury may enhance this component of the irradiation damage response. Furthermore, methods by which to harness this natural pathway and direct it, may involve enhanced marrow mobilization (G-CSF, VEGF, FLK-3 ligand administration), and homing and repopulation by engrafting cells (MnSOD-PL administration to the lung microenvironment). Such methods may prove a realistic strategy for tissue engineering to ameliorate the acute effects of irradiation lung damage.

Recent research efforts have focused on the development of superoxide dismutase mimic molecules. While MnSOD may provide an efficient antioxidant gene therapy approach for organ specific radiation

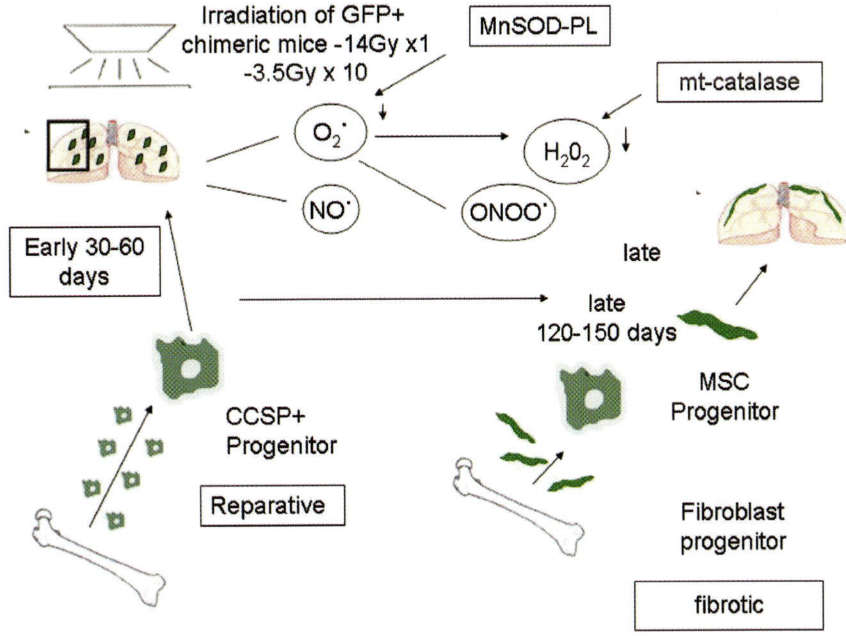

Fig. 5.3. Experimental model system to show bone marrow origin of pulmonary epithelial cells. GFP+ male marrow chimeric C57BL/6J female mice are irradiated to the lungs to 14 Gy in single dose or to 3.5 Gy daily for 10 days. Subgroups received inhalation MnSOD-PL treatments prior to first irradiation fraction, or twice weekly. Early marrow migration of GFP+ male CCSP+ marrow origin cells repopulate the functional lung. Late migration of GFP+ male marrow stromal cells (*MSC*) contribute to fibrosis [112]

protection, systemic protection may require a small molecule analog of MnSOD which could be administered either orally or by skin patch technique to facilitate irradiation repair in multiple organs. Possibly, local administration through inhalation of an aerosolized small molecule-MnSOD mimic may provide a more efficient method of prevention of acute and chronic radiation side effects to the irradiated lung.

5.3
Summary

At the present time, there is no effective way to replace significant components of the microenvironment in irradiated epithelial tissues, except by transplantation of the entire organ, and even here "bystander" damage may be sustained to the transplanted organ as a result of a continuous exposure to humoral factors including long lived free radicals that are produced for prolonged periods after irradiation [48]. Demonstrating the replacement of stem cell populations in epithelial organs, by progenitor cells derived from the bone marrow may provide a first step in understanding the role of the marrow in the pathophysiology of repair of irradiation induced tissue damage and may identify new targets for therapy. While simply transplanting new cell populations into an irradiated microenvironment, and reducing ROS production in the target organ by sustained administration of antioxidants may not reverse irradiation damage, an understanding of the consequences of these therapeutic approaches may provide valuable insights towards ameliorating the late effects of ionizing irradiation damage.

References

1. Hall EJ (1999) Radiobiology for the radiologist, 4th ed. J.B Lippincott, Inc., Philadelphia, PA
2. Rubin P, Casarett GW (1968) Clinical radiation pathology. W. B. Saunders, Philadelphia, PA
3. Mothersill C, Seymour CB (2004) Radiation-induced bystander effects – implications for cancer. Nature Reviews, Cancer, 4:158–164
4. Epperly MW, Sikora C, Defilippi S, Gretton J, Zhan Q, Kufe DW, Greenberger JS (2002) MnSOD inhibits irradiation-induced apoptosis by stabilization of the mitochondrial membrane against the effects of SAP kinases p38 and Jnk1 translocation. Radiat Res 157:568–577
5. Epperly MW, Gretton JE, Bernarding M, Nie S, Rasul B, Greenberger JS (2003) Mitochondrial localization of copper/zinc superoxide dismutase (Cu/ZnSOD) confers radioprotective functions in vitro and in vivo. Radiat Res 160:568–578
6. Miranda KM, Espey MG, Jourd'heuil D, Grisham MB, Fukuto J, Feelisch M, Wink DA (2000) The chemical biology of nitric oxide. In: Ignarro LJ (ed) Nitric oxide biology and pathobiology. Academic Press, pp 41–56
7. Epperly MW, Osipov AN, Martin I, Kawai K, Borisenko GG, Jefferson M, Bernarding M, Greenberger JS, Kagan VE (2004) Ascorbate as a "redox-sensor" and protector against irradiation-induced oxidative stress in 32D cl 3 hematopoietic cells and subclones overexpressing human manganese Superoxide dismutase. Int J Radiat Oncol Biol Phys 58:851–861
8, Daum G (1985) Lipids of mitochondria. Biochim Biophys Acta 822:1–42
9. Bevers EM, Comfurius P, Dekkers DWC, Swaal RFA (1999) Lipid translocation across the plasma membrane of mammalian cells. Biochim Biophys Acta 1439:317–330
10. Mitchell JB, Russo A, Kuppusamy P et al (2000) Radiation, radicals, and images. Ann N Y Acad Sci 899:28–43
11. Bryant PE (1985) Enzymatic restriction of mammalian cell DNA: Evidence for double-strand breaks as potentially lethal lesions. Int J Radiat Biol 48:55–60
12. Bakkenist CJ, Kastan MB (2003) DNA damage activates ATM through intermolecular autophosphorylation and dimer association. Nature 421:499–504
13. Fernandez MG, Troiano L, Moretti L et al (2002) Early changes in intramitochondrial cardiolipin distribution during apoptosis. Cell Growth Differ 13:449–455
14. Kagan VE, Tyurin VA, Jiang J et al (2005) Cytochrome c acts as a cardiolipin oxygenase required for release of proapoptotic factors. Nat Chem Biol 1:223–232
15. Petrosillo G, Casanova G, Matera M et al (2006) Interaction of peroxidized cardiolipin with rat-heart mitochondrial membranes: induction of permeability transition and cytochrome c release. FEBS Lett 580:6311–6316
16. Ott M, Robertson JD, Gogvadze V et al (2002) Cytochrome c release from mitochondria proceeds by a two-step process. Proc Natl Acad Sci USA 99:1259–1263
17. Garrido C, Galluzzi L, Brunet M et al (2006) Mechanisms of cytochrome c release from mitochondria. Cell Death Differ 13:1423–1433
18. Szewczyk A, Wojtczak L (2002) Mitochondria as a pharmacological target. Pharmacol Rev 54:101–127
19. Kowaltowski AJ, Castilho RF, Vercesi AE (1996) Opening of the mitochondrial permeability transition pore by uncoupling or inorganic phosphate in the present of Ca^{2+} is dependent on mitochondrial-generated reactive oxygen species. FEBS Lett, 378:150–152
20. Kroemer G, Reed JC (2000) Mitochondrial control of cell death. Nature Med 6:513–519
21. Stickle RL, Epperly MW, Klein E, Bray JA, Greenberger JS (1999) Prevention of irradiation-induced esophagitis by plasmid/liposome delivery of the human manganese superoxide dismutase (MnSOD) transgene. Radiat Oncol Invest Clinical & Basic Res 7:204–217

22. Till JE, McCulloch EA (1961) A direct measurement of the radiation sensitivity of normal mouse bone marrow. Radiation Research 14:213–220

23. Simmons PJ, Przepiorka D, Thomas ED, Torok-Storb B (1987) Host origin of marrow stromal cells following allogeneic bone marrow transplantation. Nature 328:429–431

24. Metcalf D (1985) The granulocyte-macrophage colony stimulating factors. Science 229:16

25. Thomas ED, Clift RA, Fefer A, Koeffler HP, Golde DW (1981) Marrow transplantation for the treatment of chronic myelogenous leukemia – new concepts. N Engl J Med 304:1201

26. Rithidech KN, Bond VP, Cronkite EP, Thompson MH (1993) A specific chromosomal deletion in murine leukemic cells induced by radiation with different qualities. Exp Hematol 21:427–431

27. Castro-Malaspina H, Gay RE, Resnik G (1980) Characterization of human bone marrow fibroblast colony forming cells (CFU-F) and their progeny. Blood 56:289–301

28. Werts ED, Gibson DP, Knapp SA, DeGowin RL (1980) Stromal cell migration precedes hematopoietic repopulation of the bone marrow after irradiation. Radiat Res 81:20–30

29. Anklesaria P, Kase K, Glowacki J, Holland CA, Sakakeeny MA, Wright JA, FitzGerald TJ, Lee CY, Greenberger JS (1987) Engraftment of a clonal bone marrow stromal cell line in vivo stimulates hematopoietic recover from total body irradiation. Proc Natl Acad Sci USA 84:7681–7685

30. Anklesaria P, FitzGerald TJ, Kase K, Ohara A, Bentley S, Greenberger JS (1989) Improved hematopoiesis in anemic S1/S1^d mice by therapeutic transplantation of a hematopoietic microenvironment. Blood 74:1144–1152

31. Gimble J, Youkhana K, Hua X, Wang C-S, Bass H, Medina K, Greenberger JS (1992) Adipogenesis in a myeloid supporting bone marrow stromal cell line. J Cell Biochem 50:73–82

32. Zhou S, Lechpammer S, Greenberger J, Glowacki J (2005) Hypoxia inhibition of adipocytogenesis in human bone marrow stromal cells requires TGFβ/Smad^3 signaling. J Biol Chem 280:22688–22696

33. Terry NH, Travis EL (1989) The influence of bone marrow depletion on intestinal radiation damage. Int J Radiat Oncol Biol Phys 17:569–573

34. Krause DS, Theise ND, Collector MI, Henegariu O, Hwang S, Gardner R, Neutzel S, Sharkis SJ (2001) Multiorgan, multi-lineage engraftment by a single bone marrow-derived stem cell. Cell 105:369–377

35. Peterson BE, Bowen WC, Patrene KD, Mars WM, Sullivan AK, Boggs SS, Greenberger JS, Goff JP (1999) Bone marrow as a potential source of hepatic oval cells. Science 284:1168–1170

36. Jang Y-Y, Collector MI, Baylin SB, Diehl AM, Sharkis SJ (2004) Hematopoietic stem cells convert into liver cells within days without fusion. Nature Cell Biology 6:532–537

37. Lagasse E, Connors H, Al-Dhalimy M, Reitsma M, Dohse M, Osborne L, Wang X, Finegold M, Weissman IL, Grompe M (2000) Purified hematopoietic stem cells can differentiate into hepatocytes in vivo. Nature Medicine 6:1229–1232

38. Camargo FD, Finegold M, Goodell MA (2004) Hematopoietic myelomonocytic cells are the major source of hepatocyte fusion partners. J Clin Invest 113:1266–1272

39. Zipori D (2004) The nature of stem cells: state rather than entity. Nature Reviews 5:873–883

40. Ishikawa F, Yasukawa M, Yoshida S, Nakamura K, Nagatoshi Y, Kanemaru T, Shimoda K, Shimoda S, Miyamoto T, Okamura J, Shultz LD, Harada M (2004) Human cord blood and bone marrow derived CD34+ cells regenerate gastrointestinal epithelial cells. FASEB 18:1958–1967

41. Spyridonidis A, Schmitt-Graff A, Tomann T, Dwenger A, Follo M, Behringer D, Finke J (2004) Epithelial tissue chimerism after human hematopoietic cell transplantation is a real phenomenon. Am J Pathol 164:1147–1155

42. Theise ND, Krause DS (2002) Toward a new paradigm of cell plasticity. Leukemia 16:542–548

43. Herzog EL, Chai L, Krause DS (2003) Plasticity of marrow-derived stem cells. Blood 102:3483–3493

44. Körbling M, Katz RL, Khanna A, Ruifrok AC, Rondon G, Albitar M, Champlin RE, Estrov Z (2002) Hepatocytes and epithelial cells of donor origin in recipients of peripheral-blood stem cells. N Engl J Med 346:738–746

45. Prindull G, Zipori D (2004) Environmental guidance of normal and tumor cell plasticity: epithelial mesenchymal transitions as a paradigm. Blood 103:2892–2899

46. Houghton JM, Stoicov C, Nomura S, Rogers AB, Carlson J, Li H, Cai X, Fox JG, Goldenring JR, Wang TC (2004) Gastric cancer originating from bone marrow-derived cells. Science 306:1568–1571

47. Epperly MW, Sikora CA, Shields DS, Greenberger JS (2004) Bone marrow origin of cells with capacity for homing and differentiation to esophageal squamous epithelium. Radiat Res 162:233–240

48. Epperly MW, Sikora CA, Defilippi S, Gretton JE, Greenberger JS (2003) Bone marrow origin of myofibroblasts in irradiation pulmonary fibrosis. Am J Respir Mol Cell Biol 29:213–224

49. Harrison DE, Astle CM, Delaittre JA (1978) Loss of proliferative capacity in immunohematopoietic stem cells caused by serial transplantation rather than aging. J Exp Med 147:1526–1531

50. Maze R, Carney JP, Kelley MR, Glassner BJ, Williams DA, Samson L (1996) Increasing DNA repair methyltransferase levels via bone marrow stem cell transduction rescues mice from the toxic effects of 1, 3-bis(2-chloroethyl)-1-nitrosourea, a chemotherapeutic alkylating agent. Proc Natl Acad Sci USA 93:206–210

51. Abedi M, Greer DA, Foster BM, Colvin GA, Harpel JA, Demers DA, Pimentel J, Dooner MS, Quesenberry PJ (2005) Critical variables in the conversion of marrow cells to skeletal muscle. Blood 106:1488–1495

52. Lapidos KA, Chen YE, Earley JU, Heydemann A, Huber JM, Chien M, Ma A, McNally EM (2004) Transplanted hematopoietic stem cells demonstrate impaired sarcoglycan expression after engraftment into cardiac and skeletal muscle. J Clin Invest 114:1577–1585

53. Nygren JM, Jovinge S, Breitbach M, Sawen P, Roll W, Hescheler J, Taneera J, Fleischmann BK, Jacobsen SE (2004) Bone marrow-derived hematopoietic cells generate cardiomyocytes at a low frequency through cell fusion, but not transdifferentiation. Nature Medicine 10:494–501

54. Jiang Y, Vaessen B, Lenvik T, Blackstad M, Reyes M, Verfaillie CM (2002) Multipotent progenitor cells can be isolated from postnatal murine bone marrow, muscle, and brain. Exp Hematol 30:896–904

55. Jackson KA, Mi T, Goodell MA (1999) Hematopoietic potential of stem cells isolated from murine skeletal muscle. Proc Natl Acad Sci USA 96:14482–14486

56. Kawada H, Ogawa M (2001) Bone marrow origin of hematopoietic progenitors and stem cells in murine muscle. Blood 98:2008–2013

57. McKinney-Freeman SL, Jackson KA, Camargo FD, Ferrari G, Mavilio F, Goodell MA (2002) Muscle-derived hematopoietic stem cells are hematopoietic in origin. Proc Natl Acad Sci USA 99:1341–1346

58. Lee JY, Qu-Peterson Z, Cao B, Kimura S, Jankowski R, Cummins J, Usas A, Gates C, Robbins P, Huard J (2000) Clonal isolation of muscle derived cells capable of enhancing muscle regeneration and bone healing. J Cell Biol 150:1085–1099

59. Bruscia EM, Price JE, Cheng EC, Weiner S, Caputo C, Ferreira EC, Egan M, Krause DS (2006) Assessment of cystic fibrosis transmembrane conductance regulator (CFTR) activity in CFTR-null mice after bone marrow transplantation. Proc Natl Acad Sci USA 103:2965–2970

60. Shamblott MJ, Axelman J, Littlefield JW, Blumenthal PD, Huggins GR, Cui Y, Cheng L, Gearhart JD (2001) Human embryonic germ cell derivatives express a broad range of developmentally distinct markers and proliferate extensively in vitro. Proc Natl Acad Sci USA 98:113–118

61. Schuliner M, Yanuka O, Itskovitz-Eldor J, Melton DA, Benvenisty N (2000) Effects of eight growth factors on the differentiation of cells derived from human embryonic stem cells. Proc Natl Acad Sci USA 97:11307–11312

62. Vallier M, Mancip J, Markossian S, Lukaszewicz A, Dehay C, Metzger D, Samarut J, Savatier P (2001) Efficient system for conditional gene expression in embryonic stem cells and in their in vitro and in vivo to differentiated derivatives. Proc Natl Acad Sci USA 98:2467–2472

63. Aliotta J, Keaney P, Passero M, Dooner M, Pimentel J, Greer D, Demers D, Foster Be, Peterson A, Dooner G, Theise N, Abedi M, Colvin G, Quesenberry P (2006) Bone marrow production of lung cells: the impact of G-CSF, cardiotoxin, graded dosed of irradiation, and subpopulation phenotype. Ex Hem 34:230–241

64. Albera C, Polak JM, Janes S, Griffiths MJD, Alison MR, Wright NA, Navaratnarasah S, Poulsom R, Jeffrey R, Fisher C, Burke M, Bishop AE (2005) Repopulation of human pulmonary epithelium by bone marrow cells: a potential means to promote repair. Tissue Eng 11:1115-1121

65. Suratt BT, Cool CD, Seris AE, Chen L, Varella-Garcia M, Shpall EJ, Brown KK, Worthen GS (2003) Human pulmonary chimerism after hematopoietic stem cell transplantation. Am J Respir Crit Care Med 168:318–322

66. Mattson J, Jansson M, Wernerson A, Hassa M (2004) Lung epithelial cells and type II pneumocytes of donor origin after allogeneic hematopoietic stem cell transplantation. Transplantation 78:154–157

67. Kleeberger W, Versmold A, Rothamel T, Glockner S, Bredt M, Haverich A, Lehmann U, Kreipe H (2003) Increased chimerism of bronchial and alveolar epithelium in human lung allografts undergoing chronic injury. Am J Pathol 162:1487–1494

68. Spencer H, Rampling D, Aurora P, Bonnet D, Hart SL, Jaffe A (2005) Transbronchial biopsies provide longitudinal evidence for epithelial chimerism in children following sex mismatched lung transplantation. Thorax 60:60–62

69. Bittmann I, Dose T, Baretton GB, Muller C, Schwaiblmair M, Kur F, Lohrs U (2001) Cellular chimerism of the lung after transplantation: an interphase cytogenetic study. Am J Clin Pathol 115:525–533

70. Prigozhina TB, Gurevitzh O, Slavin S (1999) Nonmyeloablative conditioning to induce bilateral tolerance after allogeneic bone marrow transplantation in mice. Exp Hematol 27:1503–1510

71. Blomberg M, Rao S, Reilly J, Tiarks C, Peters S, Kittler E, Quesenberry P (1998) Repetitive bone marrow transplantation in nonmyeloablated recipients. Exp Hematol 26:320–324

72. Chao NF, Koh L-P, Long GD, Gasparetto C, Horwitz M, Morris A, Lassiter M, Sullivan KM, Rizzieri DA (2004) Adult recipients of umbilical cord blood transplants after nonmyeloablative preparative regimens. Biol Blood Marrow Transplant 10:569–575

73. Koh L-P, Chao NF (2004) Umbilical cord blood transplantation in adults using myeloablative and nonmyeloablative preparative regimens. Biol Blood Marrow Transplant 10:1–22

74. Cowan CM, Jiang X, Hsu T, Soo C, Zhang B, Wang JZ, Kuroda S, Wu B, Zhang Z, Zhang X, Ting K (2007) Synergistic effects of Nell-1 and BMP-2 on the osteogenic differentiation of myoblasts. J Bone Miner Res 22:918–930

75. Qu CQ, Zhang GH, Zhang LJ, Yang GS (2007) Osteogenic and adipogenic potential of porcine adipose mesenchymal stem cells. In Vitro Cell Dev Biol Anim 43:95–100

76. Hidaka M, Su GN, Chen JK, Mukaisho K, Hattori T, Yamamoto G (2007) Transplantation of engineered bone tissue using a rotary three-dimensional culture system. In Vitro Cell Dev Biol Animal 43:49–58

77. Oka K, Oka S, Sasaki T, Ito Y, Bringas P, Nonaka K, Chai Y (2007) The role of TGF-β signaling in regulating chondrogenesis and osteogenesis during mandibular development. Dev Biol 303:391–404

78. Platt I, Rao LG, El-Sohemy A (2007) Isomer-specific effects of conjugated linoleic acid on mineralized bone nodule formation from human osteoblast-like cells. Exp Biol Med 232–246–252

79. Keilhoff G, Goihl A, Stang F, Wolf G, Fansa H (2006) Peripheral nerve tissue engineering: autologous Schwann cells vs. transdifferentiated mesenchymal stem cells. Tissue Eng 12: 1451–1465

80. Hwang Y-S, Randle WL, Bielby RC, Polak JM, Mantalaris A (2006) Enhanced derivation of osteogenic cells from murine embryonic stem cells after treatment with HepG2-conditioned medium and modulation of the embryoid body formation period: Application to skeletal tissue engineering. Tissue Eng 12:1381–1392

81. Shao X, Goh JCH, Hutmacher DW, Lee EH, Zigang G (2006) Repair of large articular osteochondral defects using hybrid scaffolds and bone marrow-derived mesenchymal stem cells in a rabbit model. Tissue Eng 12:1539–1551

82. Lee DH, Park BJ, Lee MS, Lee JW, Kim JK, Yang HC, Park JC (2006) Chemotactic migration of human mesenchymal stem cells and MC3T3-E1 osteoblast-like cells induced by COS-7 cell line expressing rhBMP-7. Tissue Eng 12:1577–1586

83. Greenberger JS, Epperly MW, Gretton J, Jefferson M, Nie S, Bernarding M, Kagan V, Guo HL (2003) Radioprotective gene therapy. Curr Gene Ther 3:183–195

84. Greenberger JS, Epperly MW (2004) Radioprotective antioxidant gene therapy: potential mechanisms of action. Gene Ther Mol Biol 8:31–44

85. Greenberger JS, Epperly MW (2007) Antioxidant therapeutic approaches toward amelioration of ionizing irradiation – induced pulmonary injury. Curr Respir Med Rev 7:29–37

86. Greenberger JS, Epperly MW (2007) Antioxidant gene therapeutic approaches to normal tissue radioprotection and tumor radiosensitization. In Vivo 21:141–146

87. Guo, HL, Seixas-Silva JA, Epperly MW, Gretton JE, Shin DM, Greenberger JS (2003) Prevention of irradiation-induced oral cavity mucositis by plasmid/liposome delivery of the human manganese superoxide dismutase (MnSOD) transgene. Radiat Res 159:361–370

88. Epperly MW, Wegner R, Kanai AJ, Kagan V, Greenberger EE, Nie S, Greenberger JS (2007) Irradiated murine oral cavity orthotopic tumor antioxidant pool destabilization by MnSOD-plasmid liposome gene therapy mediates tumor radiosensitization. Radiat Res 267:289–297

89. Epperly MW, Carpenter M, Agarwal A, Mitra P, Nie S, Greenberger JS (2004) Intra-oral manganese superoxide dismutase plasmid liposome radioprotective gene therapy decreases ionizing irradiation-induced murine mucosal cell cycling and apoptosis. In Vivo 18:401–410

90. Coppes RP (2007) Stem cell therapy to reduce normal tissue damage. CL 18, p. 68, Proceeding of the 13th International Congress of Radiation Research, San Francisco, CA

91. Epperly MW, Sikora C, Defilippi S, Bray J, Koe G, Liggitt D, Luketich JD, Greenberger JS (2000) Plasmid/liposome transfer of the human manganese superoxide dismutase (MnSOD) transgene prevents ionizing irradiation-induced apoptosis in human esophagus organ explant culture. Int J Cancer (Radiat Oncol Invest) 90:128–137

92. Friedenstein AJ, Petrakova KV, Kurolesova AL, Frolova GP (1968) Heterotopic of bone marrow. Analysis of precursor cells for osteogenic and hematopoietic tissues. Transplantation 6:230–247

93. Epperly MW, Gretton JA, Defilippi SJ, Sikora CA, Liggitt D, Koe G, Greenberger JS (2001) Modulation of radiation-induced cytokine elevation associated with esophagitis and esophageal stricture by manganese superoxide dismutase-plasmid/liposome (SOD-PL) gene therapy. Radiat Res 155:2–14

94. Epperly MW, Kagan VE, Sikora CA, Gretton JE, Defilippi SJ, Bar-Sagi D, Greenberger JS (2001) Manganese superoxide dismutase-plasmid/liposome (MnSOD-PL) administration protects mice from esophagitis associated with fractionated irradiation. Int J Cancer (Radiat Oncol Invest) 96:221–233

95. Epperly MW, Shen H, Jefferson M, Greenberger JS (2004) In vitro differentiation capacity of esophageal progenitor cells with capacity for homing and repopulation of the ionizing irradiation damaged esophagus. In Vivo 18:675–685

96. Epperly MW, Zhang X, Nie S, Cao S, Kagan V, Tyurin V, Greenberger JS (2005) MnSOD-plasmid liposome gene therapy effects on ionizing irradiation induced lipid peroxidation of the esophagus. In Vivo 19:997–1004

97. Epperly MW, Shen H, Zhang X, Nie S, Cao S, Greenberger JS (2005) Protection of esophageal stem cells from ionizing irradiation by MnSOD-plasmid liposome gene therapy. In Vivo 19:965–974

98. Niu Y, Epperly MW, Shen H, Smith T, Wang H, Greenberger JS (2008) Intraesophageal MnSOD-plasmid liposome administration enhances engraftment and self-renewal capacity of bone marrow derived progenitors of esophageal squamous epithelium. Gene Ther 15:347–356

99. Herzog EL, Van AJ, Hu B, Zhang J, Chen Q, Haberman AM, Krause DS (2007) Lung-specific nuclear reprogramming is accompanied by heterokaryon formation and Y chromosome loss following bone marrow transplantation and secondary inflammation. FASEBJ 21:2592–2601

100. Greenberger JS (2008) Gene therapy approaches for stem cell protection. Gene Ther 15:100–108

101. Epperly MW, Epstein CJ, Travis EL, Greenberger JS (2000) Decreased pulmonary radiation resistance of manganese superoxide dismutase (MnSOD)-deficient mice is corrected by human manganese Superoxide dismutase-plasmid/liposome (SOD2-PL) intratracheal gene therapy. Radiat Res 154:365–374

102. Epperly MW, Travis EL, Whitsett JA, Epstein CJ, Greenberger JS (2001) Overexpression of manganese superoxide dismutase (MnSOD) in whole lung or alveolar type II (AT-II) cells of MnSOD transgenic mice does not provide intrinsic lung irradiation protection. Radiat Oncol Invest 96:11–21

103. Epperly MW, Bray JA, Kraeger S, Zwacka R, Engelhardt J, Travis E, Greenberger JS (1998) Prevention of late effects of irradiation lung damage by manganese superoxide dismutase gene therapy. Gene Ther 5:196–208

104. Carpenter M, Epperly MW, Agarwal A, Nie S, Hricisak L, Niu Y, Greenberger JS (2005) Inhalation delivery of manganese superoxide dismutase-plasmid/liposomes (MnSOD-PL) protects the murine lung from irradiation damage. Gene Ther 12:685–690

105. Epperly MW, Guo HL, Jefferson M, Wong S, Gretton J, Bernarding M, Bar-Sagi D, Greenberger JS (2003) Cell phenotype specific duration of expression of epitope-tagged HA-MnSOD in cells of the murine lung following intratracheal plasmid liposome gene therapy. Gene Ther 10:163–171

106. Epperly MW, Defilippi S, Sikora C, Gretton J, Kalend K, Greenberger JS (2000) Intratracheal injection of manganese superoxide dismutase (MnSOD) plasmid/liposomes protects normal lung but not orthotopic tumors from irradiation. Gene Ther 7:1011–1018

107. Epperly MW, Sikora CA, Defilippi SJ, Gretton JE, Bar-Sagi D, Carlos T, Guo HL, Greenberger JS (2002) Pulmonary irradiation-induced expression of VCAM-1 and ICAM-1 is decreased by MnSOD-PL gene therapy. Biol Blood Bone Marrow Transplant 8:175–187

108. Guo H, Epperly MW, Bernarding M, Nie S, Gretton J, Jefferson M, Greenberger JS (2003) Manganese super-

oxide dismutase-plasmid/liposome (MnSOD-PL) intratracheal gene therapy reduction of irradiation-induced inflammatory cytokines does not protect orthotopic lewis lung carcinomas. In Vivo 17:13–22

109. Hong KU, Reynolds SD, Giangreco A, Hurley CM, Stripp BR (2001) Clara cell secretory protein-expressing cells of the airway neuroepithelial body microenvironment include a label-retaining subset and are critical for epithelial renewal after progenitor cell depletion. Am J Respir Cell Mol Biol 24:671–681

110. Reynolds SD, Giangreco A, Hong KU, McGrath KE, Ortiz LA, Sripp BR (2004) Airway injury in lung disease pathophysiology: selective depletion of airway stem and progenitor cell pools potentiates lung inflammation and alveolar dysfunction. Am J Physiol Lung Cell Mol Physiol 287:L1256–1265

111. Greenberger JS (1991) The hematopoietic microenvironment. Crit Rev Oncol Hematol 11:65–84

112. Greenberger JS (2008) Gene therapy approaches for stem cell protection. Gene Therapy 15:100–108

6

Development of a Queriable Database for Oncology Outcome Analysis

Thomas J. FitzGerald

* Keith White, Joel Saltz, Ashish Sharma, Eliot Siegel, Marcia Urie, Ken Ulin, James Purdy, Walter Bosch, John Matthews, Joseph Deasy, Geoffrey Ibbott, Fran Laurie, Richard Hanusik, Jeff Yorty, Maryann Bishop-Jodoin, Sandy Kessel, M Giulia Cicchetti, Kathleen McCarten, Nancy Rosen, Richard Pieters, Stephan Voss, Gregory Reaman, Mitchell Schnall, Richard Schilsky, Michael Knopp, Lawrence Schwartz, Laurence Baker, Robert Comis, Larry Kun, James Boyett, Uma Ramamurthy, Matthew Parliament, Heidi Nelson, and David Ota

CONTENTS

6.1 Introduction

Clinical trials and oncology data management have undergone considerable change in the past decade. Imaging has become a key tool for clinical trials management and a biomarker for clinical trial validation as imaging technologies improve and become more precise. Images have become extremely helpful in determining staging/eligibility, treatment response, and outcome determination including disease recurrence and progression. In modern protocols, images are often reviewed in real time to validate these points in order to improve compliance to study requirements and create uniform patient populations for clinical trials analysis. Data acquisition and management systems are currently in use to acquire and display images in electronic digital formats for view by both on site and off site radiology reviewers. As clinical trials become more global in focus, the ability for databases to accommodate diverse imaging acquisition strategies will become increasingly important for information review. It will likewise become increasingly important for tools to be created that support facile digital image transfer and review including image annotation clinical trial validation.

Imaging has become the key vehicle in radiation oncology in order to define and validate the fields of radiation therapy to use in clinical trials as well as to determine which areas receive full dose or lower dose of radiation treatment. Radiation therapy planning systems are now fully image based for tumor target definition and sparing of normal tissue. Radiation treatment execution is rapidly becoming image guided in order to accommodate for changes in position and target motion during therapy. The fusion of metabolic and anatomic images may significantly alter target volume definition at presentation and subsequent imaging on treatment may help validate deformable changes in the target volume as a function of treatment. This may improve tumor targeting and further serve to decrease radiation dose to normal tissue.

Moving forward, clinical protocols are collecting patient serum and tumor tissue at presentation and at later time points. Microarray analyses for genomics and proteomics are Dicom objects and can be thought of as images, therefore the potential exists for these objects to reside side by side with both imaging and radiation therapy objects as part of a queri-

T. J. FitzGerald, MD
Chair, Department of Radiation Oncology, Quality Assurance Review Center (QARC), University of Massachusetts Memorial Medical Center, 55 Lake Avenue North, Worcester, MA 01655, USA

* *complete authors' addresses see* List of Contributors

able database for clinical oncology analysis. Linking this information with patient outcome would greatly facilitate the development of clinical translational science. This can be accomplished with established databases housed within the cooperative groups or by creating prospective patient registries to track treatment administration and patient outcomes.

With improvements in patient outcome documented in many disease sites including breast, pediatrics, and prostate, patients are now available for analysis of normal tissue function. Although the primary clinical endpoint remains tumor control, normal tissue tolerance, both as an acute and late effect of therapy, is becoming of increasing importance in evaluation of the effects of therapy including the genesis of second malignancies which may be treatment driven. In many disease sites we are learning how to adjust and subtract therapies as well as decrease the duration of treatment. For example, in Hodgkin's disease treatment protocols are designed to reflect response to initial chemotherapy with secondary randomization points built into protocols based on chemotherapy treatment response validated by both metabolic and anatomic imaging performed and reviewed in real time. A patient determined to have a rapid early response to chemotherapy will have a shorter course of chemotherapy and possibly not undergo radiation therapy based on the completeness of their response to induction therapy. Outcome images are obtained and incorporated as part of protocol evaluation. This strategy requires real time review of images and radiation therapy treatment objects for protocol compliance. Previous iterations of protocols in Hodgkin's disease have demonstrated a discordance of 37% in site versus central review of images with respect to response and an equal rate of discordance in compliance to radiation therapy treatment schema. This could have considerable influence on study analysis and outcome. Central real time review of objects has had a considerable impact in improving the discrepancy between site and central evaluation with deviation rates on study now at or below 5% in many studies. Resolving these issues prior to randomization and pre-therapy has become an important aspect of clinical trials moving forward, and promoting these processes is expected to improve uniformity of data for clinical trials. A key objective in improving clinical trials is to promote facile data acquisition strategies and display data in a uniform database format for queriable research. Promoting media for off site clinical review strategies and establishing electronic vehicles for query will be crucial to improving access to data and will significantly enhance the productivity and quality of our translational science. Integrating information germane to clinical trials including imaging, radiation therapy, genomics/proteomics, treatment, and clinical outcome will be the objective for improving the quality of translational science. Making this information available through a single electronic format will promote clinical investigation for outcome analysis for patients treated for malignancy.

Physicians and scientists participating in the CURED effort are interested in the late effects of therapy management including the effect of treatment on normal tissue function and the generation of second malignancies [1]. The protocols in development by this group intend to capture data including images, radiation therapy treatment objects, microarray, and patient outcome data and house the information in a database that can be queried for analysis. The intent is to also collect data on cancer survivors. These patients may/may not have been treated on previous clinical trials. Integrating this data and objects including outcome into a uniform database is an important objective for this group. Incorporating existing platforms into this effort may provide the appropriate efficiency of scale to provide a robust platform for clinical research.

6.2
Efforts to Date

6.2.1
Quality Assurance Review Center

The Quality Assurance Review Center (QARC) has a long-standing interest in developing processes and initiating process improvements in imaging and radiation therapy for both clinical cooperative group and industry clinical trials. QARC became independently funded through CTEP in 1980 with initial mission focus in radiation therapy planning for both children and adults enrolled on cooperative group protocols. As radiation therapy became image based in target definition, QARC began a process in 1985 for diagnostic image acquisition to validate the fields of radiation therapy. As part of study review investigators required that the diagnostic images and the radiation therapy treatment objects resided in a side-by-side format for protocol object review. During the past decade institutions preferred to forward objects to QARC via many forms of electronic media and QARC has established a diverse portfolio for data acquisition including images in order to create a facile and all inclusive strategy for data acquisition. Institutions worldwide forward objects in many diverse electronic formats to QARC. This is often dependent on the informatics expertise and equipment at each site. Radiation therapy digital data is submitted to QARC in multiple formats and media including RTOG objects. The submitted objects, including images and radiation therapy treatment data, reside in a uniform format in the QARC database housed in a facile retrievable format. Imaging and radiation therapy objects reside in a side-by-side format for object review. The database is the central aspect of QARC function and serves as the epicenter of activities with each division of QARC using the platform for data management including real time review of objects and world-wide inter-institutional communication for problem solving [1–3].

6.2.2
Database Function

QARC: This report of the QARC Information Systems is organized in the following sections: I. Network Infrastructure; II. Web Interface and Security; III. MAX Database Operating System; IV. Digital Data Management; and V. Data Integrity and Backups.

I. Network Infrastructure

The QARC network includes 17 servers, 46 PCs, 16 laptops and 10 printers. Every node on the network connects to one of five central switches running at 1 Gigabit per second. The server group consists of Windows 2003 Enterprise Server, one Red All desktop and portable systems at QARC run Windows XP Professional Service Pack 2.

II. Web Interfaces and Security

QARC is responsible for managing its own network security. QARC has full T1 1.5 megabits per second connection to the internet. Security is implemented using Cisco 2821 IOS and Checkpoint NG Firewall. Three "demilitarized zones" (DMZs) allow protected access to QARC information. One public DMZ serves general internet users and the other two DMZ's are used to collaborate with external organizations and Cooperative Groups. Virtual Private Network (VPN) is supported using both Cisco and Checkpoint technologies.

III. MAX Database System

QARC's database, called MAX, is a validated relational operating system with its foundations in SQL server in 2005 Enterprise. It includes query by form functionality that allows any user to intuitively query data on any field or set of fields in the database. MAX includes over 300 tables, over 600

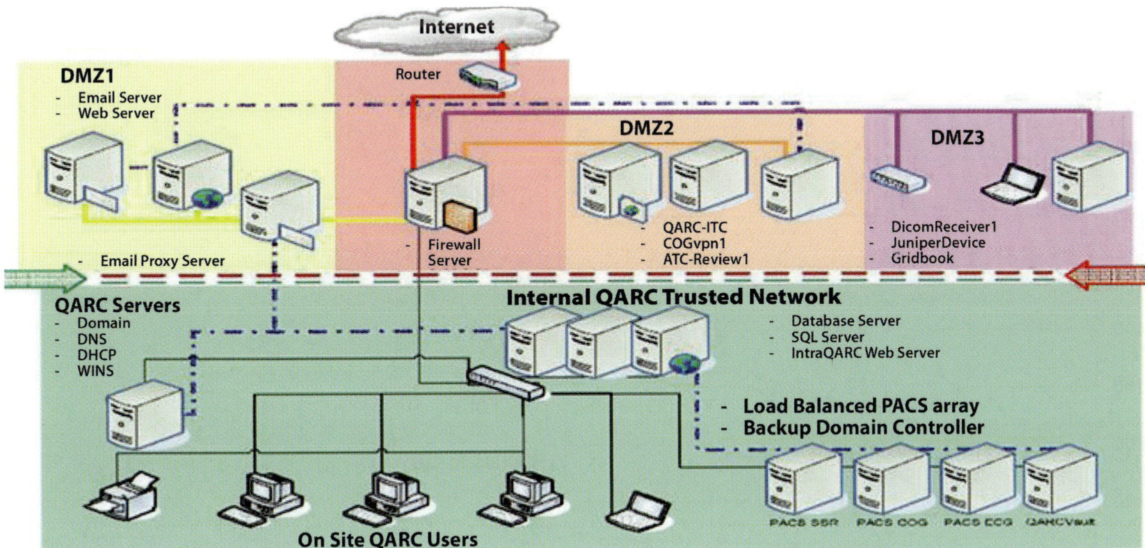

Fig. 6.1. QARC network

and approximately 200 customized reports. There are over 40,000 patient records in MAX. Within the patient record are links to the tables that include information about the cooperative group and institution contacts and benchmarks, protocols, correspondence, DICOM and non-DICOM digital data. MAX features integrated messaging systems which allow users to communicate with each other, the IS Department and with external contacts at all institutions. Patient data is routinely extracted from MAX and sent to the statistical centers of the Cooperative Groups and Pharmaceutical companies via password-protected e-mail and data files.

Internal to MAX, the QKB is an indexed help facility and library tailored for QARC staff. It is a repository of knowledge specific to QARC. MAX creates multiple audit trails of stored data and user activity within the database. QARC has undergone a systematic validation process of its information systems to be compliant with 21 CFR Part 11. A standard operating procedure (SOP) generator has been incorporated into the MAX system and is used to produce the QARC SOPs. QARC follows standard procedures to assure maintenance of compliance, including multiple auditing mechanisms, documentation templates, regular backups of the database and associated files, and strict adherence to a change management processes.

IV. Digital Data Management

The MAX system manages all electronic media received at QARC. Electronic media is divided into three categories in MAX: (a) DICOM imaging which refers to all diagnostic digital imaging that conforms to the DICOM standard and (b) DICOM RT data or RTOG data exchange data which is submitted via FTP, imported into the database and viewed using either the ATC remote review tool (RRT) or the computational environment for radiotherapy research (CERR) program; and (c) eMaterial which encompasses all electronic data that is not DICOM compliant. The growth of the acquisition of digital imaging and electronic data is demonstrated in the graph below. MAX has evolved into a PACS system which resolves patient imaging to patient records, stores out the imaging onto four PACS servers which are built and maintained onsite, and facilitates the transfer and viewing of all digital imaging. There approximately 25,000 diagnostic studies with over 6 million images archived in the QARC PACS.

DICOM Imaging: MAX is fully integrated with a software program, Dicommunicator, which was initially written by Dr. Keith White of Primary Children's Medical Center (Salt Lake City, Utah) and is used at institutions around the world to facilitate the submission of DICOM imaging to QARC. Dicommunicator was donated by Dr. White for use in the clinical trials process in 2000 and has since been managed and developed at QARC. Successful transfer has occurred between QARC and the following PACS systems: Agfa, GE, Integrad Web by Dynamic Imaging, Kodak, Philips, Siemens, Stentor. In addition to 35 installations, major accomplishments include streamlining the interface of the software to increase ease of use and improving the remote installation process.

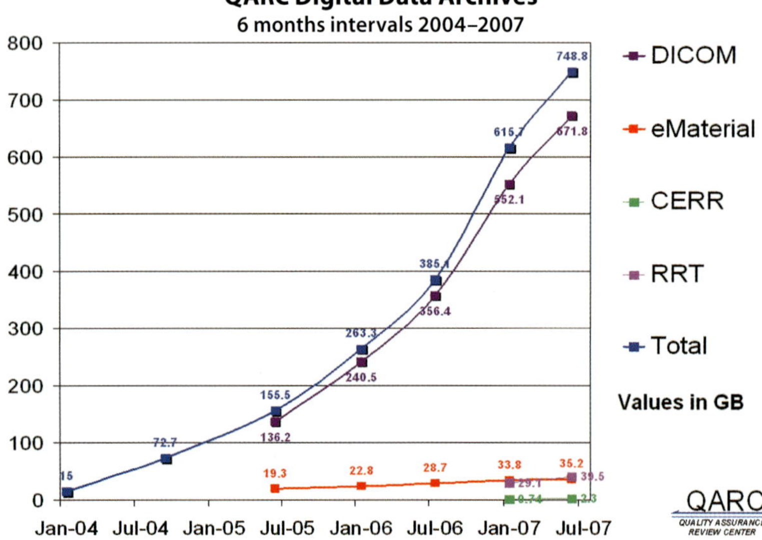

Fig. 6.2. QARC digital data archives

The Dicommunicator software is a critical component in managing digital DICOM data at QARC. Dicommunicator is used to import DICOM studies into the MAX database and match them to the appropriate patient. A CRA reviews this imaging and resolves it to the patient's diagnostic record where it can be launched and viewed by a physician. The workflow process for receiving, identifying, logging and importing digital imaging has become completely digital and is managed through a MAX utility called the "Dicommunicator Import Form Administrator" [4].

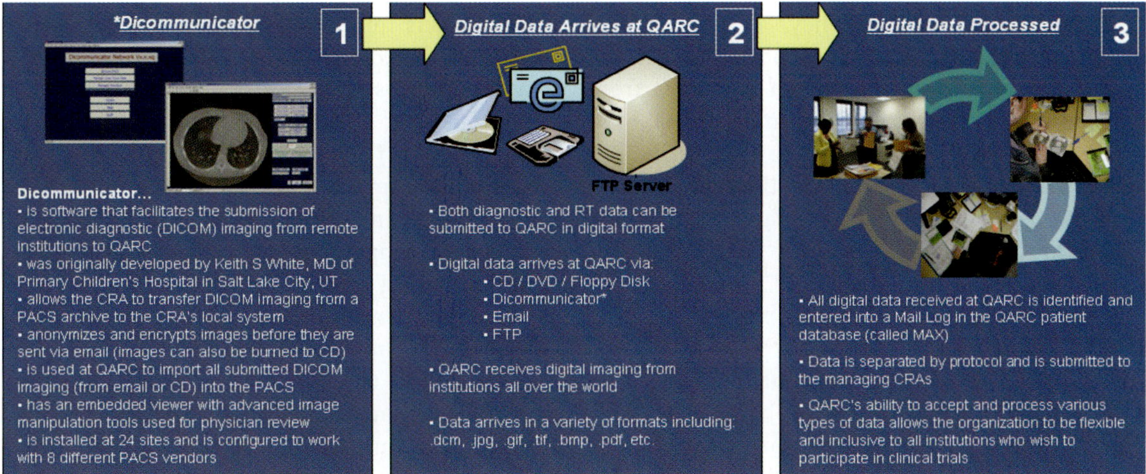

Fig. 6.3. Dicommunicator at site to submit imaging to QARC

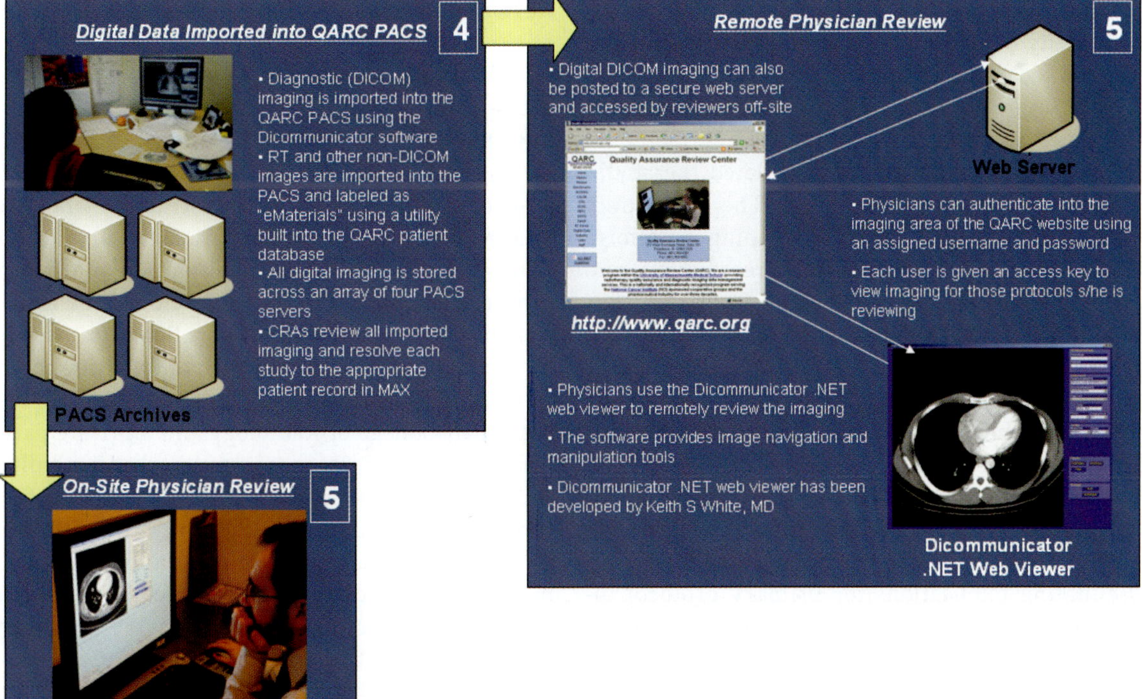

Fig. 6.4. Dicommunicator at QARC to manage imaging and facilitate reviews

V. Data Integrity/Backups

Regular backups of systems and data are realized in a number of ways. Redundant array of independent disks (RAID) is implemented on all servers. Tape Backups are performed on all servers weekly, using Symantec BackupExec Suite 10 and a robotic tape drive. These backups have been successfully utilized in the past to rebuild two servers during tests of QARC's Disaster Recovery Policy.

Peer-to-peer (P2P) routines occur at various times throughout each day, which copy data from servers and PCs to other systems and external hard drives. Database files are written to DVD disks each weeknight. For increased security the backup tapes, external hard drives and DVDs are taken offsite weekly to rotating locations.

6.2.3
Advanced Technology Consortium

The advanced technology consortium (ATC) is composed of the image guided therapy center (ITC), the Radiation Therapy Oncology Group (RTOG), the Radiological Physics Center (RPC), and QARC. The principal investigator of the grant/consortium is Dr. James Purdy, currently the Director of Physics and Vice Chair of Radiation Oncology at the University of California at Davis. The consortium has worked over the past decade to provide uniform credentialing mechanisms for institutions using advanced technology radiation therapy including image guided and intensity modulated therapy in clinical cooperative group trials. The consortium has had significant success developing a uniform data acquisition strategy for full three-dimensional radiation oncology data sets. Drs. Purdy and Bosch developed RTOG objects in collaboration with CMS planning system (St. Louis, Mo.) and this is the platform used by the RTOG for volumetric data acquisition in all clinical trials involving advanced technology treatment execution. Three-dimensional data sets including dose volume histograms are available for web based protocol review for radiation therapy objects. Aside from their efforts in facilitating publications for primary protocol intent, Dr. Purdy and the ITC group have generated many secondary endpoint publications using the database. Many of these publications have included remote review strategies including re-drawing of unintended treatment objects for radiation target

dose definition. ATC members have shared expertise and informatics process improvements. They have collaborated on many projects for process improvement strategies. One of the most successful projects was the introduction of RTOG objects into the QARC portfolio for data transfer. This permitted institutions to forward objects for review in a transparent manner independent of cooperative group membership. QARC, in turn, imbedded RTOG objects into the database housed at QARC. The RTOG objects reside in a side-by-side format with the diagnostic images at QARC linked to each specific patient. Therefore investigators can view, using on and off site mechanisms, both image and radiation therapy objects through the same database. Outcome images can be linked directly to the patient and compared to radiation therapy objects thus facilitating analysis of outcome and late effects of anti-cancer therapy in cancer survivors. One objective moving forward is to migrate the QARC database to ATC partners to share the platform for image and radiation therapy object review, thus creating a uniform platform for object review for investigators in clinical trials [5–9].

6.2.4
American College of Radiology Imaging Network (ACRIN)

ACRIN began as a clinical cooperative group in 1999 with an outstanding portfolio of trials as well as significant interactions with other cooperative groups. During this period of time ACRIN has established a well tested informatics infrastructure and has become a very strong organization for conducting multi-center clinical trials with a particular focus on cancer screening. ACRIN has developed the infrastructure to promote and support image transfer as well as successfully enhance the quality assurance of imaging. ACRIN developed, in partnership with the American College of Radiology and a private partner, an electronic image transfer mechanism called Preview 32. This system has many of the same features of Dicommunicator at QARC. It has a robust infrastructure that supports image anonymization, transmission, and quality assurance. It has been successfully deployed at more than 150 sites with engagement of PACS and IT infrastructure at participating sites. The system has acquired images on 76,000 patients including more than 13 million images on clinical trials [10, 11].

As part of the process improvement strategy, ACRIN recognized that Preview 32 required effort at the site to maintain; therefore a key focus was to evaluate an alternative image transfer strategy moving forward. Similar to QARC, Preview was built on proprietary software platforms, thus limiting interoperability with the caBIG workspace. As a response to this challenge, ACRIN, in partnership with the American College of Radiology, has developed a new generation of imaging management software. This new platform is called TRIAD. The ACR is providing the programming resources for this effort as the ACR intends to use this platform for education and credentialing strategies moving forward as well as being made available to ACRIN. TRIAD is a thin client web-based system that can be easily installed over the web on computers currently in use at sites and connected to the Internet. The advantage to TRIAD is that it will promote review of in vivo objects image related issues in a direct fashion through the Internet. As will be discussed in the following section, integrating TRIAD into the QARC database is an objective moving forward which will promote and facilitate data review.

ACRIN has developed processes similar to QARC to conduct in house reader assessments through the deployment of diagnostic quality workstations at the ACRIN headquarters local network as well as establish a mechanism for distributed assessments via image transfer to the reader's home institution. These strategies have greatly facilitated review of data for clinical trials and have served to promote the uniformity and quality of the data used for clinical trials analysis.

6.2.5
Virtual Imaging Evaluation Workspace (VIEW)

Imaging has evolved to become an important biomarker for clinical endpoints in for both industry and cooperative group clinical trials [12–14]. A challenge, however, has been to acquire, archive and centrally review, in an independent fashion, the images obtained on cooperative group treatment trials. The NCI has supported formation of a consortium for this purpose. Consortium members include those members of the cooperative groups that had electronic infrastructure in place for digital image transfer and ability to generate the audit trails necessary for regulatory compliance. The consortium consists of ACRIN, QARC, and the imaging core lab of the CALGB housed at the Ohio State University directed by Dr. Michael Knopp. The members of the consortium are in the process of developing an inter-operative IT infrastructure transparent to VIEW members and the cooperative groups served by the consortium. This infrastructure will be 21 CFR Part 11 compliant and compatible with caBIG. The consortium will develop standard operating procedures for data acquisition and assessment of imaging endpoints for cancer clinical trials for both anatomic and functional imaging as well as develop an assessment strategy for newer advanced technologies moving forward. This will include both institutional credentialing for participation in clinical trials as well as the development of standardized quality assurance metrics for reviewer assessment. The consortium will work with the FDA and clinical trials sponsors to develop imaging charters compatible with regulatory guidelines and data management standards. The consortium will further explore strategies to advance the science of alternative imaging strategies and establish database functions that can be mined for queriable research. As these ideas mature and gain strength, integration of imaging databases with both patient outcome data and other therapy objects will further promote the field of translational science. VIEW will play a key role in the integration of imaging science with translational science and further serve to help integrate imaging objectives with clinical research strategies.

6.2.6
CaBIG

In recognition of the need to develop integrative database structure and the paucity of tools to achieve this objective, the National Cancer Institute developed a strategy to move this science forward through the development of the cancer biomedical informatics grid initiative (caBIG) in February 2004. The overarching responsibility of the caBIG initiative was to develop an informatics infrastructure to facilitate exchange of information among clinical cancer centers and other institutions and develop databases for research. The caBIG community is adopting and in some cases, developing informatics standards and policies using an open source approach. The "informatics grid" strategy was established as the vehicle of choice for this purpose using open source software platforms and takes advantage of the power of grid computing and the excellent open source software developed by this community. One of the most important developments of the caBIG project is the establishment of the in vivo imaging workspace. Eliot Siegel, MD of the University of Maryland (clinical lead) and Paul Mulhern of Booz Allen Hamilton (administrative lead) coordinate this effort. One of the most important participants is Joel Saltz, MD. Dr. Saltz is the chair of Biomedical Informatics at the Ohio State University and a pathologist and computer scientist by training. Dr. Saltz has been instrumental in the development of the in vivo imaging middleware project, which provides inter-operability between computer systems that historically, have not been integrated. One of his responsibilities has been to help develop a software strategy to integrate these diverse systems for data storage into the national archive. Dr. Saltz and his team are responsible for analytical service, security infrastructure, and grid-service platforms compatible with caBIG infrastructure. The in vivo imaging middleware library supports interoperability between caGrid and DICOM data models and exposes DICOM aware data resources as caGrid compliant services.

The informatics toolkit developed by the middleware project focuses on federated data potentially arriving for archival from diverse sources and permits this data to be formatted and reviewed with multiple query functions. The middleware project makes use of the caGRID informatics infrastructure, which will be attractive to the cooperative groups, and quality assurance centers because it can be used to enhance data review and integrate diverse data platforms by exploiting the semantics of the data rather than the representative formats of the data. The transition of legacy data archives to strongly typed grid data services is one of the key thrust areas of the in vivo imaging workspace moving forward. Access to the QARC database was demonstrated via the grid architecture during the 2006 Radiological Society of North American meeting. The effort of integrated metabolic imaging formats with the CALGB imaging core service, directed by Michael Knopp MD, was demonstrated by the caBIG team as well. These are examples of legacy databases with which the in vivo imaging workspace group has begun the process of integration. The next key decision for caBIG, the cooperative group statistical data centers, and the quality assurance centers will be to decide whether caBIG efforts should be the primary data acquisition model or to integrate on the back end with existing systems for data management. Both approaches have merit, therefore an integrated plan may be strategic and provide flexibility for an all inclusive data acquisition strategy including worldwide institutions with diverse informatics

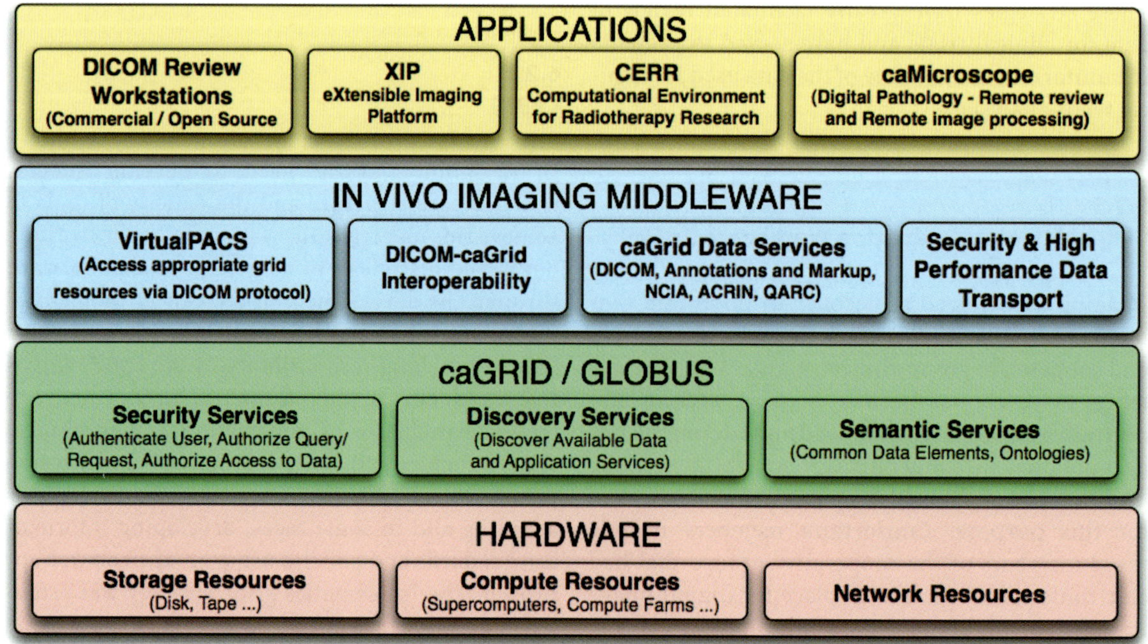

Fig. 6.5. IVI middleware

platforms. This will become especially important as clinical trials become more international in practice [15–19].

6.3
Future Strategies for Cancer Clinical Trials

The key objective for clinical trials is to promote the development of queriable databases for clinical research. Housed within the database available for query should be all information required for the evaluation of translational science including patient characteristics, imaging, radiation therapy treatment objects, treatment information, microarray for genomics and proteomics, and patient outcome. This information currently is available, however it is housed in segregated legacy informatics formats without integration. A strategy for integration is a key objective to improve our clinical science and provide an infrastructure for validating clinical trials in a facile manner.

Clinical trials are becoming more complex in scope and have multiple endpoints embedded into each trial that include images and tissue acquisition and use this information to assess secondary endpoints as part of the study. Often trials require real time review of images and object data as part of the protocol to trigger secondary and tertiary study endpoints. In COG protocol AHOD 0031 (intermediate risk Hodgkin's disease), anatomic and metabolic images are reviewed after two cycles of chemotherapy in order to determine the rapidity of response. This evaluation triggers a randomization to the duration and type of chemotherapy. Images are reviewed again after four cycles of chemotherapy as patients who had rapid early responses to chemotherapy and are deemed in complete response after four cycles are then randomized to involved field radiation therapy or no further treatment. For those who receive radiation therapy on this trial the planned fields are centrally reviewed pre-therapy for protocol compliance. Outcome images are collected on this protocol in order to confirm location of relapse and its relationship to previous sites of disease. Real time review of imaging objects is used on many adult and pediatric cancer clinical trials including trials with international participation. At QARC the database is used as the format for site and investigator review of objects in both a real time and retro-spective format. Therefore future database strategies must have the nimble functionality to permit real time review of objects and integrative strategies to permit mid-cycle evaluation of data for adaptive statistics. Query function that is diverse is important in order to review data in a complete and thorough manner [3, 4, 20].

For potential protocols for CURED, functionality that is diverse, adaptive, and complete will be very important. Because the focus of CURED will be on patient outcome and normal tissue function, data acquisition must focus on diverse strategies as patient treatment occurred using varied informatics platforms with years of informatics transition. The protocols under development by CURED include the evaluation of breast MR for patients treated for Hodgkin's disease and the use of helical computer tomography of the chest to evaluate the risk of lung cancer in patients treated for Hodgkin's disease. It will be important in these protocols to acquire patient information including imaging, radiation therapy treatment objects, and treatment programs in order to perform appropriate risk hazard analysis for these important secondary events. Likewise it is anticipated that tissue/blood analysis for these patients will also be important, particularly for assessment of germline polymorphisms that might increase the risk of late adverse events. If these patients were treated on previous cooperative group clinical trials, it will be important to link this data, including imaging and biospecimens, from established databases housed in cooperative group data centers. Because imaging and radiation therapy treatment objects on these patients would have been established at diverse time points, it will be important for the integrated database to accept data in multiple formats using a uniform strategy for data review likely through a web based mechanism. For many CURED patients their cancer therapy may have been delivered in a pediatric protocol and the patients are evaluated as adults. Therefore a strategy integrating all data centers for the cooperative groups will be an important feature for this initiative as a long-term strategy [21–24].

Quality assurance groups and data centers have the potential of meeting the objective of integration. It will require cooperation by all interested parties with active use of middleware integration platforms and the caBIG in vivo imaging database system. Each area of interest including imaging, radiation therapy objects, microarray, and patient outcome will require a different approach for data integration with integrated display available for queriable research on a uniform display platform.

Imaging will be accomplished with integration of the informatics infrastructure between ACRIN, QARC, and the CALGB through the VIEW initiative. ACRIN has developed a strategy for uniform data acquisition with both the PREVIEW and TRIAD systems. This has been a very successful strategy. The image acquisition strategy at QARC has included a uniform image transfer system (Dicommunicator) as well as a platform to accept computer disc and display the objects in a uniform data set. The South West Oncology Group has a partnership with AG Mednet for image transfer and review. This program can be integrated into the developing process as well. Each center involved in the VIEW consortium will be able to receive and accept images from each member. Therefore each member will have both CD and direct image transfer capability. QARC, in turn, will be able to integrate and launch TRIAD through the QARC database for display review.

Display of radiation therapy objects has progressed very well through the Advanced Technology Consortium. RTOG objects are available at QARC and are launched side by side to the image objects for review of protocol patients. These objects are reviewed in real time and in retrospect by QARC staff and investigators either through Webex or distributed through the .net service featured by Dicommunicator. Web based strategies for off site review of radiation therapy objects are currently used by the RTOG. Integration with VIEW investigators will insure image integration with the radiation therapy objects for simultaneous display.

In collaboration with Dr. Foran at the University of Medicine and Dentistry in New Jersey, the Saltz group has developed caGrid enabled infrastructure to support Pathology virtual slide and tissue microarray image management and analysis. This effort is now supported by R01 funding from the National Library of Medicine. This virtual slide infrastructure effort is now over 10 years old; the current virtual image management infrastructure is caGrid compliant and leverages the in vivo imaging middleware library [25, 26].

The Ohio State University houses tissue banks for the COG and the CALGB through the efforts of Drs. Qualman and Jewel. Each has considerable experience in housing microarray data in digital formats as well as establish platforms for distributed review of pathology objects. The next iteration of this strategy will be incorporating the objects into a uniform file format housed with imaging and radiation therapy objects for queriable research. In the first generation of this platform the QARC database will be modified to incorporate pathology objects and this will be further developed through cooperation of caBIG for enterprise function and archive [27–29].

Linking this information with patient outcome will be the next step in establishing the platform for queriable research. The data could be retrieved by the cooperative group from the QARC database for internal use by investigators in the cooperative groups as a first step in the development of this strategy. The QARC database is relational with each cooperative group statistical center; therefore the informatics base for initiating this objective is in place. It can be significantly improved with integration of the caBIG middleware software. For patients treated on cooperative group clinical trials a long-term strategy may include specific protocol information with outcome data potentially made available with permission from the sponsoring cooperative group including data on relapse and normal tissue toxicity. At the appropriate time point and with permission from the cooperative group, the patient outcome data could be made available to the national archive for queriable research linked to the specific patient in the QARC database for review of images, radiation therapy objects, and microarray and other biological data. This may create database utilization across protocols with similar disease site orientation.

As stated previously, patients entered on CURED protocols may/may not have been treated on cooperative group trials. If so, data may exist on the patient that could be mined for outcome analysis. Thus images, treatment objects, and tissue may be housed within the established database. Tissue and images obtained as part of the CURED protocol could be linked to the previous platforms for outcome analysis. Likewise, the database can be used to acquire and display information for CURED patients who were not treated on cooperative group protocols as needed.

Thus cooperation between established centers for quality assurance in clinical trials and cooperative group data centers can lead to a new strategy for clinical translational research. Integrating imaging, radiation therapy objects, biological data, and patient treatment/outcome data may help facilitate patient analysis and help navigate the development of new protocols and initiatives. The database at QARC currently links images and radiation therapy objects in a side-by-side format with a plan to link microarray objects to this data through cooperation with tissue banks of the cooperative groups. Middleware software generated through caBIG can be used to support this process and perhaps permit links to the established data centers of the existing cooperative groups to permit analysis of outcome events. It is possible that tissue/germline DNA may be obtained on patients treated/evaluated on separate clinical trials housed in separate databases on patients evaluated by CURED. Middleware linkages will facilitate review of these objects and promote interactions between data centers as this may become important for patients on CURED protocols. These patients may have diverse data acquisition platforms for data entry and have been treated at different time points in cancer management, however display in a common uniform file format for queriable research is possible with expertise currently at hand. Promoting this strategy may help facilitate improvements in cancer patient management, improve the outcome for cancer patients and generate new insights into the pathogenesis of cancer that can be tested in the next generation of clinical trials.

References

1. FitzGerald TJ, Aronowitz J, Giulia Cicchetti M et al (2006) The effect of radiation therapy on normal tissue function. Hematol Oncol Clin North Am 20:141–163
2. Fitzgerald TJ, Urie M, Ulin K et al (2008) Processes for quality improvements in radiation oncology clinical trials. Int J Radiat Oncol Biol Phys 71:76–79
3. Mendenhall NP, Meyer J, Williams J et al (2005) The impact of central quality assurance review prior to radiation therapy on protocol compliance: POG 9426, a trial in pediatric Hodgkin's disease. Blood 106:753
4. Laprise NK, Hanusik R, Fitzgerald TJ, Rosen N, White KS (2007) Developing a multi-institutional PACS archive and designing processes to manage the shift from a film to a digital-based archive. J Digit Imaging (in press)
5. Purdy JA (2007) From new frontiers to new standards of practice: advances in radiotherapy planning and delivery. Front Radiat Ther Oncol 40:18–39
6. Bosch W, Matthews J, Straube W, Purdy J (2007) QuASAR: quality assurance submission, archive, analysis, and review system for advanced technology clinical trials in radiation therapy. In the Proceedings of the XVth International Conference on the Use of Computers in Radiation Therapy. Oakville, Ontario (Canada). Novel Digital Publishing, pp 98–102
7. Harms WB, Bosch WR, Purdy JA (1997) An interim digital data exchange standard for multi-institutional 3D conformal radiation therapy trials. In the Proceedings of XII International Conference on the use of Computers in Radiation therapy, Madison (WI). Medical Physics Publishing, pp 465–468
8. Purdy JA, Harms WB, Michalski JM, Bosch WR (1998) Initial experience with quality assurance of multi-institutional 3D radiotherapy clinical trials. Strahlenther Onkol 174[Suppl 2]:40–42
9. Bosch W, Matthews J, Ulin K et al (2006) Implementation of ATC method 1 for clinical trials data review at the quality assurance review center. Med Phys 33:2109
10. Hillman BJ, Schnall MD (2003) American College of Radiology Imaging Network: future clinical trials. Radiology 227:631–632
11. Aberle DR, Chiles C, Gatsonis C et al (2005) American College of Radiology Imaging Network. Imaging and cancer: research strategy of the American College of Radiology Imaging Network. Radiology 235:741–751
12. Avril N, Propper D (2007) Functional PET imaging in cancer drug development. Future Oncol 3:215–228
13. Jeswani T, Padhani AR (2005) Imaging tumor angiogenesis. Cancer Imaging 5:131–138
14. Meisamy S, Bolan PJ, Baker EH et al (2004) Neoadjuvant chemotherapy of locally advanced breast cancer: predicting response with in vivo (1) H MR spectroscopy – a pilot study at 4 T. Radiology 233:424–431
15. Erdal S, Catalyurek UV, Payne PR, Saltz J, Kamal J, Gurcan MN (2007) A knowledge-anchored integrative image search and retrieval system. J Digit Imaging 2007 (in press)
16. Prior FW, Erickson BJ, Tarbox L (2007) Open source software projects of the caBIG In Vivo Imaging Workspace Software special interest group. J Digit Imaging 20[Suppl 1]:94–100
17. Sharma A, Pan T, Cambazoglu BB, Gurcan M, Kurc T, Saltz J (2007) VirtualPACS – a federating gateway to access remote image data resources over the grid. J Digit Imaging 2007 (in press)
18. Pan TC, Gurcan MN, Langella SA et al (2007) Informatics in radiology: GridCAD: grid-based computer-aided detection system. Radiographics 27:889–897
19. Gurcan MN, Pan T, Sharma A et al (2007) GridIMAGE: a novel use of grid computing to support interactive human and computer-assisted detection decision support. J Digit Imaging 20:160–171
20. Pieters RS, Laurie F, Wagner H et al (2007) Management of adolescent patients with Hodgkin's disease in cooperative group trials. Int J Radiat Oncol Biol Phys 69:578
21. Hassan S, Ferrario C, Mamo A, Basik M (2007) Tissue microarrays: emerging standard for biomarker validation. Curr Opin Biotechnol 19:19–25
22. Fujii H, Cuvelier G, She K et al (2008) Biomarkers in newly diagnosed pediatric extensive chronic graft-versus-host disease: a report from the Children's Oncology Group. Blood 111:3276–3285
23. Jani AB, Davis LW, Fox TH (2007) Integration of databases for radiotherapy outcomes analyses. J Am Coll Radiol 4:825–831
24. Harari PM, Allen GW, Bonner JA (2007) Biology of interactions: antiepidermal growth factor receptor agents. J Clin Oncol 25:4057–4065
25. Cambazoglu BB, Sertel O, Kong J, Saltz JH, Gurcan MN, Catalyurek UV (2007) Efficient processing of pathological images using the grid: computer-aided prognosis of neuroblastoma. In Proceedings of the International Work-

shop on Challenges of Large Applications in Distributed Environments (CLADE 07)

26. Cambazoglu BB, Pan TC, Sharma A et al (2007) A grid-enabled image processing infrastructure for large pathology images. APIII 2007; Pittsburg, PA

27. Vickers AJ, Ballen V, Scher HI (2007) Setting the bar in phase II trials: the use of historical data for determining "go/no go" decision for definitive phase III testing. Clin Cancer Res 13:972–976

28. Hornbrook MC, Hart G, Ellis JL et al (2005) Building a virtual cancer research organization. J Natl Cancer Inst Monogr 35:12–25

29. Chung CH, Wong S, Ang KK, Hammond EH, Dicker AP, Harari PM, Le QT (2007) Strategic plans to promote head and neck cancer translational research within the radiation therapy oncology group: a report from the translational research program. Int J Radiat Oncol Biol Phys 69[Suppl 2]:67–78

7

Post-Radiation Dysphagia

Bharat Mittal and Avraham Eisbruch

CONTENTS

B. Mittal, MD
Professor and Chairman, Department of Radiation Oncology,
Northwestern University Feinberg School of Medicine, 251 E.
Huron, LC-178 Chicago, IL 60611, USA
A. Eisbruch, MD
Professor and Associate Chair for Clinical Research,
Department of Radiation Oncology, University of Michigan
Medical Center, Ann Arbor, MI 48109–0010, USA

Swallowing is a complex process that begins with the placement of food in the mouth and ends when the food enters the stomach. It involves voluntary and involuntary stages which are coordinated through several cranial nerves and a multitude of muscles that control the function of the oral cavity, the pharynx (skull base to the lower border of the cricoid), the larynx, hyoid bone, and esophagus [1, 2].

Swallowing is initiated by the stimulation of receptors in the oropharyngeal area. Sensory impulses reach the brain stem through cranial nerves VII, IX, and X, while motor control is exercised through cranial nerves IX, X, and XII. The cricopharyngeal sphincter (CPS) relaxes as the bolus reaches the posterior pharyngeal wall before it reaches the CPS. Cranial nerve V contains both sensory and motor fibers and is important to chewing.

Swallowing physiology consists of three phases [3]:

1. Oral phase (1 s): The oral tongue and teeth reduce the food to a bolus. As the food is transported back toward the pharynx, receptors in the oropharyngeal mucosa trigger the pharyngeal phase.

2. Pharyngeal phase (1 s): During this stage, the velopharyngeal port closes to prevent food from entering the nose. The hyoid bone and larynx begin their forward and superior ascent, the epiglottis is folded down to an inverted position, the tongue base moves toward the posterior pharyngeal wall, and pressure is generated by the top-to-bottom contraction of the pharyngeal constrictor muscles, which push the bolus of food toward the esophagus. Lastly, through laryngeal and hyoid elevation and anterior movement, the cricopharyngeus muscle relaxes, resulting in the opening of the CPS.

3. Esophageal phase: When the CPS opens, the bolus of food enters the upper esophagus and is transported down to the stomach through peristalsis.

Patients with head and neck cancer tend to be elderly. With advanced age, swallowing physiology becomes compromised, resulting in increased bolus "holding", delayed onset of swallow, slower pharyngeal transit time, and reduced generation of pharyngeal pressure [4, 5].

7.1
Evaluation of the Swallowing Mechanism

7.1.1
Objective Evaluation: Instrumental Assessment

- Videofluorography (VFG) is the most commonly used procedure to assess swallowing dysfunctions. VFG, including modified barium swallow and esophagogram, can visualize the oral, pharyngeal, and esophageal phases of swallowing. During VFG, the patient is given food in measured volumes and viscosities. Swallowing physiology is viewed in the lateral and anteroposterior planes and temporal measures are made. The duration of physiologic events during the entire swallow can be measured as they change during swallows of boluses of various volumes and viscosities. Oropharyngeal residue and aspiration can be quantified. Oropharyngeal swallow efficiency (OPSE), a global measure of the safety and speed of swallow, is calculated by measuring the total oral and pharyngeal transit time of the bolus divided by the percentage of the bolus swallowed [6–9].
- Manometry, in which the patient swallows a soft tube containing pressure sensors, measures pressures generated in the mouth, pharynx, and esophagus during swallowing. Manometry is used primarily to measure pressure changes in the esophagus and has value for studying oropharyngeal swallowing dysfunctions [10, 11].
- Functional endoscopic evaluation of swallowing (FEES) provides views of the laryngopharynx different from those seen with VFG. This procedure, which is easy to perform, uses fiberoptic endoscopy (FE) to view mucosal and anatomical integrity, pharyngeal residue, swallowing with sensory testing, and aspiration [12]. Wu et al. [13] have discussed the advantages and disadvantages of using the fiberoptic endoscope vs VFG to evaluate patients with swallowing disorders.

- Ultrasonography can be used to study tongue physiology during swallowing [14]. However, this procedure has no value for assessing other phases of deglutition.

7.1.2
Objective Evaluation: Observer-Assessed

Several tools are available to assess short- and long-term cancer treatment-induced swallowing dysfunctions. Common Terminology Criteria for Adverse Events (CTCAE) are frequently used to assess acute toxicity. Late toxicities can be assessed using the Radiation Therapy Oncology Group (RTOG)/European Organization for Research and Treatment of Cancer (EORTC) criteria and the Subjective Objective Management Analytic (SOMA) scale [15–17].

7.1.3
Subjective Evaluation: Patient-Reported Quality of Life

Some of the instruments used to assess quality of life (QOL) in patients with head and neck cancer, including swallowing dysfunctions, include: the University of Washington Quality of Life tool (UWQOL) [18]; the M.D. Anderson Dysphagia Symptom Inventory (MADSI-HN) [19]; the EORTC-QLQ H&N [20]; the Performance Status Scale for Head and Neck Cancer patients (PSS-H&N) [21]; the Radiation Therapy Instrument Head and Neck (QOL-RTI/H&N) [22]; the Functional Assessment of Cancer Therapy-H&N (FACT-H&N) [23]; and the Head and Neck Radiotherapy Questionnaire (HNRQ) [24]. While these instruments all measure some aspects of head and neck cancer–related QOL, it is not clear which one best applies to the assessment of swallowing dysfunctions in patients with head and neck cancer and to various treatment modalities.

7.2
Baseline Swallowing Function in Patients with Head and Neck Cancer

PAULOSKI et al. [25] compared 352 patients with head and neck cancer with 104 controls. Pretreatment, 59% of patients complained of dysphagia. On VFG study, the majority of these patients had functional study suggesting inconsistency in perception of swallowing and actual swallowing ability. However, compared to controls, patients had significantly longer oral and pharyngeal transit time, greater oropharyngeal residue, and lower swallowing efficiency. Swallow function worsened with increased tumor stage and in patients with oral and pharyngeal lesions compared to those with laryngeal lesions. It is not clear if the swallowing decrement was the result of tumor infiltration of muscles and nerves or of pain and ulceration.

7.3 Swallowing Disorders Induced by Radiation Alone

Radiation-induced late toxicities, including swallowing disorders, are unevenly distributed, with some patients exhibiting more cellular radiosensitivity. Conflicting data have emerged related to target-tissue sensitivity (fibroblast vs DNA repair capacity vs lymphocytic chromosomal damage) and late radiation damage [26–28]. DENHAM et al. [29] have categorized radiation-induced normal tissue injury as direct, indirect, and functional, in addition to resulting from genetic susceptibility. A number of tumor and radiation variables [30–35] also influence the incidence of late damage. Several investigators have documented cervical and pharyngeal fibrosis and laryngeal dysfunction resulting in swallowing disorders following standard or accelerated radiation schemes [36–41]. Therefore, it is essential to understand the biomechanics of swallowing disorders and to know the anatomical organs that are critical for swallowing and the radiation dose–volume relationship of these organs in order to prevent and reduce the incidence of swallowing disorders and devise effective rehabilitation techniques [42].

Radiation of the head and neck area produces xerostomia and short-term laryngopharyngeal edema, resulting in acute dysphagia. Radiation-induced swallowing disorders can manifest months to years later as a result of extensive fibrosis and vascular and neural damage [43]. The biomechanics of these disorders have been studied by LAZARUS et al. [44] using VFG in a group of patients with dysphagia 10 years following radiation. These patients demonstrated a number of oropharyngeal motility disorders, including reduced tongue-base contact with the posterior pharyngeal wall, reduced laryngeal elevation, and compromised vestibule and true vocal cord closure. These disorders resulted in pharyngeal residue, which was aspirated after swallow. Despite different tumor sites, all patients exhibited similar altered biomechanics, which most likely resulted from the large radiation doses and volumes that encompassed the orolaryngopharyngeal area during treatment. In 1995, a similar observation was made by DEJAEGER et al. [43] who used manofluorography in a patient 5 years following radiotherapy for a pharyngeal carcinoma. KENDALL et al. [45, 46] used VFG to evaluate 20 patients with head and neck cancer previously treated with radiation. These patients were able to maintain nutrition and none complained of dysphagia. When compared with 60 normal subjects, all 20 patients demonstrated abnormal swallow mechanics and prolonged oropharyngeal time for all bolus sizes. The onset of aryepiglottic fold closure relative to the onset of swallow was delayed and there was a trend toward delayed hyoid elevation. In this study, there was a trend toward earlier opening of the upper-esophageal sphincter relative to the arrival of the bolus, most likely as a compensatory mechanism. Patients with base-of-tongue cancer had worse swallow mechanics compared to patients with pharyngolaryngeal cancers.

To assess pharyngeal dysfunctions following radiation, WU et al. [12] used fiberoptic endoscopic examination in 31 patients with dysphagic nasopharyngeal cancer, with a mean follow-up of 8.5 years following radiation. They observed pharyngeal retention (93.5%), post-swallow aspiration (77.4%), atrophic changes in the tongue with or without fasciculation (54.8%), vocal cord paralysis (29%), velopharyngeal incompetence (58%), delay or absence of swallow reflex (87.1%), and poor pharyngeal constriction (80.6%).

JENSEN et al. [47] made a similar observation using functional endoscopic evaluation of swallowing (FEES) and EORTC-QOL questionnaires in 25 patients with pharyngeal cancer treated with radiation alone and followed up for a minimum of 2.5 years (mean 5 years). Of these patients, 83% had subjective swallowing complaints. The most frequent objective finding was reduced sensitivity in the oropharynx (94%) and reduced range of motion at the tongue base (79%). Pharyngeal residue appeared in 88% of these patients, 59% experienced laryngeal penetration, and 18% aspirated. Penetration and aspiration were observed primarily with thin liquids. All of the six patients with aspiration were smokers.

7.4
Surgery and Radiation-Induced Swallowing Dysfunctions

Surgery-related swallowing disorders usually occur during the first few months following surgery. Abnormal swallowing biomechanics depend on the site of surgery, the extent of resection, and the type of reconstruction [1, 48, 49].

PAULOSKI et al. [50, 51] studied the effect of postoperative RT in a surgical resection-matched patient population. Patients receiving postoperative radiation had increased oral transit time, greater pharyngeal residue, lower OPSE, and shorter duration of cricopharyngeal opening. Patients without postoperative radiation demonstrated improvement in swallowing efficiency up to 12 months post-surgery, while patients with adjuvant radiation did not show any improvement in swallow function.

7.5
Chemoradiation-Induced Swallowing Dysfunctions

Over the past two decades, the intensity of treatment using chemotherapy and radiation has increased, resulting in better tumor control and organ preservation. However, acute and late toxicities have also increased [52, 53]. FORASTIERE et al. [54] reported RTOG 91-11 data where 1 year post-treatment only 9% of patients treated with radiation alone needed liquid or soft food, compared to 23% of patients in the chemoradiation group.

In two separate studies, LAZARUS et al. [55, 56] reported that the swallowing mechanics in head and neck cancer patients treated with concomitant chemoradiation protocols and compared the results with age-matched controls. A large percentage of patients exhibited abnormal swallow mechanics similar to those seen in patients treated with radiation alone; also seen were reduced tongue-base movement toward the posterior pharyngeal wall, reduced tongue strength, reduced laryngeal elevation, lower OPSE, an increased number of swallows needed to clear the bolus, and a high incidence (89%) of aspiration of liquids.

NEUMAN et al. [57] compared the effects of treatment using high-dose intra-arterial cisplatinum with radiation vs intravenous chemotherapy and radiation. A large percentage of patients exhibited abnormal swallow measures that were similar in both groups, except that the intra-arterial group exhibited less aspiration with 1–3 ml of liquids.

EISBURCH et al. [31], KOTZ et al. [58], MITTAL et al. [30], and NGUYEN et al. [59] have also reported a high incidence of oropharyngeal dysfunctions following concomitant chemoradiation. Most of these patients exhibited some degree of aspiration, base-of-the-tongue weakness, pharyngeal residue, reduced laryngohyoid movement, decreased epiglottic inversion, swallow reflex delay, and velopharyngeal incompetence. Upper esophageal stricture was also observed in several patients.

Disorders resulting from radiation and chemotherapy can affect both oral and pharyngeal phases of swallowing. Swallowing biomechanics are altered as a result of reduced lingual manipulation and propulsion of bolus, reduced tongue strength, delayed triggering of the pharyngeal motor response, impaired tongue-base motion, pharyngeal contraction, laryngohyoid motion, laryngeal vestibule closure, and cricopharyngeal opening [60].

Over time (3–12 months), these disorders may reduce in severity [61], although this is not always the case. A substantial number of patients experience deterioration of swallowing function over time as a result of vascular damage and fibrosis [44, 62–64]. This discrepancy highlights the importance of objective evaluation of swallow physiology before and at several points following treatment. Additional research is needed on the measurement and treatment of swallowing disorders after various chemoradiation protocols [3]. The confounding effects of tumor site and stage, pre-existing dysphagia, dental status, smoking history, and other comorbidities also need to be studied.

Dysphagia resulting from radiation and chemotherapy could also be a result of stricture formation in the hypopharyngeal or upper esophageal area. There is evidence to support the increased incidence and severity of stricture formation following treatment with radiation plus chemotherapy compared to radiation alone. LAURELL et al. [65] reported a 3.4% incidence of stricture formation in head and neck cancer patients treated with radiation alone compared to an incidence of 21% observed by LEE et al. [66] in a group of patients treated with radiation plus chemotherapy. This study reported a higher incidence of stricture formation in patients receiving hyperfractionation, in patients with hypopharyngeal primary tumors, and in women.

7.6
Organ at Risk and the Dose–Volume–Effect Relationship

Laryngopharyngeal disorders resulting in late dysphagia and aspiration are not regimen-specific and are the result of edema and fibrosis [51]. To correlate the relationship of radiation dose–volume–effect, it is critical to know the relative importance of the organs involved in swallowing physiology. PAULOSKI et al. [67] used VFG to evaluate the "organ at risk" in 170 patients. Laryngeal elevation, tongue-base retraction, and the cricopharyngeal opening consistently predicted patients' ability to swallow different food consistencies. EISBRUCH et al. [68] reviewed the literature and identified the structures that, if damaged, could potentially cause abnormal swallowing physiology. From their study of 26 patients assessed with VFG, direct endoscopy, and CT scan they identified pharyngeal constrictors (PC) and glottic and supraglottic larynx (GSL) as dysphagia- and/or aspiration-related structures (DARS). In a prospective study, FENG [69] established the dose–volume–effect relationship for DARS and the esophagus in 36 patients with stage 3/4 head and neck cancers treated with chemoradiation. For intensity-modulated radiation therapy (IMRT) dose optimization, planning treatment volume (PTV) was excluded from the target organ (swallowing structures, major salivary glands, and oral cavity). However, the entire organ was used to establish the dose–volume–effect relationship. A strong correlation was observed between the mean dose to DARS and dysphagia endpoints. Aspiration was observed when the PC mean dose exceeded 60 Gy and the dose–volume threshold was V40 = 90%, V50 = 80%, V60 = 70%, and V65 > 50%. For aspiration to occur, the GSL dose–volume threshold was V50 > 50% (> 50% of volume receiving 50 Gy). For stricture, a mean dose of ≥ 66 Gy and a dose–volume threshold of V50 = 85%, V60 = 70%, and V65 = 60% for PC was observed. For stricture formation to occur, no relationship between mean dose to the GSL and esophagus was observed. The mean dose to the PC and esophagus was correlated with liquid swallowing, while only the mean dose to PC was correlated with solid swallowing on patient-reported and observer-rated swallowing scores.

In a retrospective study of 25 patients managed with radiation alone, JENSEN et al. [47] studied the dose–volume–effect relationship using FEES and the QOL questionnaires EORTC C30 and H&N 35. In this study, radiation dose to base-of-tongue and PC did not correlate with swallowing endpoints. However, doses < 60 Gy to the supraglottic area, larynx, and upper esophageal sphincter resulted in a low risk of aspiration.

DORNFELD et al. [70] reported on 27 patients with head and neck cancer who were treated with IMRT radiation + chemotherapy and free of disease for at least 1 year following treatment. Swallowing difficulties and the type of diet tolerated (Diet Score) decreased progressively with radiation doses > 50 Gy to the aryepiglottic folds, false vocal cords, and lateral pharyngeal walls near the false cord.

LEVENDAG et al. [71] reported on 81 patients with oropharyngeal carcinoma treated with three-dimensional CRT or IMRT with or without brachytherapy ± chemotherapy. A significant correlation was observed between the mean dose to the superior and middle pharyngeal constrictor muscles and patient complaints of severe dysphagia. A median dose of 50 Gy predicted a 20% probability of dysphagia. This probability increased significantly beyond a mean dose of 55 Gy, with an increase of 19% associated with each additional 10 Gy to superior and middle constrictors.

DOORNAERT et al. [72], using RTOG and EORTC-QOL questionnaires in 81 patients with head and neck cancer, correlated the mean dose to the pharyngeal wall structures (PWS), including mucosa and pharyngeal constrictor muscles and swallowing outcome. They reported a steep dose–effect relationship beyond 45 Gy to PWS and concluded that a mean dose of 45 Gy is the optimal threshold dose for predicting swallowing difficulties.

COGLAR et al. [73], in a study of 96 patients with head and neck cancer treated using IMRT ± chemotherapy, observed no aspiration when the mean radiation dose to the larynx and inferior pharyngeal constrictor was ≤ 48 Gy and ≤ 54 Gy, respectively. A dose–volume effect was observed. At V50 = 21% for the larynx and V50 = 51% for the inferior constrictor, no aspiration or stricture were observed. No stricture was observed if the mean dose to the inferior constrictors was kept below 54 Gy. The mean dose to the larynx did not correlate with stricture formation.

O'MEARA et al. [74] retrospectively reviewed the data of head and neck cancer patients treated with two-dimensional radiation + concurrent chemotherapy. They observed an association between the median dose to the inferior hypopharynx (pharyn-

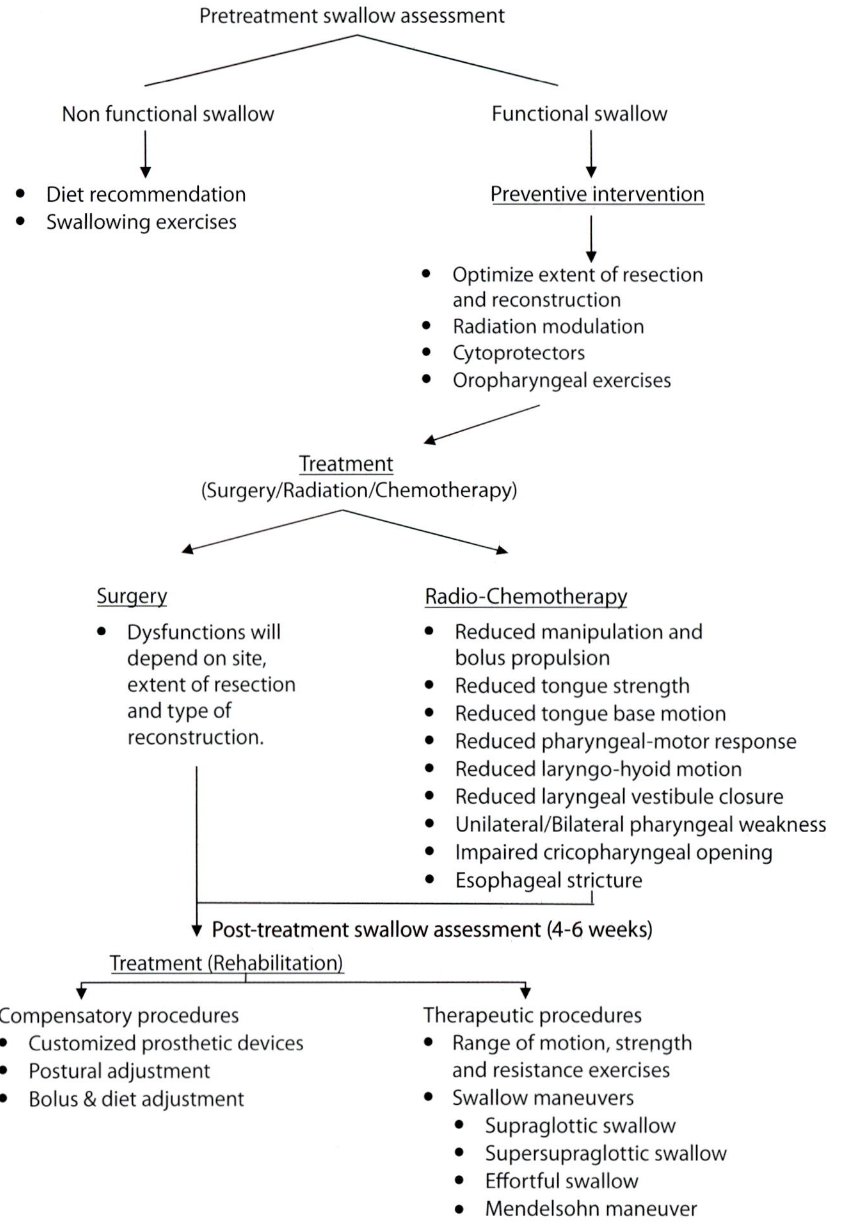

Fig. 7.1. Algorithm for the evaluation and treatment of swallowing dysfunctions in patients with head and neck cancers

goesophageal inlet) and severe late toxicity (grade ≥ 3 pharyngolaryngeal dysfunction). The incidence was 46%. The median dose to the inferior hypopharynx was 58 Gy among patients with severe late dysphagia, compared to 50 Gy in patients without severe dysphagia.

There is a paucity of dose/volume data about hypopharyngeal/upper esophageal stricture in head and neck cancer patients treated with radiation + chemotherapy. LAURELL et al. [65] compared radiation dose–volume data in 22 patients with proximal esophageal stricture vs 22 reference patients with no stricture following radiation. They recommend a mean dose of <65 Gy to the first 2 cm of proximal esophagus and a mean dose of <60 Gy to the first 5 cm of proximal esophagus as a tolerance dose below which the incidence of esophageal stricture is low. However, further studies are needed to establish the dose-modifying effect of chemotherapy given concurrently with radiation.

Table 7.1. Organs at risk and dose–volume relationship above which swallowing dysfunctions increases significantly

Reference	No. of patients	Critical organs	Dose (Gy)		Volume data (%)			End point	Evaluation method
			Mean	Median	V50	V60	V65		
[68, 69] • IMRT • RT + Chemo	26/36	Larynx			50			Aspiration	VFG
		PC	>60		80	70	50	Aspiration	
		PC	>66		85	70	60	Stricture	
[73] • IMRT • RT ± Chemo	96	Larynx	<48[a]		21			Aspiration and stricture	VFG
		IC	<54		51				
[72] RT ± Chemo	81	Pharyngeal Mucosa and constrictors	45					QOL	• RTOG • EORTC C-30 & H/N 35
[74] 2DRT + Chemo	148	Pharyngoesoph-ageal inlet		50				Grade 3 + Pharyngoe-sophageal dysfunction	RTOG late toxicity
[71] 3DCRT/IMRT ± Brachy ± Chemo	81	Superior and middle constrictors	55					• Grade ≥ 3 • EORTC • PSS – H&N • MDADI	• RTOG • QOL • QOL
[70] • IMRT • RT ± Chemo	27	Aryepiglottic fold False cord Lateral pharyngeal Wall near false cord	50					• Diet score • H & N QOL • Weight loss • PEG Tube	• QOL • Clinical Assessment
[47] • 3DCRT • RT alone	25	Larynx Upper esophageal sphincter	60					• Aspiration • QOL	• EORTC • QOL • FEES

[a] No correlation with stricture formation
PC, pharyngeal constrictors; IC, inferior constrictor; FEES, functional endoscopic evaluation of swallowing

Table 7.1 summarizes some of the published data for organs at risk and the radiation dose–volume relationship resulting in objective and/or subjective swallowing disorders. The differences between dose–volume–effect relationship and organs at risk between various studies could be due to lack of uniformity in dose reporting, differences in organ contouring, use of 2D vs 3D data for treatment planning, dose optimization, and the endpoints used to measure swallowing dysfunctions.

tional studies suggest that with the use of physical, technical, and biochemical agents and exercise of the oropharyngeal muscles it is possible to reduce the incidence and severity of swallowing disorders [42].

7.8
Radiation Modulation

Using current technologies, it is possible to reduce the radiation doses and the volume of critical structures involved in swallowing without compromising the target. EISBRUCH et al. [68] identified the larynx and PC as playing an important role. By decreasing radiation to these structures using IMRT, they were able to reduce the incidence of aspiration and swallowing disorders [69]. Similarly, MITTAL et al. [30] were able to decrease swallowing disorders with the

7.7
Preventive Intervention to Reduce Swallowing Disorders

There are no large phase 3 trials to suggest that prevention is possible. However, several single-institu-

use of static multisegmental IMRT. The incidence of early and late feeding tube placement was also decreased with IMRT [75]. However, Milano et al. [76] and Garden et al. [77] observed no difference in swallowing disorders with the use of IMRT. Garden [78] and Chao [79] also observed no difference in the need for a feeding tube when IMRT was used.

IMRT is time-consuming and organs at risk need to be defined to prevent excessive doses to the larynx and postcricoid esophagus, which can be spared using conventional radiation techniques with a small midline shield [80]. The use of this technique is also supported by the dosimetry study of Fua et al. [81]. They were able to decrease the pharyngoesophageal axis (PEA) mean dose from 55.2 Gy to 27.2 Gy using junctional IMRT (J-IMRT) with a midline shield as opposed to whole-field IMRT (WF-IMRT). The incidence of dysphagia and the duration of a feeding tube requirement were significantly less when the J-IMRT technique was used. However, the PEA can be classified as a dose-avoidance structure during WF-IMRT in order to decrease the radiation dose to the PEA. Further studies are needed to identify the dose–volume relationship to the critical organs and neuromuscular systems involved in swallowing.

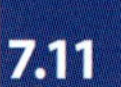

7.9
Oral Feeding vs Feeding Tube

More than 70% of patients treated with intensive concurrent chemoradiation for head and neck cancer required a feeding tube by the end of treatment [66, 82, 83]. At 1 year following treatment, at least 20% of patients still required a feeding tube to supplement their oral intake [70, 82, 83]. The use of a prophylactic feeding tube is controversial [84]. Rosenthal et al. [85] support the use of oral feeding to the maximally tolerated food viscosity as long as possible even if the patient already has a feeding tube. Gillespie et al. [86] reported a worse swallowing outcome in patients who had not had oral intake for more than 2 weeks. Patients should continue oral intake to reduce the risk of long-term tube dependency and dysphagia [87]. Rosenthal et al. [85] and Mikhal et al. [88] suggest that a nasogastric (NG) feeding tube decreases the need for esophageal dilatation vs a percutaneous endoscopic gastrostomy (PEG) tube. They hypothesized that the NG tube serves as a stent to prevent stricture

formation. However, when using the NG tube, it is necessary to take care to avoid trauma to the PEA. We also support continual oral feeding so long as it does not compromise the patient's nutritional status and increase the risk of aspiration.

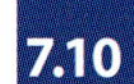

7.10
Cytoprotectors

Amifostine (WR 2721) is the most commonly used cytoprotector for reducing the incidence of xerostomia and mucositis [89–91]. However, there is no data to support its role in decreasing late swallowing disorders. Further studies are needed.

7.11
Oropharyngeal Exercises

Oropharyngeal exercises are designed to improve swallowing biomechanics by increasing the excursion of swallowing organs and strengthening the musculature involved in deglutition. Range-of-motion exercises are available for the oral tongue, base of tongue, and the hyoid-laryngeal complex [1, 3, 92]. Isometric resistance exercises are used to strengthen the tongue, jaw, larynx, and lips [93]. Some exercises can facilitate opening of the upper esophageal sphincter [94].

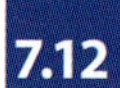

7.12
Therapeutic Intervention to Improve Swallowing Disorders

Rehabilitation of swallowing disorders should be started as soon as possible following treatment. Logemann [1] suggests less benefit with delay in swallowing therapy. Waters et al. [95] report that the extent of swallowing dysfunctions at 6 months post-treatment predicts long-term function. Kotz et al. [96] recommend treatment for oropharyngeal dysphagia as soon as possible post-chemoradiation. Rehabilitation techniques can be categorized broadly as compensatory and specific therapy procedures.

Compensatory procedures are used to manipulate the bolus flow and reduce aspiration, which can be accomplished by:

- Postural adjustments such as chin down, head tilt, head back, and head rotation toward the weak side; lying down can be effective in decreasing aspiration [97, 98].
- Bolus adjustment and dietary modification [1, 99–101]; patients with decreased awareness of food in the oropharyngeal area may benefit from a larger bolus, while patients requiring multiple swallows to clear a bolus may benefit from smaller bolus size.
- Customized oropharyngeal prosthetic devices [102–108] should be used to compensate for the loss of tissues during surgery; these devices will result in the reduction of oral residue and efficient clearance of food from the oral cavity to the oropharynx.

7.13
Therapy Procedures

Oropharyngeal exercises to improve strength and excursion range of the oral tongue, base of tongue, and the laryngohyoid complex will improve oral transit time, decrease pharyngeal residue, improve oropharyngeal swallowing efficiency, and decrease the risk of aspiration [92, 101, 109, 110]. Therapy exercises developed by SHAKER et al. [94, 111] have been shown to improve dysphagia resulting from dysfunction of the upper-esophageal sphincter.

Patients can also be taught voluntary maneuvers to improve OPSE and prevent aspiration during deglutition. Supraglottic swallow protects the airway by holding the vocal folds closer together [1]. Super-supraglottic swallow prevents aspiration by facilitating closure of the laryngeal vestibule [112]. The effortful swallow causes increased pressure in the oral cavity and pharynx, resulting in better bolus clearance [112]. The Mendelsohn maneuver works by increasing the opening of the upper-esophageal sphincter during swallow [113, 114].

Optimum rehabilitation requires pre- and post-treatment assessment of swallowing physiology and observation of modified barium swallow (MBS) changes while various therapeutic swallow procedures and maneuvers are implemented. Patient education techniques such as biofeedback using FE, MBS, and surface electromyography have been used to help patients learn various exercises and improve swallowing dysfunctions [115, 116]. Several randomized trials are in progress to assess the outcome of various treatment strategies to improve dysphagia [117].

7.14
Summary

Swallowing is a complex process involving neuromuscular coordination of several oropharyngeal muscles and cranial nerves. Swallowing physiology can be studied using VFG, FE, and oropharyngeal manometry. Patients' symptoms and treatment toxicity can be assessed using validated QOL measures and observer assessment.

Dysphagia is often present before treatment of head and neck cancer begins.

Radiation, surgery, and chemotherapy result in anatomical and functional changes in swallow mechanics. Radiation-induced xerostomia results in increased bolus transit time. Primary radiation-induced neuromuscular dysfunction causes increased oropharyngeal transit time, incoordination of bolus movement through the oropharynx, reduced tongue-base contact with the posterior pharyngeal wall, impaired laryngohyoid movement, poor vestibule and true vocal cord closure, and impaired upper esophageal sphincter function. These abnormalities result in pharyngeal residue and aspiration.

The use of radiation therapy following surgery exacerbates the damage caused by surgical resection. Surgery-related swallowing disorders usually manifest during the first few months after surgery. The additional effects of RT on swallowing are the result of neuromuscular damage, fibrosis, and uncoordinated oral and pharyngeal phases of swallowing.

Patients treated with concomitant chemoradiation protocols show a higher incidence of swallow disorders compared to patients treated with RT alone [118]. Most orolaryngopharyngeal dysfunctions are similar to those observed in patients treated with RT alone. It is not possible to quantitate the roles played individually by RT and chemotherapy in causing swallowing disorders.

Preliminary clinical and dosimetry data characterize the radiation dose–volume and toxicity relationship of some of the critical structures involved with pharyngeal swallowing. Several studies are in progress to expand this knowledge.

Further studies are needed to tease out the confounding effects of patient age, tumor location and stage, pre-existing dysphagia, dental status, xerostomia, smoking history, and other comorbidities.

Several preventive and therapeutic strategies can be implemented to reduce the incidence or prevent some swallowing disorders. Pre- and post-treatment assessment of the swallowing physiology of all head and neck cancer patients is essential to best implement these measures.

References

1. Logemann JA (1998) Evaluation and treatment of swallowing disorders. PRO-ED Inc., Austin, TX
2. Goldsmith T (2003) Videofluoroscopic evaluation of oropharyngeal swallowing. In: Som PM, Curtin HD (eds) Head and neck imaging, 4th ed. Mosby, St. Louis, pp 1727–1753
3. Logemann JA (2007) Mechanism of normal and abnormal swallowing. In: Cummings JW, Flint PW, Haughey BA, Richardson MA, Robbins KT, Thomas JR et al. (eds) Otolaryngology head and neck surgery, 5th ed. Mosby, St. Louis (in press)
4. Tracy JF, Logemann JA, Kahrilas PJ et al (1989) Preliminary observation of the effects of age on oropharyngeal deglutition. Dysphagia 4:90–94
5. Robbins J, Hamilton J, Lof G et al (1992) Oropharyngeal swallowing in normal adults of different ages. Gastroenterology 103:823–829
6. Logemann J (1993) Manual for the Videofluorographic study of swallowing, 2nd ed. PRO–ED, Inc., Austin, TX
7. Kendall KA, McKenzie SW, Leonard RJ et al (2000) Timing of events in normal swallowing: a videofluoroscopic study. Dysphagia 15:74–83
8. Kahrilas, PJ, Logemann JA, Lin S et al (1992) Pharyngeal clearance during swallow: a combined manometric and videofluoroscopic study. Gastroenterology. 103:128–136
9. Rademaker AW, Pauloski BR, Logemann JA et al (1994) Oropharyngeal swallowing efficiency as a representative measure of swallowing function. J Speech Hearing Res 37:314–325
10. Ergun GA, Kahrilas PJ, Logemann JA (1993) Interpretation of pharyngeal manometric recordings: limitations and variability. Diseases Esophagus 6:11–16
11. McConnel FMS (1988) Analysis of pressure generation and bolus transit during pharyngeal swallowing. Laryngoscope 96:71–78
12. Wu CH, Ko JY, Hsiao TY et al (2000) Dysphagia after radiotherapy: endoscopic examination of swallowing in patients with nasopharyngeal carcinoma. Ann Otol Rhinol Laryngol 109:320–325
13. Wu CH, Hsiao TY, Chen JC, Chang YC, Lee SY (1997) Evaluation of swallowing safety with fiberoptic endoscope: comparison with videofluoroscopic technique. Laryngoscope 107:396–401
14. Shawker T, Sonies JS, Stone M (1983) Real-time ultrasound visualization of tongue movement during swallowing. J Clin Ultrasound 11:485–490
15. Cox JD, Stetz J, Pajak TF (1995) Toxicity criteria of the Radiation Therapy Oncology Group (RTOG) and the European Organization for Research and Treatment of Cancer (EORTC). Int J Radiat Oncol Biol Phys 31:1341–1346
16. [No authors listed] (1995) LENT SOMA scales for all anatomic sites. Int J Radiat Oncol Biol Phys 31:1049–1091
17. Denis F, Geraud P, Bardet E et al (2003) Late toxicity results of the GORTEC 94–01 randomized trial comparing radiotherapy with concomitant radiochemotherapy for advanced-stage oropharynx carcinoma: comparison of LENT/SOMA, RTOG/EORTC, and NCI–CTC scoring system. Int J Radiat Oncol Biol Phys 55:93–98
18. Hassan SJ, Weymuller EA (1993) Assessment of quality of life in head and neck cancer patients. Head Neck 15:485–496
19. Rosenthal DI, Mendoza TR, Chambers MS et al (2007) Measuring head and neck cancer symptom burden: the development and validation of the M.D. Anderson symptom inventory, head and neck module. Head Neck 29:923–931
20. Bjordal K, Freng A, Thorvik J et al (1995) Patient self-reported and clinician-rated quality of life in head and neck cancer patients. Eur J Cancer Part B Ora Oncol 31B:235–241
21. List MA, D'Antonio LL, Cella DF et al (1996) The performance status scale for head and neck cancer patients and the functional assessment of cancer therapy – head and neck scale. Cancer 77:2294–2301
22. Trotti A, Johnson DJ, Gwede C et al (1998) Development of a head and neck companion module for the quality of life-radiation therapy instrument (QOL-RTI). Int J Radiat Oncol Biol Phys 42:257–261
23. Long SA, D'Antonio LL, Robinson EB et al (1996) Factors related to quality of life and functional status in 50 patients with head and neck cancer. Laryngoscope 106:1084–1088
24. Browman GP, Levine MN, Hodson DI et al (1993) The head and neck radiotherapy questionnaire: a morbidity/quality-of-life instrument for clinical trials of radiation therapy in locally advanced head and neck cancer. J Clin Oncol 11:863–872
25. Pauloski BR, Rademaker AW, Logemann JA, Stein D et al (2000) Pretreatment swallowing function in patients with head and neck cancer. Head Neck 22:474–482
26. Rudat V, Dietz A, Nollert J, Condradt C et al (1999) Acute and late toxicity, tumor control, and intrinsic radiosensitivity of primary fibroblasts in vitro of patients with advanced head and neck cancer after concomitant boost radiochemotherapy. Radiother Oncol 53:233–245
27. Borgmann K, Röper B, El-Awady RA et al (2002) Indicators of late normal tissue response after radiotherapy for head and neck cancer: fibroblasts, lymphocytes, genetics, DNA repair, and chromosomal aberrations. Radiother Oncol 64:141–152

28. Geara FB, Peters LJ, Kian Ang K et al (1992) Intrinsic radiosensitivity of normal fibroblasts and lymphocytes after high- and low-dose-rate irradiation. Cancer Res 52:6348–6352

29. Denham J, Hauer-Jensen M, Peters L et al (2001) Is it time for a new formalism to categorize normal tissue radiation injury? Int J Radiat Oncol Biol Phys 50:1105–1106

30. Mittal BB, Kepka A, Mahadevan A et al (2001) Tissue-dose compensation to reduce toxicity from combined radiation and chemotherapy for advanced head and neck cancers. Int J Cancer (Radiat Oncol Invest) 96:61–70

31. Eisbruch A, Lyden T, Bradford CR et al (2002) Objective assessment of swallowing dysfunction and aspiration after radiation concurrent with chemotherapy for head and neck cancer. Int J Radiat Oncol Biol Phys 53:23–28

32. Ang KK, Thames HD, Peters LJ (1997) Altered fractionation schedules. Princ Pract Radiat Oncol 3:1341–1346

33. Maciejewski B, Preuss-Bayer G, Trott KR (1983) The influence of the number of fractions and of the overall treatment time on local control and late complication rate in squamous-cell carcinoma of the larynx. Int J Radiat Oncol Biol Phys 9:321–328

34. Fu KK, Pajak TF, Marcial VA et al (1995) Late effects of hyperfractionated radiotherapy for advanced head and neck cancer: long-term follow-up results of RTOG 83–13. Int J Radiat Oncol Biol Phys 32:557–588

35. Taylor JM, Mendenhall WM, Lavey RS (1992) Dose, time, and fraction size issues for late effects in head and neck cancers. Int J Radiat Oncol Biol Phys 22:3–11

36. Delaney GP, Fisher RJ, Smee RI et al (1995) Split-course accelerated therapy in head and neck cancer: an analysis of toxicity. Int J Radiat Oncol Biol Phys 32:763–768

37. Horiot JC, Fur R, N'Guyen T et al (1992) Hyperfractionation vs conventional fractionation in oropharyngeal carcinoma: final analysis of a randomized trial of the EORTC cooperative group of radiotherapy. Radiother Oncol 25:231–241

38. Nguyen TD, Panis X, Froissart D et al (1988) Analysis of late complications after rapid hyperfractionated radiotherapy in advanced head and neck cancers. Int J Radiat Oncol Biol Phys 14:23–25

39. Olmi P, Celai E, Chiavacci A et al (1990) Accelerated fractionation in advanced head and neck cancer: results and analysis of late sequelae. Radiother Oncol 17:199–207

40. Marks JE, Bedwinek JM, Lee FA (1982) Dose-response analysis for nasopharyngeal carcinoma. Cancer 82:1042–1050

41. Cooper JS, Fu K, Marks J et al (1995) Late effects of radiation therapy in head and neck region. Int J Radiat Oncol Biol Phys 31:1141–1164

42. Mittal BB, Pauloski BR, Haraf DJ et al (2003) Swallowing dysfunction – preventative and rehabilitation strategies in patients with head and neck cancers treated with surgery, radiotherapy, and chemotherapy: a critical review. Int J Radiat Oncol Biol Phys 57:1219–1230

43. Dejaeger E, Goethals P (1995) Deglutition disorder as a late sequel of radiotherapy for a pharyngeal tumor. Am J Gastroenterol 90:493–495

44. Lazarus CL (1993) Effects of radiation therapy and voluntary maneuvers on swallow function in head and neck cancer patients. Clin Comm Disorders 3:11–20

45. Kendall KA, McKenzie SW, Leonard RJ et al (1998) Structural mobility in deglutition after single-modality treatment of head and neck carcinomas with radiation therapy. Head Neck 20:720–725

46. Kendall AK, Leonard RJ, McKenzie SW et al (2000) Timing of swallowing events after single-modality treatment of head and neck carcinomas with radiotherapy. Ann Otol Rhinol Laryngol 109:767–775

47. Jensen K, Lambertsen K, Grau C (2007) Late swallowing dysfunction and dysphagia after radiotherapy for pharynx cancer: frequency, intensity, and correlation with dose and volume parameters. Radiother Oncol 85:74–82

48. Logemann JA, Bytell DE (1979) Swallowing disorders in three types of head and neck surgical patients. Cancer 81:469–478

49. McConnel FMS, Pauloski BR, Logemann JA et al (1998) The functional results of primary closure vs flaps in oropharyngeal reconstruction: a prospective study of speech and swallowing. Arch Otolaryngol Head Neck Surg 124:625–630

50. Pauloski BR, Rademaker AW, Logemann JA et al (1998) Speech and swallowing in irradiated and nonirradiated postsurgical oral cancer patients. Otolaryngol Head Neck Surg 118:616–624

51. Pauloski BR, Logemann JA, Rademaker AW et al (1994) Speech and swallowing function after oral and oropharyngeal resections: one-year follow-up. Head Neck 16:313–322

52. Henk JM (1997) Controlled trials of synchronous chemotherapy with radiotherapy in head and neck cancer: overview of radiation morbidity. Clin Oncol (R Coll Radiol) 9:308–312

53. Adelstein DJ, Saxton JP, Lavertu P et al (1997) A phase 3 randomized trial comparing concurrent chemotherapy and radiotherapy with radiotherapy alone in resectable stage 3 and 4 squamous cell head and neck cancer: preliminary results. Head Neck 19:567–575

54. Forastiere AA, Goepfert H, Maor M et al (2003) Concurrent chemotherapy and radiotherapy for organ preservation in advanced laryngeal cancer. N Eng J Med 349:2091–2098

55. Lazarus CL, Logemann JA, Pauloski BR et al (1996) Swallowing disorders in head and neck cancer patients treated with radiotherapy and adjuvant chemotherapy. Laryngoscope 106:1157–1166

56. Lazarus CL, Logemann JA, Pauloski BR et al (2000) Swallowing and tongue functions following treatment for oral and oropharyngeal cancer. J Speech Lang Hearing Res 43:1011–1023

57. Newman LA, Robbins KT, Logemann JA et al (2002) Swallowing and speech ability after treatment for head and neck cancer with targeted intra-arterial vs intravenous chemoradiation. Head Neck 24:68–77

58. Kotz T, Abraham S, Beitler J et al (1999) Pharyngeal transport dysfunction consequent to an organ-sparing protocol. Arch Otolaryngol Head Neck Surg 125:410–413

59. Nguyen NP, Frank C, Moltz GC et al (2006) Aspiration rate following chemoradiation for head and neck cancer: an underreported occurrence. Radiother Oncol 80:302–306

60. Lazarus CL, Ward EC, Yiu EM (2007) Speech and swallowing following oral, oropharyngeal, and na-

sopharyngeal cancers. In: Ward EC, van As Brooks CJ (eds) Head and neck cancer: treatment, rehabilitation and outcomes. Plural Publishing Inc., San Diego, pp 103–122

61. Rademaker AW, Vonesh EE, Logemann JA et al (2003) Eating ability in head and neck cancer patients following chemoradiation: a 12-months follow-up study accounting for dropout. Head Neck 25:1034–1041

62. Law MP (1981) Radiation-induced vascular injury and its relation to late effects in normal tissues. In: Lett JT, Adler H (eds) Advances in radiation biology. Academic Press, New York, Vol #9, pp 37–73

63. Smith RV, Kotz T, Beitler JJ et al (2000) Long-term swallowing problems after organ preservation therapy with concomitant radiation therapy and intravenous hydroxyurea. Arch Otolaryngol Head Neck Surg 126:384–389

64. Watkin KL, Diouf I, Gallagher TM et al (2001) Ultrasonic quantification of geniohyoid cross-sectional area and tissue composition: a preliminary study of age and radiation effects. Head Neck 23:467–474

65. Laurell G, Kraepelien T, Mavroidis P et al (2003) Stricture of the proximal esophagus in head and neck carcinoma patients after radiotherapy. Cancer 97:1693–1700

66. Lee WT, Akst LM, Adelstein DJ et al (2006) Risk factors for hypopharyngeal/upper esophageal stricture formation after concurrent chemoradiation. Head Neck 28:808–812

67. Pauloski BR, Rademaker AW, Logemann JA et al (2006) Relationship between swallow motility disorders on videofluorography and oral intake in patients treated for head and neck cancer with radiotherapy with or without chemotherapy. Head Neck 28:1069–1076

68. Eisbruch A, Schwartz M, Rasch C et al (2004) Dysphagia and aspiration after chemoradiotherapy for head and neck cancer: which anatomic structures are affected and can they be spared by IMRT? Int J Radiat Oncol Biol Phys 60:1425–1439

69. Feng FY, Kim HM, Lyden TH et al (2007) Intensity-modulated radiotherapy of head and neck cancer aiming to reduce dysphagia: early dose-effect relationships for the swallowing structures. Int J Radiat Onco Biol Phys 68:1289–1298

70. Dornfeld K, Simmons JR, Karnell L et al (2007) Radiation doses to structures within and adjacent to the larynx are correlated with long-term diet- and speech-related quality of life. Int J Radiat Oncol Biol Phys 68:750–757

71. Levandag PC, Teguh DN, Voet P et al (2007) Dysphagia disorders in patients with cancer of the oropharynx are significantly affected by the radiation therapy dose to the superior and middle constrictor muscle: a dose-effect relationship. Radiother Oncol 85:64–73

72. Doornaert P, Slotman BJ, Rietveld DHF et al (2007) The mean radiation dose in pharyngeal structures is a strong predictor of acute and persistent swallowing dysfunction and quality of life in head and neck radiotherapy [Abstract #97]. Int J Radiat Oncol Biol Phys 69[Suppl]:55

73. Coglar HB, Allen AM, Othus M et al (2007) Dose to the larynx predicts for swallowing complications following IMRT and chemotherapy [Abstract #95]. Int J Radiat Oncol Bio Phys 69[Suppl]:53

74. O'Meara EA, Machtay M, Moughan J et al (2007) Association between radiation doses to pharyngeal regions and severe late toxicity in head and neck cancer patients treated with concurrent chemoradiotherapy – an RTOG analysis [Abstract #96]. Int J Radiat Oncol Biology Phys 69[Suppl]:54

75. Koneru NS, Bhate A, Logemann J, Mittal BB et al (2007) Intensity-modulated radiation treatment for head and neck cancer: the Northwestern University experience [ASTRO abstract #2486]. Int J Radiat Oncol Biol Phys 69[Suppl]:471

76. Milano MT, Vokes EE, Witt ME et al (2003) Retrospective comparison of IMRT and conventional three-dimensional RT in advanced head and neck patients treated with definitive chemoradiation [ASCO abstract]. Proc Am Soc Clin Oncol 22:499

77. Garden AS, Morrison WH, Wong S et al (2003) Preliminary results of intensity-modulated radiation therapy for small primary oropharyngeal carcinoma [ASTRO abstract #2108]. Int J Radiat Oncol Biol Phys 57:407

78. Garden A (2003) Mucositis: current management and investigations. Semin Radiat Oncol 13:267–273

79. Chao K, Ozyigit G, Blanco A et al (2004) Intensity-modulated radiation therapy for oropharyngeal carcinoma: impact of tumor volume. Int J Radiat Oncol Biol Phys 59:43–50

80. Amdur R, Li J, Liu C et al (2004) Unnecessary laryngeal irradiation in the IMRT era. Head Neck 26:257–263

81. Fua TF, Corry J, Milner AD et al (2007) Intensity-modulated radiotherapy for nasopharyngeal carcinoma: clinical correlation of dose to the pharyngoesophageal axis and dysphagia. Int J Radiat Oncol Biol Phys 67:976–981

82. Ang KK, Harris J, Garden AS et al (2005) Concomitant boost radiation plus concurrent cisplatin for advanced head and neck carcinoma; Radiation Therapy Oncology Group phase 2 trial 99-14. J Clin Oncol 23:3008–3015

83. Kies MS, Haraf DJ, Athanasiadis I et al (1998) Induction chemotherapy followed by concurrent chemoradiation for advanced head and neck cancer: improved disease control and survival. J Clinc Oncol 16:2715–2721

84. Al-Othman M, Amdur R, Morris C et al (2003) Does feeding tube placement predict for long-term swallowing disability after radiotherapy for head and neck cancer? Head Neck. 25:741–747

85. Rosenthal DI, Lewin JS, Eisbruch A (2006) Prevention and treatment of dysphagia and aspiration after chemoradiation for head and neck cancer. J Clin Oncol 14:2636–2643

86. Gillespie MB, Brodsky MB, Day TA et al (2004) Swallowing-related quality of life after head and neck cancer treatment. Laryngoscope 114:1362–1367

87. Murphy BA, Lewin JS, Ridner S et al (2006) Mechanism of weight loss in patients with head and neck cancer who were treated with chemotherapy. In: Perry MC (ed) American Society of Clinical Oncology Educational Book 2006. American Society of Clinical Oncology, Alexandria, VA, pp 340–344

88. Mekhail TM, Adelstein DJ, Rybicki LA et al (2001) Enteral nutrition during the treatment of head and neck carcinoma: is percutaneous endoscopic gastrostomy tube preferable to a nasogastric tube? Cancer 91:1785–1790

89. Brizel DM, Wasserman TH, Henke M et al (2000) Phase 3 randomized trial of amifostine as a radioprotector in head and neck cancer. J Clin Oncol 18:3339–3345

90. Büntzel J, Glatzel M, Küttner K et al (2002) Amifostine in simultaneous radiochemotherapy of advanced head and neck cancer. Semin Radiat Oncol 12:4–13

91. Sasse AD, Clark, LG, Sasse EC et al (2000) Amifostine reduces side effects and improves complete response rate during radiotherapy: results of a meta-analysis. Int J Radiat Oncol Biol Phys 64:784–791

92. Veis S, Logemann JA, Colangelo L (2000) Effects of three techniques on maximum posterior movement of the tongue base. Dysphagia 15:142–145

93. Robin DA, Goel A, Somodi LB et al (1992) Tongue strength and endurance: relation to highly skilled movements. J Speech Hearing Res 35:1239–1245

94. Shaker R, Kern M, Bardan E et al (1997) Augmentation of deglutive upper-esophageal sphincter in the elderly by exercise. Am J Physiol 272:G1518–1522

95. Waters T, Logemann J, Pauloski B et al (2004) Beyond efficacy and effectiveness: conducting economic analysis during clinical trials. Dysphagia 19:109–119

96. Kotz T, Costello R, Posner MR (2004) Swallowing dysfunction after chemoradiation for advanced squamous cell carcinoma of the head and neck. Head Neck 26:365–372

97. Logemann JA, Rademaker AW, Pauloski BR et al (1994) Effects of postural change on aspiration in head and neck surgical patients. Otolaryngol Head Neck Surg 110:222–227

98. Rasley A, Logemann JA, Kahrilas PJ et al (1993) Prevention of barium aspiration during videofluoroscopic swallowing studies: value of change in posture. AJR Am J Roentgenol 160:1005–1009

99. Lazarus CL, Logemann JA, Rademaker AW et al (1993) Effects of bolus volume, viscosity, and repeated swallows in nonstroke subjects and stroke patients. Arch Phys Med Rehabilitat 74:1066–1070

100. Logemann JA (1999) Behavioral management for oropharyngeal dysphagia. Folia Phoniatr Logopaedic 51:199–212

101. Bisch EM, Logemann JA, Rademaker AW et al (1994) Pharyngeal effects of bolus volume, viscosity, and temperature in patients with dysphagia resulting from neurologic impairment and in normal subjects. J Speech Hearing Res 37:1041–1049

102. Davis JW, Lazarus C, Logemann J et al (1987) Effect of a maxillary glossectomy prosthesis on articulation and swallowing. J Prosthet Dent 57:715–719

103. Light J (1995) A review of oral and oropharyngeal prostheses to facilitate speech and swallowing. Am J Speech Lang Pathol 4:15–21

104. Weber RS, Ohlms L, Bowman J et al (1991) Functional results after total or near-total glossectomy with laryngeal preservation. Arch Otolaryngol Head Neck Surg 117:512–515

105. DaBreo EL, Chalian VA, Lingeman R et al (1990) Prosthetic and surgical management of osteogenic sarcoma of the maxilla. J Prosthet Dent 63:316–320

106. Yontchev E, Karlsson S, Lith A et al (1991) Orofacial functions in patients with congenital and acquired maxillary defects: a fluoroscopic study. J Oral Rehab 18:483–489

107. Pauloski BR, Logemann JA, Colangelo LA et al (1996) Effect of intraoral prostheses on swallowing function in postsurgical oral and oropharyngeal cancer patients. Am J Speech Lang Pathol 5:31–46

108. Wheeler RL, Logemann JA, Rosen MS (1980) Maxillary reshaping prostheses: effectiveness in improving speech and swallowing of postsurgical oral cancer patients. J Prosthet Dent 43:313–319

109. Pauloski BR, Logemann JA, Fox JC et al (1995) Biomechanical analysis of the pharyngeal swallow in postsurgical patients with anterior tongue and floor-of-mouth resection and distal flap reconstruction. J Speech Hearing Res 38:110–123

110. Logemann JA, Paulsoki BR, Rademaker AW et al (1997) Speech and swallowing rehabilitation for head and neck cancer patients. Oncology 11:651–659

111. Shaker R, Easterling C, Kern M et al (2002) Rehabilitation of swallowing by exercise in tube-fed patients with pharyngeal dysphagia secondary to abnormal UES opening. Gastroenterology 122:1314–1321

112. Martin BJW, Logemann JA, Shaker R et al (1993) Normal laryngeal valving patterns during three-breath hold maneuvers: a pilot investigation. Dysphagia 8:11–20

113. Kahrilas PJ, Logemann JA, Krugler C et al (1991) Volitional augmentation of upper esophageal sphincter opening during swallowing. Am J Physiol 260:G450–G456

114. Lazarus C, Logemann JA, Gibbons P (1993) Effects of maneuvers on swallow functioning in a dysphagic oral cancer patient. Head Neck 15:419–424

115. Denk DM, Kaider A (1997) Videoendoscopic biofeedback: a simple method to improve the efficacy of swallowing rehabilitation of patients after head and neck surgery. J Otol Rhinol 59:100–105

116. Crary MA, Carnaby GD, Groher ME et al (2004) Functional benefits of dysphagia therapy using adjunctive sEMG biofeedback. Dysphagia 19:160–164

117. Logemann JA (2006) Update on clinical trials in dysphagia. Dysphagia 21:116–120

118. Logemann, JA, Pauloski, BR, Rademaker, AW et al (2008) Swallowing disorders in the first year post-radiation and chemoradiation. Head Neck 30:148–158

Lithium as a Differential Neuroprotector During Brain Irradiation

Luigi Moretti, Eddy S. Yang, Denis E. Hallahan, and Bo Lu

CONTENTS

L. Moretti, MD
E. S. Yang, MD, PhD
D. E. Hallahan, MD
B. Lu, MD, PhD
Department of Radiation Oncology, Vanderbilt-Ingram Cancer Center, Vanderbilt University, Nashville, TN 37232, USA

Introduction

Radiotherapy remains a major treatment modality for primary and metastatic brain tumors, as well as leukemia and lymphoma involving the central nervous system (CNS). Cranial irradiation is also used as prophylaxis for patients at high risk of involvement of the brain by neoplasia, for example small-cell lung cancer. Despite important advances in diagnosis and therapy of malignant solid tumors, brain metastases continue to present significant problems for clinicians attempting to prevent progression of disease and limit morbidity associated with therapy. Indeed, up to two thirds of all brain metastases cause clinical symptoms [1, 2]. In addition, there is evidence that the overall incidence of brain metastases is increasing because of improved systemic therapy for cancer [3]. Further, the survival rates of children with both primary [4–7], and secondary [3] brain tumors are increasing.

Although important advances have been made, cranial radiation therapy continues to present significant problems for clinicians attempting to prevent and limit morbidity associated with the therapy. The radiation dose that can be administered safely to the tumor is limited by the potential toxicity on normal surrounding CNS tissue. The primary factors influencing the likelihood of developing complications include the volume of normal brain tissue treated, the total radiation dose, and the fractionation schedule. The likelihood of brain damage also increases in the young [8, 9, 10–14], especially < 5 years old, and the elderly [10]. Furthermore, the use of concurrent or sequential chemotherapy can significantly affect the incidence and severity of radiation-induced toxicity. In addition, the tumor burden often impairs cognitive function, making it difficult to assess accurately the separate effect of radiation. These side effects impact dramatically the quality of life and are associated with decreased education and increased unemployment when these treated children reach adulthood [8, 15, 16]. Moreover, the cognitive defects occurring after radiation therapy seem to be progressive and irreversible [17, 18].

A full understanding of the potential complications such as cognitive impairments associated with cranial irradiation is needed to develop novel strategies for toxicity prevention.

8.2
Neurotoxicity from Brain Radiotherapy

The complications of radiation therapy are usually divided into acute effects that can occur during the course of radiation, early-delayed effects that appear 2–4 months after radiation, and late effects that can develop more than three months after the initiation of radiation therapy. Complications that might occur many months or even years following cranial irradiation are generally not important as a consideration for patients with brain metastases or grade IV primary brain tumors, where a median survival in the range of 6–12 months is expected. Late effects are a more important consideration for patients with a much longer life expectancy (e.g. low-grade glioma patients or pediatric patients with acute lymphocytic leukemia) [19, 20]. The distinction between early and late complications is also important since acute and early-delayed complications are usually reversible while late reactions often are not. Finally, a recent study also suggests that the ability to focus and sustain attention in children with primary brain tumors changes during the 6- to 7-week period of cranial irradiation and the subsequent 5 years, and remain relatively stable over time after irradiation [21]. The following is a brief review of potential radiation-induced side effects, with an emphasis on late neurocognitive injury.

8.2.1
Acute Complications

Acute encephalopathy generally occurs within 2 weeks of the onset of irradiation. The disorder is usually mild, characterized by headache, nausea, drowsiness, fever, and sometimes worsening of neurological signs [22]. Exceptionally, the encephal-

opathy is severe in patients who already had a syndrome of intracranial hypertension at the onset of treatment (multiple metastases, large posterior fossa tumor) or who received high-dose fractionation. In these cases, patients may develop a clinical picture of brain herniation [22]. Radiation-induced breakdown of the blood–brain barrier with increased intracranial pressure is incriminated in the pathogenesis of the syndrome. Acute encephalopathy is generally most severe following the first radiation dose and gradually lessens in severity thereafter.

8.2.2
Early-Delayed Complications

Early-delayed complications occur between 2 weeks and 3–4 months after the completion of radiotherapy and may take several forms:
- The somnolence syndrome develops in many patients (particularly children) who have received whole brain or large volume irradiation [23]. It is mainly characterized by hypersomnia, drowsiness, irritability and sometimes headache and fever [24]. At this stage, neuropsychological evaluation often demonstrates attention deficits and alteration of recent memory functions. The somnolence syndrome usually resolves spontaneously within 2–3 weeks. Corticosteroids reduce the duration of the syndrome and may prevent its development [25, 26].
- In about 15% of patients, early-delayed complications simulate local tumor recurrence. Patients may complain of recurrent focal symptoms, with headache and/or recurrence of pretreatment neurologic symptoms and signs. Improvement occurs spontaneously, but steroids accelerate its resolution [27].
- A severe leukoencephalopathy with cognitive dysfunction is a very rare early-delayed complication of cerebral irradiation, which may be transient or persistent. Reversible defects in memory also occur, and do not necessarily predict long-term impairment [28, 29].

8.2.3
Delayed Complications

Delayed complications occur 3 months to many years after completion of radiotherapy. Unlike early-delayed reactions that are usually reversible, late reactions are generally irreversible. The likelihood that the irradiation will induce delayed damage to the nervous system depends on many factors including the total dose delivered to the nervous system, the dose delivered with each treatment, and the total volume of nervous system irradiated. On the brain, a dose of 60 Gy delivered with 1.8- to 2-Gy fractions represents the upper limit of the "safe dose". Other factors that influence tolerance of the nervous system include the length of survival after completion of radiation therapy, the presence of other systemic diseases that enhance the side effects of irradiation (e.g., diabetes, hypertension), concomitant chemotherapy and other unidentifiable host factors [30]. Cognitive dysfunction/leukoencephalopathy and radionecrosis are the main delayed complications of brain irradiation.

8.2.3.1
Neurocognitive Effects

Differentiating adverse effects of cranial irradiation upon neurocognitive function from the effects of the underlying malignancy can be very difficult. Within the last decade, prospective studies have been performed to characterize accurately the effects of cranial irradiation upon neurocognitive function [31]. It is important for such studies to include long follow-up whenever feasible, because impaired neurocognitive function may become evident as a late effect of treatment [32]. Important data on the impact of radiotherapy on neurocognitive function has been derived from studies in adults treated with prophylactic cranial irradiation and low-grade gliomas, as well as in pediatric patients. Indeed, a large follow-up study of children who survive acute lymphoblastic leukemia [33] showed that men and women in the irradiated group had higher-than-average unemployment rates compared to the adults who didn't receive brain radiotherapy in their childhood (15.1% vs. 5.4% and 35.4% vs. 5.2%, respectively).

8.2.3.1.1
Cognitive Dysfunction/Leukoencephalopathy

Radiation-induced cognitive dysfunction and leukoencephalopathy without necrosis are becoming the most frequent complications in long-term survivors [34]. This clinical "entity", also called "diffuse radiation injury" or "radiation-induced leukoencephalopathy" differs from radionecrosis in clinico-radiological aspects as well as in pathology [35]. The most dramatic complication is dementia, but there is also evidence that radiotherapy can induce a less severe encephalopathy leading to subtle neuropsychological impairment [28, 36].

8.2.3.1.2
Radiation-Induced Dementia

Progressive "subcortical dementia" represents the main clinical characteristic of this disorder. At a late stage, severe cognitive deterioration is typically characterized by a severe intellectual loss, with predominant fixative memory impairment, difficulties in focusing attention, emotional lability and apathy. Productive phenomena such as delirium or hallucination are typically absent. Signs of cortical involvement, like aphasia, apraxia or agnosia, are unusual. As a consequence of preserved insight, depression is frequent, but antidepressants do not improve intellectual performance. Gait disturbances, ranging from mild retropulsion to severe ataxia, are constant features, as is incontinence at later stages [37]. The course is characterized by progressive deterioration (80% of cases), more rarely by stabilization and exceptionally by a lasting improvement. Patients become bedridden over a few weeks to months and usually die 1–48 months after the onset of symptoms. There is no effective therapy. There are at least four factors that affect the risk of developing cognitive dysfunction/dementia:

1. Radiation schedule: the risks of cognitive dysfunction are very low with "safe" doses of whole brain irradiation.
2. Volume irradiated: virtually absent for patients undergoing focal conventional radiotherapy alone (volume of radiation excluding the temporal lobes).
3. Concurrent chemotherapy: the frequency of cognitive dysfunction/dementia is increased in patients treated with radiotherapy and concurrent chemotherapy, at least when methotrexate is used.
4. Age: elderly patients appear to be much more sensitive to the diffuse neurotoxicity of radiotherapy. The pathological substrate for intellectual decline has not been clearly identified, but all authors found predominant involvement of the white matter, in agreement with neuropsychological and radiological findings. Diffuse white matter spongiosis, multiple miliary foci of necrosis, and demyelination with severe loss of oligodendrocytes have been reported.

8.2.3.1.3
Mild or Moderate Neuropsychological Impairment

This complication may occur in children (after prophylactic treatment of acute leukemia or irradiation for primary brain tumor) and in adults (after prophylactic irradiation for small cell lung cancer or in long-term survivors of primary or secondary brain tumors). The symptoms generally occur within 4 years of irradiation and are mainly characterized by attention deficits, memory dysfunction and immediate problem solving ability [38, 39]. The clinical course is usually characterized by slow decline of neuropsychological scores without decrease in performance status, but spontaneous stabilization may also occur. Intellectual dysfunctions with significant reductions in overall intelligence quotients (IQ) score have been observed in survivors of childhood acute lymphocytic leukemia in relation to therapy central-nervous-system prophylaxis consisting of cranial irradiation and intrathecal methotrexate [13]. Several factors were found to be closely associated with a lower IQ score in long-term survivors of childhood acute lymphoblastic leukemia, including a younger age at the time of radiation (in both verbal IQ and full-scale IQ) [40]. Subgroup analysis further showed a correlation between sex, age at the time of radiation, dose of cranial radiation, concomitant intrathecal methotrexate therapy, and duration of therapy with a lower level of intellectual function. Similar decreased IQ scores were found in long-term survivors of cerebellar medulloblastoma treated with surgery and irradiation, especially those children younger than 8 years at time of radiotherapy [41]. These deficits can potentially affect learning, academic performance, as well as employment rate [13, 33].

8.2.3.2
Radiation Necrosis

This disorder is a serious complication that usually begins 1–3 years after completion of radiation therapy. The symptoms depend upon the location of the lesion, and generally recapitulate those of the brain tumor or consist in new focal neurological signs simulating a tumor de novo. Radiation necrosis is caused by vascular endothelial cell damage, resulting in fibrinoid necrosis of small arterial vessels, and therefore in focal coagulative necrosis and demyelination of the brain parenchyma [42]. These patients do well when the area of radiation necrosis is resected. Corticosteroids usually produce prompt symptomatic improvement in most patients, and there are reports of prolonged responses after corticosteroid therapy without surgery at the price of a frequent dependence on corticosteroids. Anticoagulants and hyperbaric oxygen therapy have also been reported to provide benefit [43, 44]. Radiation necrosis, however, is uncommon with doses of 60 Gy or less using conventional fractionation [45, 46]. Radionecrosis is more likely to occur when high doses per fraction are administered and possibly with concurrent chemotherapy [47].

8.2.3.3
Other Adverse Consequences

Include vascular abnormalities (lesions of large blood vessels) [48], and endocrinopathies [49–51].

8.3
Mechanisms of Brain Injury

An increasing body of evidence suggests that radiation-induced brain injury is a continuous, multifactorial, and dynamic process. Pathology in the brain has been attributed to vascular injury, inflammation, and apoptosis (thoroughly reviewed in [52]). Discussion of all these mechanisms is beyond the scope of this chapter. We will particularly focus on the potentially reversible mechanisms of radiation-induced brain injury. In particular, the proposed mechanisms of cognitive deficits due to cranial irradiation will be discussed.

Clinical studies reveal that radiation-induced damage to the hippocampus plays a significant role in the cognitive decline seen in patients who have undergone cranial irradiation. The hippocampus is one of two sites in the mammalian forebrain that exhibit active neurogenesis even in adulthood and is the critical neurologic center for learning and memory [53, 54]. Problems with learning, memory, and spatial processing that have been observed in patients after cranial irradiation are related to hippocampus injury. In support of this, radiation to the hippocampus is associated with more pronounced cognitive deficits [55–58].

Ionizing radiation induces a number of cellular responses including apoptosis and cell cycle checkpoints. Radiation-induced hippocampal injury has been linked to increased apoptosis of neuronal progenitor cells within the subgranular zone of the hippocampus. This appears to involve an increase in the proapoptotic proteins p53, Bax, and caspase-3 by radiation [54, 59–61]. Interestingly, little to no apoptosis is seen in other areas of the cerebrum [62]. In addition to the increased neuronal cell apoptosis, decreased neurogenesis within this subgranular zone has been reported [59, 62–66]. This is secondary to the induction of p53-mediated cell cycle checkpoints by radiation and is associated with increased levels of phosphorylated p53 and the cell cycle regulating protein p21 [54]. Finally, decreased microvascular angiogenesis and increased microglial activation have been attributed to the loss of these pre-seen following cranial irradiation [65]. Taken together, these data suggest that radiation-induced hippocampal cell apoptosis and inhibition of neurogenesis contribute to the cognitive decline seen in patients who have undergone cranial irradiation.

8.4
Potential Neuroprotectors

In an effort to decrease neurotoxicity and improve patient quality of life following cranial irradiation, pharmacologic agents which exhibit radioprotective effects have been rigorously investigated. Since radiation-induced cellular damage has been attributed primarily to the adverse effects of free radicals, agents with direct free radical scavenging properties were studied as radioprotectors. The best known radioprotectors are the sulfhydryl compounds, such as cysteine [67] and cysteamine [68]. However, these molecules are considered to be toxic at the doses required for radioprotection, and result in significant side effects, including nausea and vomiting. Another well studied compound is amifostine [69], which has been approved by FDA as a radioprotector [70]. Indeed, amifostine, a synthetic thiol, has been used in clinical trials and it protects normal tissue, such as oral mucosa, from the unwanted effects of radiation more than tumour cells. Several mechanisms of action were proposed, including free radical scavenging, hydrogen transfer, inducing hypoxia and stabilizing DNA through direct binding [70–72]. Despite encouraging data, the use of amifostine is limited for the protection of the central nervous system. In addition, several side effects occurring with amifostine are dose-limiting and prevent maximal

radioprotection [69, 73–75], including hypotension, hypocalcaemia, nausea and vomiting, sneezing, and mild somnolence. In recent years, numerous promising agents such as immunomodulators, haemopoietic growth (i.e. oxymetholone, 5-androstendiol) and stimulating factors (i.e. EPO, interleukins), synthetic chelators and natural antioxidants (i.e. glutathione, melatonin, vitamin E) have been examined for their ability to attenuate radiation-induced injury [76–85]. So far, their clinical benefits and neuroprotective efficacy remain limited.

Therefore, there is still a need to identify novel and effective compounds to protect the brain from radiation-induced injury. One such compound is lithium, a drug which has been widely used in the treatment of bipolar mood disorder [86]. Evidence suggests that lithium protects the brain against a variety of insults to the brain such as stroke and oxidative stress [58, 61, 86–90]. However, the mechanisms of the neuroprotection by lithium are not well defined. The signal transduction pathways perturbed by lithium include phosphoinositide turnover and activation of the wnt pathway via inhibition of GSK-3. In addition, lithium suppresses pro-apoptotic proteins p53 and Bax while enhancing pro-survival proteins Bcl-2 and Akt [87, 91]. Importantly, lithium reduces brain damage in animal models of neurodegenerative diseases and stroke [92]. These actions by lithium make it an attractive candidate as a neuroprotector during cranial irradiation.

8.5
Mechanisms of Lithium-Mediated Neuroprotection Against Radiation-Induced Apoptosis

Given the neuroprotective effects of lithium, the potential of lithium as a neuroprotector during cranial irradiation was investigated using preclinical models. A decrease in radiation-induced cell death was demonstrated with a 7-day lithium prophylaxis prior to the initiation of radiation in HT-22 neuronal cells as well as in neurons within the subgranular zone of irradiated mice [61]. As shown in Figure 8.1, lithium improved clonogenic survival of irradiated HT-22 neurons but not D54 glioma cancer cells. Specifically, analysis of apoptosis via annexin V staining in these cells reveals a protection from radiation-induced apoptosis by lithium (Fig. 8.2). In irradiated

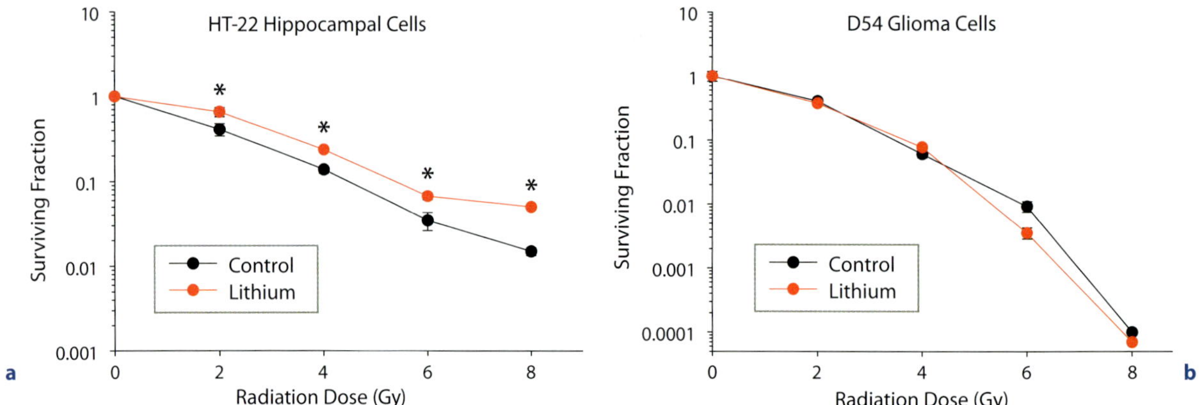

Fig. 8.1a,b. Lithium protects normal hippocampal neurons (**a**) but not D54 glioma cancer cells (**b**) from radiation-induced cell death. HT22 normal hippocampal neurons and D54 glioma cancer cells were treated with either vehicle or 3 mmol/L lithium chloride for 7 days followed by various doses of radiation. Colony-formation assays were subsequently assessed in these cells. Surviving fractions for each dose of radiation are shown relative to irradiated cells not exposed to lithium (* $p < 0.05$). (Adapted with permission from [61])

mice, lithium protects hippocampal neurons in the subgranular zone from apoptosis as evidenced by TUNEL staining (Fig. 8.3). Thus, lithium appears to decrease radiation-induced apoptosis of neurons.

More importantly, lithium also improved cognitive performance in irradiated mice. In these experiments, mice were subjected to Morris water maze studies, which involve a circular pool filled with water with an attached clear square platform beneath the water. The platform could either be visible via marking with a black flag or hidden by removing the flag and clouding the water with white paint. The study began 6 weeks following irradiation with or without lithium prophylaxis by placing the mouse into the water, and the length of time to find the platform in water was measured (average latency time). At 8 days after training, the average latency time was measured again. As shown in Figure 8.4, radiation treatment significantly increased the average latency time compared to unirradiated mice. This increase in latency is attenuated by lithium. These results indicate that lithium indeed protects hippocampal cells and neurons within the subgranular zone against radiation-induced apoptosis and preserves cognitive functions in irradiated mice compared with mice treated with radiation alone.

Optimal neuroprotection by lithium is achieved when administered for 7 days prior to irradiation. This suggests an epigenetic change by lithium. To assess the effects on gene expression by lithium during neuroprotection, microarray analysis was performed. Over 30,000 genes were examined in the

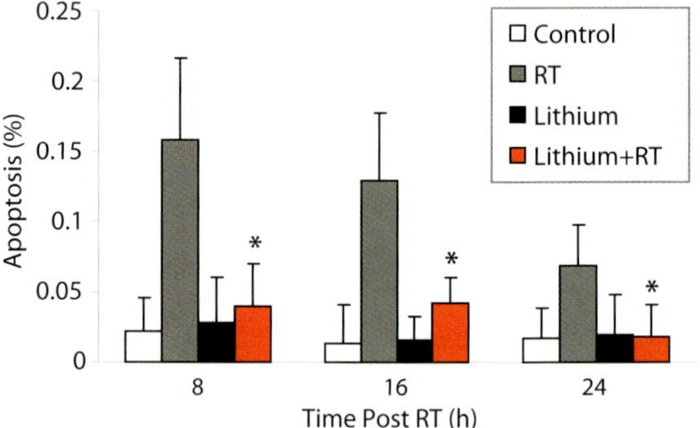

Fig. 8.2. Lithium-mediated protection of normal hippocampal neurons involves reduction of radiation-induced apoptosis. HT22 normal hippocampal neurons treated with vehicle or 3 mmol/L lithium chloride for 7 days were subjected to sham or 3-Gy irradiation. Morphologic nuclear condensation of cells was subsequently assessed via DAPI staining and analysis under microscopy. Percentage of apoptotic cells is shown (* $p < 0.05$). (Adapted with permission from [61])

HT-22 neuronal cells following 7 days of lithium. Interestingly, lithium induced a greater than two-fold expression of genes involved in anti-apoptosis signaling, neurogenesis, and DNA repair. Conversely, lithium also suppressed greater than two-fold the expression of proapoptotic genes. Verification of several of these genes confirmed microarray results. Specifically, the mRNA of the antiapoptotic proteins decorin and NAIP are induced by lithium, and a similarly increase in the protein levels of decorin and NAIP can be observed.

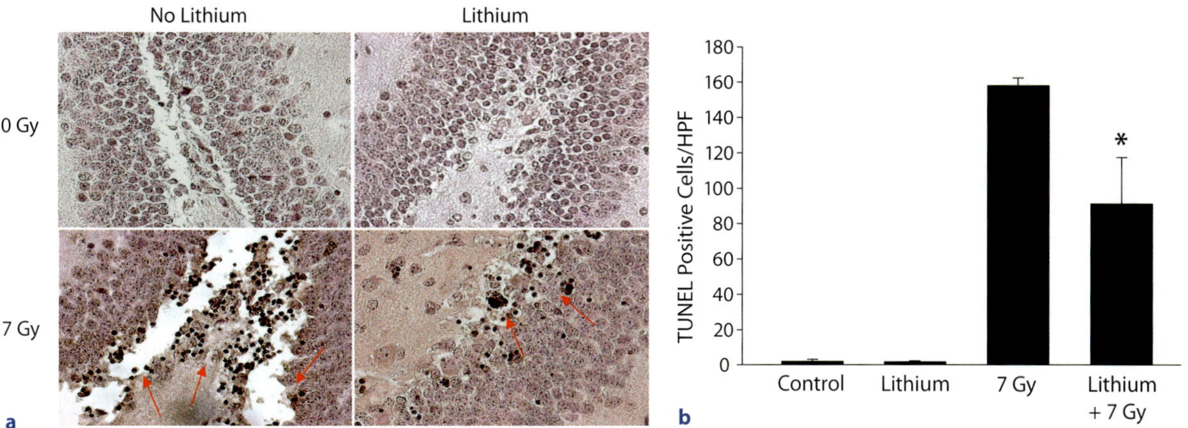

Fig. 8.3a,b. Lithium protects hippocampal neurons in vivo from radiation-induced apoptosis. (**a**) Representative histologic hippocampal sections from mice treated with and without lithium, with and without radiation. (**b**) Quantitation of apoptotic cells. Two-week-old C57/BL/6J mice pups were treated with daily i.p. injections of lithium chloride (40 mg/kg) or PBS. On the 7th day of lithium treatment, the pups were treated with 7 Gy of cranial irradiation or sham irradiation. At 10 h later, the animals were sacrificed and brains were fixed and coronally sectioned. Apoptosis of cells was assessed via TUNEL staining (* $p < 0.05$). (Adapted with permission from [61])

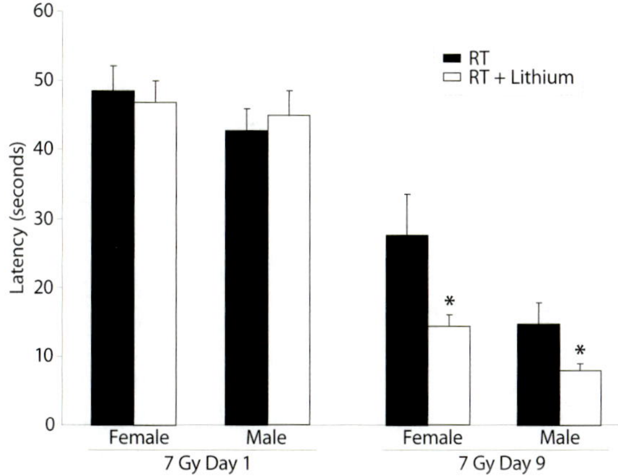

Fig. 8.4. Lithium attenuates radiation-induced cognitive decline in irradiated mice. Cognitive function following cranial irradiation was studied in C57/BL6 mice. One-week-old pups were treated with daily i.p. injections of lithium chloride (40 mg/kg) or PBS for 7 days. On the 7th day of lithium treatment, the pups were treated with 7 Gy of cranial irradiation or sham irradiation. At 6 weeks later, the animals were studied using hidden Morris water maze testing. Average latency times in male and female mice are shown in irradiated animals with or without lithium prophylaxis at day 1 and day 9 of testing (* $p < 0.05$). (Adapted with permission from [61])

To further characterize the molecular mechanism by which lithium protects neurons from radiation-induced apoptosis, several other proteins involved in the apoptotic pathway were analyzed in response to lithium. Lithium treatment correlates with activation of the pro-survival Akt pathway and enhances the levels of the antiapoptotic proteins bcl-2 and β-catenin [61]. Interestingly, lithium also suppresses the proapoptotic pathways [61]. Decreased levels of bax, whose function has been shown to be required for radiation-induced apoptosis [93], are observed with lithium. Lithium also inhibits the proapoptotic enzyme glycogen synthase kinase-3β (GSK-3β). GSK-3β activity can be regulated via activating phosphorylation at Tyr216 or inhibitory phosphorylation at Ser9. Lithium increases Ser9 phosphorylation and concomitantly decreases Tyr216 phosphorylation [61]. This is associated with accumulation of β-catenin and cyclin D, two downstream targets of GSK-3β. As the GSK-3β pathway is known to be involved in cell survival and proliferation, radioprotection by lithium could be due to lithium-mediated inhibition of GSK-3β. Our preliminary results confirm this hypothesis, as inhibition of the GSK-3β pathway using small molecule inhibitors or genetic manipulation using dominant negative GSK-3β reproduces the neuroprotective effects by lithium [94].

Our microarray results also suggest a potential role of DNA repair pathways in lithium-mediated neuroprotection. This is intriguing as the most critical lesion induced by radiation is the DNA double strand break (DSB) [95]. As few as one unrepaired DSB is lethal to the cell. Preliminary results suggest that the neuroprotective effects by lithium involve enhanced DNA repair of radiation-induced DSBs (personal communication, Fen Xia, MD, PhD). In support of this possibility, inhibition of DNA repair pathways with small molecule inhibitors attenuates lithium-mediated neuroprotection.

The actions of lithium are multifactorial but seem to converge with the inhibition of radiation-induced apoptosis. However, the exact defining mechanism to achieve neuroprotection remains to be fully elucidated. The potential of GSK-3β inhibition as a target for neuroprotection is an interesting alternative to lithium and will be discussed later in this chapter.

8.6
Future Directions

8.6.1
Clinical Phase I Trial of Lithium

Based on the promising pre-clinical results, and given that long-term neurotoxicity following cranial radiotherapy is a significant clinical problem that affects the quality of life of cancer survivors, a lithium clinical phase I trial is currently ongoing. This study tests the safety and toxicity of lithium as a neuroprotective agent during cranial radiotherapy. Patients with histologically confirmed extracranial primary malignancy and associated brain metastases received lithium treatment one week prior to as well as during whole brain radiotherapy. The dosing of lithium started at one-half (300 mg BID) of the maximal dose (300 mg QID) indicated for mood disorders. Whole brain irradiation consisted of a total of 3,000 cGy over ten fractions. Preliminary data suggests that lithium can be safely administered concurrently to whole-brain radiation therapy with minimal grade 3 toxicity, although the dosage needs to be adjusted accordingly to serum levels of lithium. A phase II clinical trial is currently planned to study functional MRI and neurocognitive function in adult patients receiving prophylactic cranial irradiation.

8.6.2
Potential Disadvantages of Lithium

Although lithium is available in multiple oral preparations (i.e. carbonate or citrate), several critical variables can limit its potential in clinical setting. First, lithium has a relatively low therapeutic index, requiring careful blood level monitoring in light of the well known toxicity of lithium [96]. Side effects from lithium are common but generally mild, especially when used for a short treatment course for radioprotection. Lithium's early potential adverse effects are gastrointestinal discomforts (nausea, vomiting, diarrhea, stomach pain), muscular weakness, thirstiness and frequent urination, feelings of being dazed, sleepy, and tired, and hand tremor [96], which can sometimes disappear in certain patients. After several days of treatment this group of early side effects normally subsides. Late side effects of lithium can occur in longer therapy, including hand tremor, constant thirst and abundant urine excretion. Another major late side effect is thyroid enlargement, which is caused by lithium's perturbation of thyroid functioning.

In addition, the therapeutic action of lithium is delayed, requiring 5–7 days prophylaxis prior to the initiation of radiation therapy to reach steady-state concentrations [97]. Lithium is renally excreted after ~ 24 h, and is a function of renal sufficiency [98]. Finally, the therapeutic efficacy of lithium may rely on the "dirty" characteristics of its multiple mechanisms of action, which non-specificity can be viewed as a potential weakness.

8.6.3
GSK-3β Inhibitors

GSK-3β belongs to a family of glycogen-synthase kinases, which is a multifunctional serine/threonine kinase implicated in multiple biological processes including apoptosis [99–102]. GSK-3β is highly enriched in the brain and has been implicated in central nervous system dysfunctions including Alzheimer's disease [103], schizophrenia [104], dopamine-associated behaviors [105], bipolar disorders [106], and Parkinson's disease [107]. Our previous data support a role of GSK-3β inhibition in lithium-mediated neuroprotection against radiation-induced apoptosis. Consistent with this hypothesis, specific inhibition of GSK-3β 16 h prior to irradiation or using dominant negative GSK-3β significantly attenuated radiation-induced apoptosis in hippocampal neurons [94].

Given lithium's requirement for a 7 day prophylaxis, its narrow therapeutic window, and its lack of specificity, the use of GSK3β inhibitors as neuroprotectors provide clear advantages over lithium. Prophylaxis with GSK3β inhibitors can start as early as

16 h (vs. 7 days for lithium) prior to starting cranial radiation, eliminating the need to wait 1 week prior to initializing radiation treatment that is necessary with lithium. In addition, increased specificity can be achieved using these inhibitors, potentially decreasing the side effects of neuroprotectors. Further investigation with these inhibitors is warranted.

8.6.4
Summary

There is strong pre-clinical rationale to support the use of lithium as a protector of radiation-associated injury to the brain. Lithium inhibits GSK3 and blocks radiation-induced apoptosis in hippocampal neurons without protecting cancer cells. Lithium also improved neurocognitive function in mice treated with whole-brain irradiation.

A phase I clinical trial currently evaluates the feasibility of neoadjuvant and concurrent lithium treatment in patients receiving whole-brain radiotherapy. Preliminary results suggest that lithium is well tolerated in patients with brain metastases treated with cranial irradiation, and support future clinical studies to evaluate the efficacy of lithium as a neuroprotector.

Acknowledgements

This research was supported in part by NIH grants R01-CA112385, R01-CA88076, R01-CA89674, R01-CA89888, and P50-CA90949; Ingram Charitable Fund; and Vanderbilt-Ingram Cancer Center grant CCSG P30-CA68485. Dr. Luigi Moretti was supported by a grant from "Yvonne and Thomas Rucquois Fund". Dr. Eddy S. Yang is a recipient of an RSNA Seed Grant ID #RR0725.

References

1. Cairncross JG, Kim JH, Posner JB (1980) Radiation therapy for brain metastases. Ann Neurol 7:529–541
2. Chao JH, Phillips R, Nickson JJ (1954) Roentgen-ray therapy of cerebral metastases. Cancer 7:682–689
3. Posner JB, Chernik NL (1978) Intracranial metastases from systemic cancer. Adv Neurol 19:579–592
4. Bailey CC, Gnekow A, Wellek S et al (1995) Prospective randomised trial of chemotherapy given before radiotherapy in childhood medulloblastoma. International Society of Paediatric Oncology (SIOP) and the (German) Society of Paediatric Oncology (GPO): SIOP II. Med Pediatr Oncol 25:166–178
5. Packer RJ, Boyett JM, Zimmerman RA et al (1994) Outcome of children with brain stem gliomas after treatment with 7,800 cGy of hyperfractionated radiotherapy. A Childrens Cancer Group Phase I/II Trial. Cancer 74:1827–1834
6. Packer RJ, Sutton LN, Elterman R et al (1994) Outcome for children with medulloblastoma treated with radiation and cisplatin, CCNU, and vincristine chemotherapy. J Neurosurg 81:690–698
7. Rousseau P, Habrand JL, Sarrazin D et al (1994) Treatment of intracranial ependymomas of children: review of a 15-year experience. Int J Radiat Oncol Biol Phys 28:381–386
8. Glauser TA, Packer RJ (1991) Cognitive deficits in long-term survivors of childhood brain tumors. Childs Nerv Syst 7:2–12
9. Anderson DM, Rennie KM, Ziegler RS et al (2001) Medical and neurocognitive late effects among survivors of childhood central nervous system tumors. Cancer 92:2709–2719
10. Christie D, Leiper AD, Chessells JM et al (1995) Intellectual performance after presymptomatic cranial radiotherapy for leukaemia: effects of age and sex. Arch Dis Child 73:136–140
11. Fletcher JM, Copeland DR (1988) Neurobehavioral effects of central nervous system prophylactic treatment of cancer in children. J Clin Exp Neuropsychol 10:495–537
12. Grill J, Renaux VK, Bulteau C et al (1999) Long-term intellectual outcome in children with posterior fossa tumors according to radiation doses and volumes. Int J Radiat Oncol Biol Phys 45:137–145
13. Meadows AT, Gordon J, Massari DJ et al (1981) Declines in IQ scores and cognitive dysfunctions in children with acute lymphocytic leukaemia treated with cranial irradiation. Lancet 2:1015–1018
14. Roman DD, Sperduto PW (1995) Neuropsychological effects of cranial radiation: current knowledge and future directions. Int J Radiat Oncol Biol Phys 31:983–998
15. Macedoni-Luksic M, Jereb B, Todorovski L (2003) Long-term sequelae in children treated for brain tumors: impairments, disability, and handicap. Pediatr Hematol Oncol 20:89–101
16. Riva D, Giorgi C (2000) The neurodevelopmental price of survival in children with malignant brain tumours. Childs Nerv Syst 16:751–754
17. Ellenberg L, McComb JG, Siegel SE et al (1987) Factors affecting intellectual outcome in pediatric brain tumor patients. Neurosurgery 21:638–644
18. Duffner PK, Cohen ME, Thomas P (1983) Late effects of treatment on the intelligence of children with posterior fossa tumors. Cancer 51:233–237
19. Borgelt B, Gelber R, Kramer S et al (1980) The palliation of brain metastases: final results of the first two studies by the Radiation Therapy Oncology Group. Int J Radiat Oncol Biol Phys 6:1–9
20. Simpson JR, Horton J, Scott C et al (1993) Influence of location and extent of surgical resection on survival of patients with glioblastoma multiforme: results of three consecutive Radiation Therapy Oncology Group (RTOG) clinical trials. Int J Radiat Oncol Biol Phys 26:239–244

21. Kiehna EN, Mulhern RK, Li C et al (2006) Changes in attentional performance of children and young adults with localized primary brain tumors after conformal radiation therapy. J Clin Oncol 24:5283–5290

22. Young DF, Posner JB, Chu F et al (1974) Rapid-course radiation therapy of cerebral metastases: results and complications. Cancer 34:1069–1076

23. Freeman JE, Johnston PG, Voke JM (1973) Somnolence after prophylactic cranial irradiation in children with acute lymphoblastic leukaemia. Br Med J 4:523–525

24. Ryan J (2000) Radiation somnolence syndrome. J Pediatr Oncol Nurs 17:50–53

25. Mandell LR, Walker RW, Steinherz P et al (1989) Reduced incidence of the somnolence syndrome in leukemic children with steroid coverage during prophylactic cranial radiation therapy. Results of a pilot study. Cancer 63:1975–1978

26. Uzal D, Ozyar E, Hayran M et al (1998) Reduced incidence of the somnolence syndrome after prophylactic cranial irradiation in children with acute lymphoblastic leukemia. Radiother Oncol 48:29–32

27. Hoffman WF, Levin VA, Wilson CB (1979) Evaluation of malignant glioma patients during the postirradiation period. J Neurosurg 50:624–628

28. Armstrong C, Ruffer J, Corn B et al (1995) Biphasic patterns of memory deficits following moderate-dose partial-brain irradiation: neuropsychologic outcome and proposed mechanisms. J Clin Oncol 13:2263–2271

29. Armstrong CL, Corn BW, Ruffer JE et al (2000) Radiotherapeutic effects on brain function: double dissociation of memory systems. Neuropsychiatry Neuropsychol Behav Neurol 13:101–111

30. Schultheiss TE, Kun LE, Ang KK et al (1995) Radiation response of the central nervous system. Int J Radiat Oncol Biol Phys 31:1093–1112

31. Regine WF, Schmitt FA, Scott CB et al (2004) Feasibility of neurocognitive outcome evaluations in patients with brain metastases in a multi-institutional cooperative group setting: results of Radiation Therapy Oncology Group trial BR-0018. Int J Radiat Oncol Biol Phys 58:1346–1352

32. Duffey P, Chari G, Cartlidge NE et al (1996) Progressive deterioration of intellect and motor function occurring several decades after cranial irradiation. A new facet in the clinical spectrum of radiation encephalopathy. Arch Neurol 53:814–818

33. Pui CH, Cheng C, Leung W et al (2003) Extended follow-up of long-term survivors of childhood acute lymphoblastic leukemia. N Engl J Med 349:640–649

34. Crossen JR, Garwood D, Glatstein E et al (1994) Neurobehavioral sequelae of cranial irradiation in adults: a review of radiation-induced encephalopathy. J Clin Oncol 12:627–642

35. Price RA, Jamieson PA (1975) The central nervous system in childhood leukemia. II. Subacute leukoencephalopathy. Cancer 35:306–318

36. Frytak S, Shaw JN, O'Neill BP et al (1989) Leukoencephalopathy in small cell lung cancer patients receiving prophylactic cranial irradiation. Am J Clin Oncol 12:27–33

37. DeAngelis LM, Delattre JY, Posner JB (1989) Radiation-induced dementia in patients cured of brain metastases. Neurology 39:789–796

38. Garcia-Perez A, Sierrasesumaga L, Narbona-Garcia J et al (1994) Neuropsychological evaluation of children with intracranial tumors: impact of treatment modalities. Med Pediatr Oncol 23:116–123

39. Chadderton RD, West CG, Schuller S et al (1995) Radiotherapy in the treatment of low-grade astrocytomas. II. The physical and cognitive sequelae. Childs Nerv Syst 11:443–448

40. Robison LL, Nesbit ME Jr, Sather HN et al (1984) Factors associated with IQ scores in long-term survivors of childhood acute lymphoblastic leukemia. Am J Pediatr Hematol Oncol 6:115–121

41. Silverman CL, Palkes H, Talent B et al (1984) Late effects of radiotherapy on patients with cerebellar medulloblastoma. Cancer 54:825–829

42. Burger PC, Mahley MS Jr, Dudka L et al (1979) The morphologic effects of radiation administered therapeutically for intracranial gliomas: a postmortem study of 25 cases. Cancer 44:1256–1272

43. Chuba PJ, Aronin P, Bhambhani K et al (1997) Hyperbaric oxygen therapy for radiation-induced brain injury in children. Cancer 80:2005–2012

44. Glantz MJ, Burger PC, Friedman AH et al (1994) Treatment of radiation-induced nervous system injury with heparin and warfarin. Neurology 44:2020–2027

45. Emami B, Lyman J, Brown A et al (1991) Tolerance of normal tissue to therapeutic irradiation. Int J Radiat Oncol Biol Phys 21:109–122

46. Leibel SA, Sheline GE (1987) Radiation therapy for neoplasms of the brain. J Neurosurg 66:1–22

47. Ruben JD, Dally M, Bailey M et al (2006) Cerebral radiation necrosis: incidence, outcomes, and risk factors with emphasis on radiation parameters and chemotherapy. Int J Radiat Oncol Biol Phys 65:499–508

48. Hirata Y, Matsukado Y, Mihara Y et al (1985) Occlusion of the internal carotid artery after radiation therapy for the chiasmal lesion. Acta Neurochir (Wien) 74:141–147

49. Constine LS, Woolf PD, Cann D et al (1993) Hypothalamic-pituitary dysfunction after radiation for brain tumors. N Engl J Med 328:87–94

50. Gleeson HK, Shalet SM (2004) The impact of cancer therapy on the endocrine system in survivors of childhood brain tumours. Endocr Relat Cancer 11:589–602

51. Shalet SM, Beardwell CG, MacFarlane IA et al (1977) Endocrine morbidity in adults treated with cerebral irradiation for brain tumours during childhood. Acta Endocrinol (Copenh) 84:673–680

52. Wong CS, Van der Kogel AJ (2004) Mechanisms of Radiation Injury to the Central Nervous System: Implications for Neuroprotection. Mol Interv 4:273–284

53. Abayomi OK (2002) Pathogenesis of cognitive decline following therapeutic irradiation for head and neck tumors. Acta Oncol 41:346–351

54. Limoli CL, Giedzinski E, Rola R et al (2004) Radiation response of neural precursor cells: linking cellular sensitivity to cell cycle checkpoints, apoptosis and oxidative stress. Radiat Res 161:17–27

55. Deweer B, Pillon B, Pochon JB et al (2001) Is the HM story only a "remote memory"? Some facts about hippocampus and memory in humans. Behav Brain Res 127:209–224

56. Enokido Y, Araki T, Tanaka K et al (1996) Involvement of p53 in DNA strand break-induced apoptosis in postmitotic CNS neurons. Eur J Neurosci 8:1812–1821

57. Xiang H, Hockman DW, Saya H et al (1996) Evidence for p53-mediated modulation of neuronal viability. J Neurosci 16:6753–6765

58. Wood GE, Young LT, Reagan LP et al (2004) Stress-induced structural remodeling in hippocampus: prevention by lithium treatment Proc Natl Acad Sci U S A 101:3973–3978

59. Fukuda H, Fukuda A, Zhu C et al (2004) Irradiation-induced progenitor cell death in the developing brain is resistant to erythropoietin treatment and caspase inhibition. Cell Death Differ 11:1166–1178

60. Achanta P, Thompson KJ, Fuss M et al (2007) Gene expression changes in the rodent hippocampus following whole brain irradiation. Neurosci Lett 418:143–148

61. Yazlovitskaya EM, Edwards E, Thotala D et al (2006) Lithium treatment prevents neurocognitive deficit resulting from cranial irradiation. Cancer Res 66:11179–11186

62. Nagai R, Tsunoda S, Hori Y et al (2000) Selective vulnerability to radiation in the hippocampal dentate granule cells. Surg Neurol 53:503–506

63. Mizumatsu S, Monje ML, Morhardt DR et al (2003) Extreme sensitivity of adult neurogenesis to low doses of X-irradiation. Cancer Research 63:4021–4027

64. Peissner W, Kocher M, Treuer H et al (1999) Ionizing radiation-induced apoptosis of proliferating stem cells in the dentate gyrus of the adult rat hippocampus. Brain Res Mol Brain Res 71:61–68

65. Monje M, Mizumatsu S, Fike J et al (2002) Irradiation induces neural precursor-cell dysfunction. Nat Med 8:955–962

66. Tada E, Parent J, Lowenstein D et al (2000) X-irradiation causes a prolonged reduction in cell proliferation in the dentate gyrus of adult rats. Neuroscience 99:33–41

67. Patt HM, Tyree EB, Straube RL et al (1949) Cysteine Protection against X Irradiation. Science 110:213–214

68. Bacq ZM, Herve A (1955) New data on the radioprotective effects of oral cystamine. C R Seances Soc Biol Fil 149:1509–1512

69. Yuhas JM, Spellman JM, Culo F (1980) The role of WR-2721 in radiotherapy and/or chemotherapy. Cancer Clin Trials 3:211–216

70. Cassatt DR, Fazenbaker CA, Bachy CM et al (2002) Preclinical modeling of improved amifostine (Ethyol) use in radiation therapy. Semin Radiat Oncol 12:97–102

71. Held KD, Biaglow JE (1994) Mechanisms for the oxygen radical-mediated toxicity of various thiol-containing compounds in cultured mammalian cells. Radiat Res 139:15–23

72. Maisin JR (1998) Bacq and Alexander Award lecture – chemical radioprotection: past, present, and future prospects. Int J Radiat Biol 73:443–450

73. Glover D, Riley L, Carmichael K et al (1983) Hypocalcemia and inhibition of parathyroid hormone secretion after administration of WR-2721 (a radioprotective and chemoprotective agent). N Engl J Med 309:1137–1141

74. Kligerman MM, Glover DJ, Turrisi AT et al (1984) Toxicity of WR-2721 administered in single and multiple doses. Int J Radiat Oncol Biol Phys 10:1773–1776

75. Schuchter LM, Luginbuhl WE, Meropol NJ (1992) The current status of toxicity protectants in cancer therapy. Semin Oncol 19:742–751

76. Harapanhalli RS, Narra VR, Yaghmai V et al (1994) Vitamins as radioprotectors in vivo. II. Protection by vitamin A and soybean oil against radiation damage caused by internal radionuclides. Radiat Res 139:115–122

77. Sarma L, Kesavan PC (1993) Protective effects of vitamins C and E against gamma-ray-induced chromosomal damage in mouse. Int J Radiat Biol 63:759–764

78. Shimoi K, Masuda S, Furugori M et al (1994) Radioprotective effect of antioxidative flavonoids in gamma-ray irradiated mice. Carcinogenesis 15:2669–2672

79. Slyshenkov VS, Omelyanchik SN, Moiseenok AG et al (1998) Pantothenol protects rats against some deleterious effects of gamma radiation. Free Radic Biol Med 24:894–899

80. Spotheim-Maurizot M, Ruiz S, Sabattier R et al (1995) Radioprotection of DNA by polyamines. Int J Radiat Biol 68:571–577

81. Srinivasan V, Weiss JF (1992) Radioprotection by vitamin E: injectable vitamin E administered alone or with WR-3689 enhances survival of irradiated mice. Int J Radiat Oncol Biol Phys 23:841–845

82. Ueda T, Toyoshima Y, Kushihashi T et al (1993) Effect of dimethyl sulfoxide pretreatment on activities of lipid peroxide formation, superoxide dismutase and glutathione peroxidase in the mouse liver after whole-body irradiation. J Toxicol Sci 18:239–244

83. Ueda T, Toyoshima Y, Moritani T et al (1996) Protective effect of dipyridamole against lethality and lipid peroxidation in liver and spleen of the ddY mouse after whole-body irradiation. Int J Radiat Biol 69:199–204

84. Uma Devi P (2001) Radioprotective, anticarcinogenic and antioxidant properties of the Indian holy basil, Ocimum sanctum (Tulasi). Indian J Exp Biol 39:185–190

85. Uma Devi P, Ganasoundari A, Vrinda B et al (2000) Radiation protection by the ocimum flavonoids orientin and vicenin: mechanisms of action. Radiat Res 154:455–460

86. Manji HK, Moore GJ, Chen G (1999) Lithium at 50: have the neuroprotective effects of this unique cation been overlooked? Biol Psychiatry 46:929–940

87. Manji HK, Moore GJ, Chen G (2000) Lithium up-regulates the cytoprotective protein Bcl-2 in the CNS in vivo: a role for neurotrophic and neuroprotective effects in manic depressive illness. J Clin Psychiatry 61 Suppl 9:82–96

88. Ren M, Senatorov VV, Chen RW et al (2003) Postinsult treatment with lithium reduces brain damage and facilitates neurological recovery in a rat ischemia/reperfusion model Proc Natl Acad Sci USA 100:6210–6215

89. Chen RW, Chuang DM (1999) Long term lithium treatment suppresses p53 and Bax expression but increases Bcl-2 expression. A prominent role in neuroprotection against excitotoxicity. J Biol Chem 274:6039–6042

90. Bauer M, Alda M, Priller J et al (2003) Implications of the neuroprotective effects of lithium for the treatment of bipolar and neurodegenerative disorders. Pharmacopsychiatry 36[Suppl 3]:S250–254

91. Ghribi O, Herman MM, Spaulding NK et al (2002) Lithium inhibits aluminum-induced apoptosis in rabbit hippocampus, by preventing cytochrome c translocation, Bcl-2 decrease, Bax elevation and caspase-3 activation. J Neurochem 82:137–145

92. Chuang DM, Chen RW, Chalecka-Franaszek E et al (2002) Neuroprotective effects of lithium in cultured

cells and animal models of diseases. Bipolar Disord 4:129–136

93. Chong MJ, Murray MR, Gosink EC et al (2000) Atm and Bax cooperate in ionizing radiation-induced apoptosis in the central nervous system. Proc Natl Acad Sci USA 97:889–894

94. Thotala D, Linkous A, Hallahan DE et al (2008) Inhibition of glycogen synthase kinase 3-beta attenuates neuronal progenitor cell death in the irradiated brain. Cancer Research (Conditional Acceptance)

95. Rich T, Allen RL, Wyllie AH (2000) Defying death after DNA damage. Nature 407:777–783

96. Marini JL, Sheard MH (1976) Sustained-release lithium carbonate in double-blind study: serum lithium levels, side effects, and placebo response. J Clin Pharmacol 16:276–283

97. Keck PE Jr, McElroy SL (2002) Clinical pharmacodynamics and pharmacokinetics of antimanic and mood-stabilizing medications. J Clin Psychiatry 63 Suppl 4:3–11

98. Birch NJ, Greenfield AA, Hullin RP (1980) Pharmacodynamic aspects of long-term prophylactic lithium. Int Pharmacopsychiatry 15:91–98

99. Embi N, Rylatt DB, Cohen P (1980) Glycogen synthase kinase-3 from rabbit skeletal muscle. Separation from cyclic-AMP-dependent protein kinase and phosphorylase kinase. Eur J Biochem 107:519–527

100. Frame S, Cohen P (2001) GSK3 takes centre stage more than 20 years after its discovery. Biochem J 359:1–16

101. Jope RS, Johnson GV (2004) The glamour and gloom of glycogen synthase kinase-3. Trends Biochem Sci 29:95–102

102. Grimes CA, Jope RS (2001) The multifaceted roles of glycogen synthase kinase 3beta in cellular signaling. Prog Neurobiol 65:391–426

103. Bhat RV, Budd Haeberlein SL, Avila J (2004) Glycogen synthase kinase 3: a drug target for CNS therapies. J Neurochem 89:1313–1317

104. Emamian ES, Hall D, Birnbaum MJ et al (2004) Convergent evidence for impaired AKT1-GSK3beta signaling in schizophrenia. Nat Genet 36:131–137

105. Beaulieu JM, Sotnikova TD, Yao WD et al (2004) Lithium antagonizes dopamine-dependent behaviors mediated by an AKT/glycogen synthase kinase-3 signaling cascade. Proc Natl Acad Sci USA 101:5099–5104

106. Klein PS, Melton DA (1996) A molecular mechanism for the effect of lithium on development. Proc Natl Acad Sci USA 93:8455–8459

107. Kozikowski AP, Gaisina IN, Petukhov PA et al (2006) Highly potent and specific GSK-3beta inhibitors that block tau phosphorylation and decrease alpha-synuclein protein expression in a cellular model of Parkinson's disease. ChemMedChem 1:256–266

Risks and Surveillance of Second Malignant Tumors in Prostate and Bladder Cancer Survivors

ANDRE KONSKI

CONTENTS

A. KONSKI, MD, MBA, MA, FACR
Director Clinical Research, Department of Radiation Oncology, Fox Chase Cancer Center, 333 Cottman Avenue, Philadelphia, PA 19111, USA

9.1 Introduction

The relative proportion of men surviving prostate cancer has increased as a consequence of a combination of aggressive screening, resulting in an earlier stage cancer at presentation, and improvements in treatment. Administrative databases, such as the Surveillance, Epidemiology, and End Results Program (SEER) database, have been useful in determining the incidence of second malignant tumors in patients treated with either external beam radiotherapy or interstitial seed implants. What cannot be determined, however, from a review of administrative databases is whether second malignant tumor development was a result of treatment or other causes such as genetic susceptibility resulting in increases in tumor development. Guidelines, such as the National Comprehensive Cancer Network (NCCN) guidelines, offer little guidance as to which surveillance tests are appropriate for patients once they are considered "cured" of their cancer.

This chapter will review the incidence of second malignant tumors in patients with prostate and bladder cancer and attempt to develop principles for second malignant tumor surveillance.

9.2 Risk of Second Malignant Tumors after Prostate Cancer

An increased risk of second malignancies after curative radiotherapy has been reported with other cancers, such as breast cancer, but the literature is mixed as to whether an increased risk is observed for patients undergoing radiation for prostate cancer [1–3]. Single institution reports with small numbers of patients have concluded an increased rate of second malignancies is not seen after radiotherapy while other mostly large studies using administrative data bases such as SEER, have concluded otherwise [4–8]. The overall incidence of second malignant tumors may be low and second malignant tumor development could be related to anatomic location for some malignant tumors, such as bladder or rectal cancer being in close geographic proximity to the radiation field [8].

9.3
Rectal Cancer

Studies using the SEER database have reported an increased incidence of rectal cancer after external beam radiation for prostate cancer. BRENNER et al. [7] were among the first to use SEER data, from 1973–1993, to report an increased risk of rectal cancer after radiation when compared to surgery. The higher risk of rectal cancer development after radiotherapy for prostate cancer increased for patients surviving $\geq$ 10 years.

More recently, BAXTER et al. [9] reported an increase in colorectal cancer in irradiated sites but not in the remainder of the colon from an analysis of SEER registry data from 1973–1994. The adjusted hazards ratio for rectal cancer development was 1.7 (95% CI, 1.4–2.2) when compared to the surgery only group. The analysis was limited to men 18–80 years old and only men with invasive, non-metastatic microscopically confirmed cancer. In addition only men alive 5 years after diagnosis were included and excluded men who had developed rectal cancer within the 5-year period after the completion of radiotherapy. The investigators used the International Classification of Disease Oncology 2 (ICD 0 2) to classify the location of the rectal cancer in relation to the radiation field. This method is imprecise at locating the second malignancy in relation to the radiation field as field sizes are not specified in the SEER database.

In another study using SEER data from patients treated between 1973 and 1999, MOON and colleagues [8] reported a statistically significant increased risk of rectal cancer in men treated with external beam radiation therapy as their only form of therapy [adjusted odds ratios (OR) 1.6; 95% CI, 1.29–1.99]. Men receiving radiation of an unspecified type had higher odds of secondary rectal cancer (OR, 2.34; 95% CI, 1.50–3.65). Interestingly, men receiving implants, either alone or in combination with external beam radiation did not have significant different odds of secondary cancer occurring at any of the 20 most common sites reported. This could be a result of less exposure of normal tissues to radiation by the implant and lower external beam doses used when combined with prostate seed implants. Similarly, LIAUW et al. [10] also did not find an increased risk of rectal cancer in patients treated with either brachytherapy alone (n = 125) or combined with external beam radiation (n = 223). But small numbers of patients in this study may limit the ability to detect a small increased risk of second cancer if one does exist. In addition, an analysis of over 1351 consecutive patients treated with brachytherapy alone (n = 652) or combined with external beam radiation (n = 699) found an equal distribution of colorectal cancer before (n = 23) or after brachytherapy (n = 25) [11]. The majority of the cancers (73%), however, were diagnosed within 5 years of brachytherapy with a peak incidence 1 year after implant. The contribution of external beam radiation to the development of colorectal tumors could not be made as the authors did not separate the incidence of second malignant tumors by treatment.

A similar finding of increased risk of colorectal cancer was reported by PICKLES and PHILLIPS [12] from patients with prostate cancer treated with external beam radiation in British Columbia between 1984–2000. They, however, included second primary tumors starting 2 months after the conclusion of the radiation which could have overestimated the true incidence of second malignant rectal cancers.

In contrast, an increased risk of rectal cancer after prostate radiotherapy was not reported by KENDAL and colleagues [13] using SEER registry data for patients treated between 1973 and 2001 controlling for age effects and differences between the surgical and untreated cohorts. Cancers of the rectosigmoid colon were excluded in this study because the authors stated the rectosigmoid colon would not uniformly fall within the usual radiation treatment fields used for prostate cancer treatment. The rate of rectal cancer development was more than twice that of surgical controls, similar to the rate BAXTER et al. [9] reported. Furthermore, BRENNER [14], in an editorial to the KENDAL et al. [13] article, highlighted differences between the Kendal and the Baxter analyses, which showed an increased risk of rectal cancer. A number of single institution studies have not detected an increased risk of rectal cancer development after prostate radiation suffering from insufficient number of patients and lacking statistical power to show an increased risk of rectal cancer development [4–6]. The large database studies are summarized in Table 9.1.

9.4
Bladder Cancer

The bladder's close proximity to the prostate makes it an organ at significant risk for development of a second malignancy after radiotherapy. A 77% increase in risk of bladder cancer development > 10 years after completion of treatment compared to patients with prostate cancer treated with surgery was reported by BRENNER et al. [7]. NEUGENT et al. [15] only found an increased risk of bladder cancer, and not other cancers, after radiotherapy when an analysis of the SEER database was performed. NEUGENT et al. did not restrict their analysis to patients < 60 years old as BRENNER et al. did which may account for not finding an increased risk of other malignancies. LEVI at al., using a smaller database, did not find an increased risk of bladder cancer after radiotherapy for prostate cancer. MOON et al. [8], using SEER data, also found an increased risk of bladder cancer in patients treated with radiotherapy. Interestingly, men who had an interstitial implant, alone or in combination with external beam radiotherapy, did not have an increased incidence of second malignant tumors. Total bladder dose may be important etiologic factor in bladder cancer development after radiotherapy since patients receiving an interstitial implant receive a lower external beam dose when combined with an implant.

Cigarette smoking was identified as the single most important etiologic factor for bladder cancer development after 1421 men were treated with radiotherapy for prostate cancer [16]. In another analysis, patients treated with radical prostatectomy were approximately half as likely to have post-treatment bladder cancer compared to patients who underwent radiation [17]. A second bladder cancer, however, was defined as a cancer developing only 30 days after the end of radiation compared to 5 years in SEER database studies. Patients receiving radiation were 1.59 times more likely to develop bladder cancer compared to patients receiving any other treatment [17]. Similar to WEGNER et al., patients who smoked

cigarettes had an independent two-fold increase in the risk of bladder cancer over non-smokers. CHROUSER et al. [18], in an analysis of patients receiving radiotherapy for prostate cancer at the Mayo Clinic, found a higher rate of bladder cancer development after external beam radiotherapy in patients who also smoked cigarettes.

The biologic behavior of bladder cancer developing in patients receiving radiotherapy compared to de novo bladder cancer has not been studied extensively. Bladder cancer screening programs may be beneficial for patients having undergone radiotherapy for prostate cancer if the cancers that develop after radiotherapy are more aggressive and are potentially less curable compared to de novo bladder cancers. In an analysis of the University of Miami cystectomy database, BOSTROM et al. [19] found most bladder cancers in patients with a history of radiation for prostate cancer presented as locally advanced tumors and had poorer survival than age and stage matched controls. CHOUSER et al. [18] found while patients developing bladder cancer after radiotherapy had fewer recurrences, 20% had progressed to invasion compared to 10% progressing to invasion in the sporadic population. The pertinent large database studies are outlined in Table 9.2.

9.5
Sarcoma

Post-radiation sarcomas usually develop many years after the completion of radiation and are located in the high dose radiation region. Single institution studies have reported the development of post-radiation sarcomas within the radiation field many years after prostate cancer irradiation [20–22]. Large database analyses have also reported an increased risk of sarcoma development. PICKLES and PHILLIPS reported an increased risk of sarcomas comparing patients receiving radiation to those not receiving radiation with a relative risk of 2.49 but did not mention where the sarcomas developed in relation to the radiotherapy field [12]. In addition, BRENNER et al. [7] reported an increased risk of sarcomas developing within the treatment field in patients receiving radiation when compared to patients not receiving radiation but did not find a significant difference in sarcoma development outside the radiation field when comparing the two groups.

Table 9.1. Second rectal cancers after radiation for prostate cancer

Author	Data Type	Patients	Second malignant tumor development risk	
BRENNER et al. [7]	SEER	122,123	OER (RT compared to surgery) ≥ 5 years 35%; 95% CI (−1,86) ≥ 10 years 105%; 95% CI (9,292)	$p = 0.06$ $p = 0.03$
BAXTER et al. [9]	SEER	85,815	HR 1.7;	$p < 0.0001$ compared to surgery
KENDAL et al. [13]	SEER	237,773	RR (RT compared to surgery) 0–10 years – 2.16; 95% CI (2.0–2.33) > 10 years – 15.62; 95% CI (12.01–19.83)	
PICKLES and PHILLIPS [12]	British Columbia Registry	39,261	SIR (RT compared to no RT) > 5 years 32% > 10 years 53%	
MOON et al. [8] EBRT EBRT/Iimplant Implant	SEER	297,069	AOR 1.6; 95% CI (1.29–1.99) 1.59 0.3	$p < 0.05$
NEUGUT et al. [15]	SEER	141,761	RR < 5 years 0.7 (0.5–0.9) 5–8 years 0.8 (0.5–1.2) > 8 years 0.8 (0.4–1.3)	

OER, observed to expected ratio; HR, hazard ratio; RR, relative risk; AOR, adjusted odds ratios; EBRT, external beam radiation therapy; RT, radiation therapy; SIR, standardized incidence ratios

Table 9.2. Second bladder cancers after radiation for prostate cancer

Author	Data Type	Patients	Second malignant tumor development risk	
BRENNER et al. [7]	SEER	122,123	OER (RT compared to surgery) ≥ 5 years 55%; 95% CI (24,92) ≥ 10 years 77%; 95% CI (14,163)	$p = 0.0001$ $p = 0.01$
LIAUW et al. [10]	Single institution	348	OER 5–10 years 2.33 (0.6–4.06) 10.1–20 years 2.35 (0.05–4.66)	
BOORJIAN et al. [17]	CaPSURE	9,780	HR 1.59; 95% CI (0.97–2.6)	
PICKLES and PHILLIPS [12]	British Columbia Registry	39,261	SIR (RT compared to no RT) > 5 years 8% > 10 years 89%	
MOON et al.[8] EBRT EBRT/implant Implant	SEER	297,069	AOR 1.63; 95% CI (1.44–1.84) 1.08 1.4	$p < 0.05$
NEUGUT et al. [15]	SEER	141,761	RR < 5 years 1.0 (0.8–1.2) 5–8 years 1.3 (1.0–1.7) > 8 years 1.5 (1.1–1.2)	

OER, observed to expected ratio; HR, hazard ratio; RR, relative risk; AOR, adjusted odds ratios; EBRT, external beam radiation therapy

9.6
Lung Cancer

Although not geographically in close proximity to the prostate, SEER database analyses have reported an increased incidence of lung cancer in patients with prostate cancer treated with radiation. BRENNER et al. [7] and MOON et al. [8], both using SEER data, found a statistically significant radiation-associated increase relative risk in lung cancer after radiotherapy for prostate cancer. An increasing risk of lung cancer correlated with increasing survival time, meaning the longer the patients lived the greater the chance they would develop lung cancer. LEVI on the other hand, using a smaller database, did not find an increased risk of lung cancer in patients with prostate cancer treated with radiation. PICKLES and PHILLIPS [12] reported a significant increased risk of tumors of the pleura in men with prostate cancer receiving radiation. What is not explicitly stated in their report is what is meant by tumors of the pleura and whether this also includes lung cancer.

A history of tobacco abuse could be one explanation of the higher rate of lung cancer in men with prostate cancer treated with radiation. There was, however, no difference in the proportion of men who smoked or ever smoked between men who had surgery or radiation in a Canadian case controlled study [23]. In an attempt to explain the increased risk, BRENNER et al. [7] hypothesized given the treatment techniques of the time the lung would have received 0.6 Gy, almost two orders of magnitude less than the bladder and rectum would have received. The increased incidence of lung cancer may be as a result of the low radiation dose which is supported by the increase in relative risk of lung cancer development from 5% in the 0–5 year time period after radiation compared to 42% $\geq$ 10 years after radiation.

9.7
Male Breast Cancer

Male breast and prostate cancer are hormonally driven cancers, therefore sharing a common thread. A 5% coincidence of male breast cancer with prostate cancer exists but it is important to distinguish between metastatic spread of cancer [24]. A few sin-gle institution case reports have documented male breast cancer being diagnosed a number of years after the diagnosis of prostate cancer in patients receiving hormone therapy leading to speculation of the role of estrogen in the development of male breast cancer [25, 26]. None of the reports using SEER information, however, reported an increase in male breast cancer after prostate radiation [7, 8]. An increased risk of male breast cancer after a diagnosis of prostate cancer was found in a review of the Swedish Cancer Registry [27]. The mode of treatment was not mentioned in the report and development of male breast cancer was hypothesized to be related to estrogen therapy the men may have received although some of the increased risk could be related to a BRCA2 mutation in some patients [28].

9.8
Pancreas Cancer

Like lung, the pancreas is not located in geographic proximity to the prostate therefore it can be difficult to explain the exact mechanism for second malignancy development in the pancreas as a result of radiotherapy for prostate cancer. Using SEER data from 1973 to 1990, NEUGUT et al. [29] found an increased relative risk (1.2, 95% CI 1.1–1.3) of pancreas cancer as a second malignancy in men who were treated for prostate cancer. This has been the only study, SEER based or single institution, to report an increase in pancreatic cancer in patients with prostate cancer. Inclusion of synchronous pancreatic tumors may be the reason for the finding since the authors only excluded the first 6 months after diagnosis. This may point to a role of other etiologies such as a relationship to other tobacco-related malignancies or an undiscovered genetic susceptibility in a certain patient population.

9.9
Leukemia

Using SEER data, NEUGET et al. [15] reported a radiotherapy associated risk of acute myelocytic leukemia of 0.1% in 10 years. The mean bone marrow dose for 14 prostate cancer patients treated with conformal radiotherapy ranged from 3.5 Gy to 7.7 Gy [30]. This dose range is similar to that calculated for patients treated with radiation for ankylosing spondylitis and for women with cervical cancer treated with radiation [31, 32]. An increased risk of 1% in the 10 years following radiation was reported for patients with ankylosing spondylitis treated with radiation and 0.3% for women with cervical cancer treated with radiation. A higher risk of leukemia within the first 5 years was not detected by other researchers when compared to atomic bomb survivors, but BRENNER et al. did find a non-significant 5% increased relative risk for leukemia during the first 5 years after diagnosis [5, 7, 12]. The impact of treatment with intensity modulated radiation therapy (IMRT) on the development of second malignant tumors including leukemia will need to be investigated in the future since IMRT spreads lower doses of radiation over greater areas of non-cancerous tissue [33, 34].

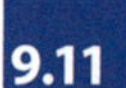

9.10
Surveillance Strategies for Prostate Cancer Patients Treated with Radiotherapy

Surveillance strategies should target patients at increased risk for second malignancy development and start approximately 5 years after completion of treatment. It is unclear whether screening should occur only in patients who are without evidence of biochemical failure or should all patients regardless of disease status be screened. Screening recommendations should be developed for detection of lung, rectal and bladder cancer since these are the tumors determined to be more prevalent after treatment for prostate cancer. More aggressive screening recommendations should be considered for patients who have abused tobacco because the incidences of lung and bladder cancers are higher in this patient population. The data are not clear at this point, which screening tests would be best for identification of second malignant tumors in patients > 5 years from the end of treatment. Urine cytology is a non-invasive test while cystoscopy visualizes the entire bladder but is invasive. Chest X-rays are an inexpensive method of evaluating the lungs but may not be able to detect smaller tumors compared to a high resolution CT scan. Further studies are necessary to determine the most appropriate screening tests in this patient population.

9.11
Second Malignant Tumors after Treatment for Bladder Cancer

An increased risk of second tumors has also been reported after bladder cancer treatment [35–42]. Secondary upper urinary tract tumors were reported in 3.1% of patients following treatment of primary transitional cell carcinoma of the bladder [37]. The mean latency between initial treatment and development of bladder cancer was 80 months and a significant difference in the development of a second malignant tumor was not seen regardless of initial treatment. A higher incidence of lung cancer, standardized incidence ratio (SIR) of 1.3 among males and 2.6 among females, was noted in a report of > 10,000 patients treated for bladder cancer in Finland [39]. An increased SIR was also found for larynx caner in males, SIR 1.7, and kidney cancer in females, SIR 3.6. A greater risk of second cancers was seen among patients < 60 years of age at the time of diagnosis of the bladder cancer compared to patients > 60 years of age. Using the same patients, SALMINEN et al. [38] investigated the role of tobacco-related products in the development of second malignancy and found 44% of the second malignancies were smoking related. Lung cancer was the most frequent occurring second malignancy followed by larynx cancer in men, SIR 1.67, and kidney cancer in women, SIR 3.55. An excess risk was noted up to 20 years after diagnosis. In an analysis of patients with early stage bladder cancer treated on a prospective trial of bacillus Calmette-Guerin, HERR et al. [40] found 21% of patients developed upper tract tumors after a median interval of 7.3 years. The majority of the cancers were invasive with ⅓ of patients dying of the upper tract tumors. Multiple primary superficial bladder tumors increased the risk of upper urinary tract cancers in an analysis of > 1500 patients treated for superficial bladder tumors [41]. The increased risk of upper tract tumors probably represents the multifocal nature of this disease as opposed to the adverse effects of treatment. FABBRI et al. [42] found a relatively constant high incidence of prostate cancer and kidney cancer in patients with bladder cancer over time [42]. The authors, however, included cases of second cancer diagnosed within 6 months after the diagnosis of bladder cancer making it difficult to know if the cancers were synchronous or metachronous.

Second malignant tumors developing after treatment for bladder cancer may not be related to the treatment received, as was seen in patients treated with radiotherapy for prostate cancer, but may be related to the etiologic agent causing the bladder cancer initially. Post-treatment follow-up strategies should be monitor not only for bladder cancer recurrence but also other tobacco-related malignancies.

9.12
The Effect of Technology on Second Malignant Tumor Development after Prostate Radiotherapy

Technologic advances such as improved target localization by CT treatment planning and sophisticated treatment planning algorithms have improved the ability of radiation oncologists to shrink the treatment field for patients with prostate cancer undergoing radiotherapy. Normal tissue exposure from radiation would be decreased as radiation oncologist move away from conventional radiotherapy to three dimensional conformal radiotherapy (3-D CRT).

Radiation technique and delivered dose cannot be determined from SEER data and only one paper mentioned radiation technique in reporting second malignant tumors of the bladder after radiotherapy for prostate cancer [18]. The importance of radiation dose and field size can be inferred from the studies not reporting an increased risk of second malignancy in patients having an interstitial implant as part of the management for their prostate cancer. These patients received external beam radiation doses lower than that received by patients treated with external beam radiotherapy alone. The volume of tissue receiving high radiation doses should decrease as treatment progresses from 3D CRT to IMRT. The result of this, however, will be a larger volume of normal tissue exposed to lower doses of radiation. In addition, total body exposure will be increased, secondary to the increased number of monitor units used to deliver the modulated treatment, due to leakage radiation [34].

HALL and WUU have estimated IMRT is likely to almost double the incidence of second malignancies compared with conventional radiotherapy with the number being higher for younger patients. KRY et al. [33] estimated a conservative maximal risk of fatal secondary malignancy associated with six IMRT and one conventional treatment plans for prostate cancer. Depending upon treatment energy and type of linear accelerator, IMRT treatments required 3.5–4.9 times as many monitor units to deliver the prescribed treatment compared to the conventional plan. The conservative maximal risk of a fatal second malignancy varied depending upon beam energy and linear accelerator.

The use of proton beam therapy in the treatment of prostate cancer is increasing with an increasing number of proton beam centers planned for the United States. The risk of second malignancies in patients treated with proton beam therapy is hypothesized to be lower than for patients treated with X-rays because of the unique physical properties of the proton beam. An incidence rate of 82 second cancers per 100,000 person-years was reported in patients with ≥ 5 years of follow-up who received proton therapy [43]. The contribution of proton beam therapy to the development of second malignancies could not be determined from this study since all patients who developed second malignancies had a combination of photons and protons. Further studies are needed with the expected increase in the use of proton beam therapy in the future.

9.13
Cost-Effectiveness of Screening for Second Malignant Tumors

Currently, there are no studies evaluating the cost-effectiveness of screening for second malignant tumors after prostate cancer radiation. Studies evaluating the cost-effectiveness of surveillance strategies for breast cancer survivors have been recommended while CT screening for lung cancer in Hodgkin's lymphoma survivors may increase overall and disease-free survival, especially for patient who smoke cigarettes [44, 45].

Any screening program should utilize non-invasive means for detecting a tumor with as low as a false negative rate as possible. General screening for many of the urologic malignancies, however, do not meet the criteria for a successful cancer screening program namely, high prevalence, availability of a sensitive and specific screening test, ability to detect clinically important cancers at an early stage, and cost-effectiveness [46]. A screening program for bladder cancer in a high risk population utilizing a urinary dipstick for hematuria, the nuclear matrix proten-22 (NMP-22)test (BladderChek, Matritech, Inc., Newton, MA) voided urine cytology and a molecular cytology test (UroVysion, Abbott Molecular Inc., Des Plaines, Il) detected a 3.3% rate of bladder cancer [47]. The authors reported the most efficient screening tool was the combination of UroVysion, cytology and urinary dipstick testing. Urinary NMP-22 was found to be a cost-effective marker for early detection of bladder cancer in patients with hematuria or other indications for risk of bladder cancer [48].

References

1. Brown LM, Chen BE, Pfeiffer RM et al (2007) Risk of second non-hematological malignancies among 376,825 breast cancer survivors. Breast Cancer Res Treat 106:439–451

2. Kirova YM, Gambotti L, De Rycke Y et al (2007) Risk of second malignancies after adjuvant radiotherapy for breast cancer: a large-scale, single-institution review. Int J Radiat Oncol Biol Phys 68:359–363

3. Virtanen A, Pukkala E, Auvinen A (2007) Angiosarcoma after radiotherapy: a cohort study of 332,163 Finnish cancer patients. Br J Cancer 97:115–117

4. Movsas B, Hanlon AL, Pinover W et al (1998) Is there an increased risk of second primaries following prostate irradiation? Int J Radiat Oncol Biol Phys 41:251–255

5. Levi F, Randimbison L, Te VC et al (1999) Second primary cancers in patients with lung carcinoma. Cancer 1999;86:186–190

6. Johnstone PA, Powell CR, Riffenburgh R et al (1998) Second primary malignancies in T1-3N0 prostate cancer patients treated with radiation therapy with 10-year followup. J Urol 159:946–949

7. Brenner DJ, Curtis RE, Hall EJ et al (2000) Second malignancies in prostate carcinoma patients after radiotherapy compared with surgery. Cancer 88:398–406

8. Moon K, Stukenborg GJ, Keim J et al (2006) Cancer incidence after localized therapy for prostate cancer. Cancer 107:991–998

9. Baxter NN, Tepper JE, Durham SB et al (2005) Increased risk of rectal cancer after prostate radiation: a population-based study. Gastroenterology 128:819–824

10. Liauw SL, Sylvester JE, Morris CG et al (2006) Second malignancies after prostate brachytherapy: incidence of bladder and colorectal cancers in patients with 15 years of potential follow-up. Int J Radiat Oncol Biol Phys 66:669–673

11. Gutman SA, Merrick GS, Butler WM et al (2006) Temporal relationship between prostate brachytherapy and the diagnosis of colorectal cancer. Int J Radiat Oncol Biol Phys 66:48–55

12. Pickles T, Phillips N (2002) The risk of second malignancy in men with prostate cancer treated with or without radiation in British Columbia, 1984–2000. Radiother Oncol 65:145–151

13. Kendal WS, Eapen L, Macrae R et al (2006) Prostatic irradiation is not associated with any measurable increase in the risk of subsequent rectal cancer. Int J Radiat Oncol Biol Phys 65:661–668

14. Brenner DJ (2006) Induced second cancers after prostate-cancer radiotherapy: no cause for concern? Int J Radiat Oncol Biol Phys 65:637–639

15. Neugut AI, Ahsan H, Robinson E et al (1997) Bladder carcinoma and other second malignancies after radiotherapy for prostate carcinoma. Cancer 79:1600–1604

16. Wegner HE, Meier T, Klan R et al (1994) Bladder cancer following prostate cancer – an analysis of risk factors. Int Urol Nephrol 26:43–51

17. Boorjian S, Cowan JE, Konety BR et al (2007) Bladder cancer incidence and risk factors in men with prostate cancer: results from Cancer of the Prostate Strategic Urologic Research Endeavor. J Urol 177:883–887; discussion 887–888

18. Chrouser K, Leibovich B, Bergstralh E et al (2005) Bladder cancer risk following primary and adjuvant external beam radiation for prostate cancer. J Urol 174:107–110; discussion 110–101

19. Bostrom PJ, Soloway MS, Manoharan M et al (2008) Bladder cancer after radiotherapy for prostate cancer: detailed analysis of pathological features and outcome after radical cystectomy. J Urol 179:91–95; discussion 95

20. McKenzie M, MacLennan I, Kostashuk E et al (1999) Postirradiation sarcoma after external beam radiation therapy for localized adenocarcinoma of the prostate: report of three cases. Urology 53:1228

21. Chandan VS, Wolsh L (2003) Postirradiation angiosarcoma of the prostate. Arch Pathol Lab Med 127:876–878

22. Prevost JB, Bossi A, Sciot R et al (2004) Post-irradiation sarcoma after external beam radiation therapy for localized adenocarcinoma of the prostate. Tumori 90:618–621

23. Rohan TE, Hislop TG, Howe GR et al (1997) Cigarette smoking and risk of prostate cancer: a population-based case-control study in Ontario and British Columbia, Canada. Eur J Cancer Prev 6:382–388

24. Leibowitz SB, Garber JE, Fox EA et al (2003) Male patients with diagnoses of both breast cancer and prostate cancer. Breast J 9:208–212

25. Coard K, McCartney T (2004) Bilateral synchronous carcinoma of the male breast in a patient receiving estrogen therapy for carcinoma of the prostate: cause or coincidence? South Med J 97:308–310

26. Khalbuss WE, Ambaye A, Goodison S et al (2006) Papillary carcinoma of the breast in a male patient with a treated prostatic carcinoma diagnosed by fine-needle aspiration biopsy: a case report and review of the literature. Diagn Cytopathol 34:214–217

27. Thellenberg C, Malmer B, Tavelin B et al (2003) Second primary cancers in men with prostate cancer: an increased risk of male breast cancer. J Urol 169:1345–1348

28. Karlsson CT, Malmer B, Wiklund F et al (2006) Breast cancer as a second primary in patients with prostate cancer – estrogen treatment or association with family history of cancer? J Urol 176:538–543

29. Neugut AI, Ahsan H, Robinson E (1995) Pancreas cancer as a second primary malignancy. A population-based study. Cancer 76:589–592

30. Gershkevitsh E, Rosenberg I, Dearnaley DP et al (1999) Bone marrow doses and leukaemia risk in radiotherapy of prostate cancer. Radiother Oncol 53:189–197

31. Darby SC, Doll R, Gill SK et al (1987) Long term mortality after a single treatment course with X-rays in patients treated for ankylosing spondylitis. Br J Cancer 55:179–190

32. Boice JD, Jr., Blettner M, Kleinerman RA et al (1987) Radiation dose and leukemia risk in patients treated for cancer of the cervix. J Natl Cancer Inst 79:1295–1311

33. Kry SF, Salehpour M, Followill DS et al (2005) The calculated risk of fatal secondary malignancies from intensity-modulated radiation therapy. Int J Radiat Oncol Biol Phys 62:1195–1203

34. Hall EJ, Wuu CS (2003) Radiation-induced second cancers: the impact of 3D-CRT and IMRT. Int J Radiat Oncol Biol Phys 56:83–88

35. Greven KM, Spera JA, Solin LJ et al (1992) Secondary malignant neoplasms in patients with bladder carcinoma. Urology 39:204–206

36. Xu YM, Cai RX, Wu P et al (1993) Urethral carcinosarcoma following total cystectomy for bladder carcinoma. Urol Int 50:104–107

37. Schwartz CB, Bekirov H, Melman A (1992) Urothelial tumors of upper tract following treatment of primary bladder transitional cell carcinoma. Urology 40:509–511

38. Salminen E, Pukkala E, Teppo L (1994) Bladder cancer and the risk of smoking-related cancers during follow-up. J Urol 152:1420–1423

39. Salminen E, Pukkala E, Teppo L et al (1994) Subsequent primary cancers following bladder cancer. Eur J Cancer 30A:303–307

40. Herr HW, Cookson MS, Soloway SM (1996) Upper tract tumors in patients with primary bladder cancer followed for 15 years. J Urol 156:1286–1287

41. Millan-Rodriguez F, Chechile-Toniolo G, Salvador-Bayarri J et al (2000) Upper urinary tract tumors after primary superficial bladder tumors: prognostic factors and risk groups. J Urol 164:1183–1187

42. Fabbri C, Ravaioli A, Bucchi L et al (2007) Risk of cancer of the prostate and of the kidney parenchyma following bladder cancer. Tumori 93:124–128

43. Chung C, Yock T, Johnson J, Esty B, Tarbell N (2007) Proton Radiation Therapy and the Incidence of Secondary Malignancies. Int J Radiat Oncol Biol Phys 69:S178

44. Tolaney SM, Winer EP (2007) Follow-up care of patients with breast cancer. Breast 16 Suppl 2:S45–50

45. Das P, Ng AK, Earle CC et al (2006) Computed tomography screening for lung cancer in Hodgkin's lymphoma survivors: decision analysis and cost-effectiveness analysis. Ann Oncol 17:785–793

46. Stephenson AJ, Kuritzky L, Campbell SC (2007) Screening for urologic malignancies in primary care: pros, cons, and recommendations. Cleve Clin J Med 74 Suppl 3:S6–14

47. Steiner H, Bergmeister M, Verdorfer I et al (2008) Early results of bladder-cancer screening in a high-risk population of heavy smokers. BJU Int [Epub ahead of print]

48. Zippe C, Pandrangi L, Potts JM et al (1999) NMP22: a sensitive, cost-effective test in patients at risk for bladder cancer. Anticancer Res 19:2621–2623

Cardiotoxic Effects of Radiation Therapy in Hodgkin's Lymphoma and Breast Cancer Survivors and the Potential Mitigating Effects of Exercise

Karen M. Mustian, M. Jacob Adams, Ronald G. Schwartz, Steven E. Lipshultz, and Louis S. Constine

CONTENTS

10.1 Introduction

Radiation-induced cardiovascular disease can compromise the quality of life of cancer survivors. Aerobic exercise training is an intervention that offers the potential to modify the expression and possibly the physiologic severity of cardiac injury. In this chapter, we review evidence supporting this approach to helping our growing survivorship population.

Historically the heart was considered to be resistant to radiation injury. However, cardiovascular disease resulting from radiation therapy that incidentally includes portions of the heart is now known to initiate, augment, or precipitate a spectrum of sequelae. Numerous reports over the last four decades document the cardiac damage which can accompany treatment for Hodgkin's lymphoma (HL) and breast cancer (BC). The delayed sequelae stemming from this cardiovascular disease dramatically increases the potential loss of productive life years among these cancer survivors by increasing morbidity and mortality [3, 4]. Most dramatically, this is illustrated by the fact that cardiac disease is the third leading cause of death in HL survivors treated with mediastinal radiotherapy, ranking below only disease recurrence and secondary cancers [7, 33, 53]. Just as importantly, cardiopulmonary compromise may be related to the persistent fatigue that is often seen in cancer survivors [42, 61, 67]. After years of concern that exercise was dangerous to people in the general population who had heart failure, it has now been shown to be safe and to improve cardiac function and fatigue. However, it is not clear whether exercise regimens are safe and effective for improving fatigue and cardiac function in cancer survivors treated with thoracic radiotherapy.

The purpose of this discussion is to review the potential cardiac sequelae of chest irradiation, the evidence linking cardiac function to fatigue and quality of life and finally the published evidence showing exercise is safe and effective in patients and survivors treated with chest irradiation. Because the most common cancers treated with chest radiotherapy with a significant number of survivors are HL and BC, we focus on the evidence from these two populations.

K. M. Mustian, PhD
Assistant Professor, Department of Radiation Oncology, Department of Community and Preventive Medicine, Susan B. Anthony Institute for Women and Gender Studies, Center for Future Health, University of Rochester School of Medicine and Dentistry, 601 Elmwood Avenue, Box 704, Rochester, NY 14642, USA

complete authors' adresses see list of Contributors

10.2
Cardiopulmonary Sequelae

All of the structures of the heart including the pericardium, myocardium, valves, conduction system, and coronary arteries can be damaged by radiation therapy. Therefore the spectrum of radiation-induced cardiac disease is quite broad and includes both direct (Table 10.1) and indirect effects (Table 10.2) [1]. This range of possible manifestations draws largely from reports on HL survivors, while the risk in BC survivors has only been unequivocally demonstrated for ischemic disease through epidemiologic studies of myocardial infarction risk and perfusion scan data. The latter potentially also relates to the risk of restrictive cardiac changes affecting function. Furthermore the risk in BC survivors is likely restricted to patients treated with radiotherapy that included the internal mammary nodes on the left side.

Hodkin`s: Three reports representing a combined 4553 survivors treated between the 1960s and 1990 with mediastinal radiotherapy demonstrated that cardiovascular disease (CVD) accounted for between 9.4% and 16% of all deaths [3, 4, 6, 33, 53]. Absolute excess mortality from cardiovascular disease ranged from 11.9 to 48.9 per 10,000 patient years. This excess CVD mortality is predominantly caused by the increased risk of fatal myocardial infarction. Studies of HL survivors treated with mediastinal radiotherapy have estimated that they are 2.2 to 7.6 times more likely to die from MI than the general population [31, 53, 49]. This risk becomes statistically significant 5–10 years after treatment [7].

A recent update of a Dutch cohort of 1474 HL survivors, treated before age 41 between 1965 and 1995, established that CVD incidence as well as mortality is increased [6] among this group. HL survivors had a three- to five-fold increased incidence of CVD compared with the general population, with a 24%

Table 10.1. Spectrum of radiation-induced cardiovascular disease. (Modified from [2] with permission)

Manifestation	Comments
Pericarditis	1. During therapy: Associated with mediastinal tumor and some chemotherapy agents such as cyclophosphamide [83] 2. Post-therapy: Acute effusion, chronic effusion, pericarditis, constrictive pericarditis. Seen with high doses of RT and large volumes of heart within the RT field [83]
Myocardial fibrosis	1. Fibrosis secondary to microvasculature changes [83] 2. Frequently with normal left ventricular dimensions, ejection fraction and fractional shortening as measured by radionuclide scan or echocardiogram [50] 3. Progressive, restrictive cardiomyopathy with fibrosis may occur. This can lead to pulmonary vascular disease and pulmonary hypertension [50] 4. Diastolic dysfunction may occur alone as well as with systolic dysfunction [50]
Coronary artery disease	1. The structural changes in the coronary arteries associated with radiation therapy are essentially the same as those of ordinary atherosclerosis [83] 2. Premature fibrosis may accelerate atherosclerosis [12, 86] 3. Distribution of arteries affected tends to be anterior with anterior weighted RT 4. ↑ Rates of silent ischemia (see autonomic effects) [31]
Valvular disease	1. Predominantly mitral valve and aortic valve [15] 2. ↑ Regurgitation and stenosis with ↑ time since therapy [15]
Conduction system / arrhythmia	1. Complete or incomplete right bundle branch block is suggestive of right bundle branch fibrosis [80] 2. Initial conduction abnormalities may progress to complete heart block and cause congestive heart failure, requiring a pacemaker [80] 3. Complete heart block rarely occurs without other radiation-associated abnormalities of the heart [80]
Autonomic dysfunction	1. Frequent cardiac dysfunction with tachycardia, loss of circadian rhythm and respiratory phasic heart rate variability [32] 2. Signs listed in #1 are similar to a denervated heart. This raises the question of whether such changes in survivors are related to autonomic nervous system damage [32] 3. ↓ Perception of anginal pain [32]

Table 10.2. Indirect effects of mediastinal radiation on the cardiovascular system. (Modified from [2] with permission)

Manifestation	Comments
Mediastinal fibrosis	↓ Success of cardiovascular surgery [38]
Lung fibrosis	Chronic, restrictive and can be progressive [19]
Scoliosis and ↓ skeletal muscle	↓ Cardiovascular and lung function [19]
Thyroid	Usually hypothyroid [74] Affects cardiovascular function and lipid profile. May cause pericarditis
Thoracic duct fibrosis	Chylothorax-late onset and extremely rare [85]

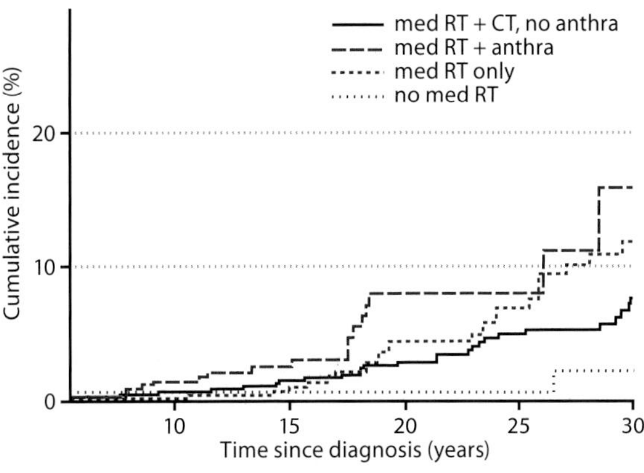

Fig. 10.1. Cumulative incidence of all CVDs combined by treatment group with death from any cause as competing risk (including CVDs) (reproduced from [6]). *med RT*, Mediastinal RT; *CT*, chemotherapy; *anthra*, anthracyclines; *MI*, myocardial infarction; *AP*, angina pectoris; *CHF*, congestive heart failure

cumulative incidence after a median follow-up of 18.7 years. The relative risk for myocardial infarction (MI) and congestive heart failure (CHF) was 3.6 and 4.9, respectively, which translated into 35.7 excess cases of MI and 25.6 excess cases of CHF per 10,000 patient-years. The researchers estimated that HL therapy accounted for 66%–80% of all CVD events in survivors (Fig. 10.1).

Breast: Relative risk estimates of fatal MI after left-sided radiotherapy for BC range as high as 2.2 compared with women who were treated for right-sided BC [71]. Further evaluation has revealed that the increased risk appears limited to those who received the highest dose-volumes of cardiac radiation, which would be women who had their internal mammary lymph nodes irradiated. Convincing evidence that ischemic heart disease is correlated with RT was reported in the Early Breast Cancer Trialists' Collaborative Group meta-analysis of randomized clinical trials. The update in 2005 showed an increased relative risk (RR) of mortality from heart disease among women treated with RT versus no RT (RR = 1.27) [18]. Long-term cardiac outcomes from randomized clinical trials of post-mastectomy RT have been reported [48, 76]. These reveal an increased risk of cardiac mortality (RR ≈ 2.5) in association with left-sided IMN RT. Retrospective population-based investigations have compared mortality endpoints by laterality or by left-side RT versus surgical controls. Two recent investigations showed an increased risk of cardiac mortality (HR ≈ 1.5) among left versus right-side cancers treated

with RT in the 1970s, but no apparent increased risk with more modern treatments [22, 28]. However, most studies have demonstrated a significant increase in CAD and/or non-fatal MI associated with left compared to either right-sided RT or no RT [11, 43].

Studies using clinical imaging of the heart underscore the danger of prematurely concluding that the newer methods of RT pose no risk to the heart. Investigators from several institutions have evaluated the heart in patients treated for BC with cardiac perfusion imaging. Researchers at Duke University have accumulated the largest series of patients. Between 1998 and 2001, 114 patients with left-sided BC underwent pre- and serial post-RT single photon emission computed tomography (SPECT) gated cardiac perfusion scans. Studies published on this cohort of patients demonstrate that: (1) radiotherapy to the left chest wall/breast using modern techniques causes perfusion defects in 50%–63% of women 6–24 months post-RT [34]; (2) that the incidence of perfusion defects is associated with the volume of left ventricle irradiated; (3) that the perfusion defects generally persist 3–5 years post-RT [87]; and (4) that the perfusion defects are associated with abnormalities in regional wall motion, subtle reductions in ejection fraction, [52] and episodes of chest pain [87].

Based on the available evidence from research with HL patients, which may translate for BC patients as well, the severity and types of manifestations depend upon the presence of risk factors such as higher total dose (> 35–40 Gy), higher fractionated dose ($\geq$ 2.0 Gy per day), increased volume of heart exposure, relative amounts of radiation delivered to specific parts of the heart, lack of subcarinal blocking, tumor located next to the heart, younger age at exposure, length of time since exposure, type of radiation source, use of adjuvant cardiotoxic chemotherapy, and additional known risk factors for cardiovascular disease [3, 4]. While certain cardiac sequelae have been greatly reduced by the use of modern techniques, such as acute pericarditis, the effect on the incidence of other events such as myocardial infarction is not as clear.

It should also be noted that both clinically discernible cardiac complications and subclinical abnormalities with cardiac screening modalities such as echocardiogram or nuclear perfusion imaging occur in Hodgkin's and BC survivors after radiation therapy with the presence of asymptomatic abnormalities being much higher among these survivors [73]. The clinical manifestations of radiation-induced heart disease are listed in Table 10.3. The symptoms of a particular cardiac abnormality in survivors is similar to the same problem in the general population. One significant exception may be the fact that survivors treated with chest irradia-

Table 10.3. Signs, symptoms, evaluation and treatment of patients at risk for late effects of thoracic radiotherapy. (Modified from [19] with permission)

Late effects	Treatment[a]	Signs and symptoms	Screening and diagnostic tests	Management and intervention
Pericarditis	>35 Gy	Fatigue, dyspnea on exertion, chest pain, cyanosis, ascites, peripheral edema, hypotension, friction rub, muffled heart sounds, venous distension, pulses paradoxus, Kussmaul's Sign	Electrocardiogram Chest X-ray, Echocardiogram	Pericardiocentesis Pericardiectomy
Cardiomyopathy (Myocardial disease)	>35 Gy or >25 Gy and anthracycline	Fatigue, cough, dyspnea on exertion, peripheral edema, hypertension, tachypnea, rales, tachycardia, murmur, extra heart sounds, hepatomegaly, syncope, palpitations	Echocardiogram and/or radionuclide ventriculography – Evaluate diastolic and systolic function	Education regarding risks of: alcohol, isometric exercise, smoking and other drug use, pregnancy, and anesthesia Afterload reducers, beta-blocker, antiarrhythmics, diuretics, digoxin Cardiac transplant
Coronary heart disease	>30 Gy	Chest pain, dyspnea, diaphoresis, hypotension, pallor, nausea, arrhythmia	Exercise or dobutamine stress test with radionuclide perfusion imaging, or echocardiography (Frequency depends on risk factor profile and symptoms)	Risk factor modifications including diet and conditioning regimens Cardiac medications and lipid lowering agents Coronary artery bypass graft or angioplasty
Valvular disease	>30 Gy	Cough, weakness, dyspnea on exertion, new murmur, rales, peripheral edema or any other sign of congestive heart failure	Echocardiogram Cardiac catheterization	Ampicillin prophylaxis for dental or surgical procedures Replacement of valve
Arrhythmia		Palpitations, light-headedness, syncope	Electrocardiogram and 24-h ECG Evaluation for other abnormalities	Pacemaker

[a] Treatment: cumulative radiation exposure of the mediastinum at this level or higher clearly indicates increased risk for the specific complication and thus the need to screen for it; however, the complication may also occur at lower doses

tion are more likely to suffer asymptomatic myocardial ischemia and infarction. This would be due to the fact that radiation has been shown to damage the nerves innervating the heart as suggested by the increased risk of autonomic dysfunction in these survivors [5]. The increased risk of myocardial infarction and its devastating consequences, along with the fact that it is more likely to occur without warning in this population, makes it that much more important to screen for traditional risk factors for coronary heart disease, such as hypertension and hypercholesterolemia, and treat them aggressively.

Additionally, the cardiomyopathy and cardiac failure associated with thoracic radiation is significantly different than that occurring most commonly in the general population and that due to anthracycline therapy. The last two are associated with a dilated cardiomyopathy and characterized by systolic dysfunction. In contrast, because radiation causes fibrosis of the myocardium, restrictive cardiomyopathy characterized by diastolic dysfunction, predominates in survivors treated with RT alone. Although clinically evident heart failure is rare in survivors treated with radiotherapy alone, studies evaluating survivors with imaging technologies show that subclinical changes are common and may be progressive. The concern is that these subclinical diastolic abnormalities may progress over the long-term to systolic dysfunction, congestive heart failure or both. In either case, one of the most common, albeit non-specific, symptoms of heart failure is fatigue

10.3
Fatigue and Its Relationship to Cardiopulmonary Sequelae

10.3.1
Cancer Related Fatigue

The most prevalent problem reported by all cancer survivors is fatigue; commonly referred to as cancer-related fatigue (CRF) [16, 37, 41, 42, 46, 61, 67, 77]. Cancer survivors report that CRF is first noticed with diagnosis. This CRF worsens during treatment and can persist for months and even years after treatments are complete [37, 41, 42, 61, 67]. It is common to see CRF persist even when the survi-

vor's cancer is undetectable or in remission [37, 41, 42, 61, 67].

CRF is reported by 60%–100% of patients, with 41% or more reporting severe CRF (a score > 7 on an 11-point Likert scale where 0 = no CRF and 10 = CRF incapacitating) during treatment [17, 41, 46, 55, 36, 37, 63]. As many as 81% of cancer survivors report that CRF persists, with 17%–38% reporting persistent CRF at 6 months or longer after completing treatment as severe [9, 42, 61, 63, 67, 75]. This persistent and sometimes severe CRF may be a strong clinical indicator of portending cardiovascular disease resulting from radiation therapy to the chest.

CRF is typically defined as a multifaceted, subjective, physiological state characterized by persistent, overwhelming exhaustion and a decreased capacity for physical and mental work. The nature of CRF in cancer survivors makes it a symptom that is difficult to define well. In general, CRF is differentiated from the fatigue experienced by healthy individuals because of its severity, its impact on the quality of life of cancer survivors, the fact that it is not alleviated by rest, and its association with cardiovascular toxicity resulting from therapeutic radiation to the chest [3, 42, 61, 67]. The impact of CRF is far reaching because of its day-to-day impact on quality of life. Cancer survivors endure tremendous distress as a result of CRF because of the inability to prevent or alleviate this debilitating side-effects and the co-morbidities like cardiovascular disease that are associated with its presence [3, 42, 61, 67, 77].

10.3.2
Fatigue in HL Patients and Possible Associations with Cardiopulmonary Status

In HL survivors, fatigue is one of their most common complaints, with one investigator finding that 30% reported symptoms consistent with chronic fatigue, compared to 12% of the general population [51]. Recent studies from the Netherlands [60], Norway [39, 40] and the Dana Farber Cancer Institute [69] have reaffirmed that fatigue, quality of life, or both, are worse in HL survivors than in the general public or sibling controls. In HL survivors, fatigue may be associated with other known late effects such as hypothyroidism, cardiovascular disease, pulmonary dysfunction, muscle atrophy and/or psychological sequelae [69].

In the Norwegian cohort, about half of the subjects were assessed 8 years earlier [51]. Subjects with chronic fatigue at baseline continued to have worse fatigue than those who did not. The association between B-symptoms at diagnosis and chronic fatigue revealed in the original study was also reaffirmed in the larger sample [39], and suggests a relationship with the cytokines responsible for systemic symptoms ("B") in HL. A second report from this cohort suggested chronic fatigue in HL survivors was more related to physical problems than psychological [40].

At least two studies have demonstrated a possible association between fatigue or quality of life and cardiac status. In the Dana Farber study, multivariate analysis revealed that self-reported cardiac disease, history of tobacco use, psychiatric conditions, and low exercise frequency were all associated with worse fatigue [69]. ADAMS et al. [5] in a study of 48 survivors of adolescent or young adulthood HL treated with mediastinal radiotherapy showed that the physical composite score (PCS) on the SF36 quality of life scale correlated with peak oxygen consumption on exercise stress testing, a measure of cardiopulmonary function. Results suggested that cardiopulmonary function explained 30% of the variation in PCS (r-squared = 0.30, $p < 0.001$) and 13% of the variation in fatigue (r-squared = 0.13, $p < 0.021$). Unpublished data by this group demonstrated the same correlation with PCS measured a median 5 years later. This relationship is unsurprising because fatigue may be an early clinical indicator of heart failure, especially heart failure due to diastolic dysfunction which often does not present in the classic manner of systolic heart failure.

10.4
Exercise Interventions for Fatigue and Cardiopulmonary Function Among Cancer Survivors

10.4.1
Rationale for Exercise Interventions in Cancer Survivors Treated with Mediastinal Radiotherapy

Although evidenced-based guidelines exist for the treatment of heart failure and myocardial infarction, the treatment of diastolic heart failure in general is not well studied and no reports exist that specifically address radiation associated cardiac disease.

Consequently, prevention is the clearest approach to "treating" radiation-induced cardiotoxicity. By definition, prevention suggests that effective interventions need to be initiated and continued prior to, during and after radiation therapy. Modern radiotherapy techniques decrease the dose-volume of the heart irradiated and probably decrease the risk of most types of cardiac disease. Modern techniques include using three-dimensional treatment planning, a linear accelerator as a radiation source, equally weighted anterior/posterior portals each treated daily, and a conformal blocking to minimize cardiac exposures. However, these methods do not eliminate cardiovascular sequelae. Thus effective non-invasive and non-pharmacologic therapy targeting improvements in cardiorespiratory function could prevent or delay the onset of cardiovascular disease. Through this mechanism or independently by reducing CRF, exercise might significantly reduce the symptoms and co-morbidity burden among survivors of HL and BC.

Exercise training leads to several adaptive responses involving both central (i.e., heart and lungs) and peripheral (e.g., vascular function, skeletal muscle oxidative capacity) cardiovascular systems. Central adaptations, such as reductions in left ventricular cavity dilation, increased ejection fraction, improved stroke volume and cardiac output and New York Heart Association functional class, are strongly associated with enhanced global cardiovascular functioning, improvements in quality of life and clinical symptoms, and an overall survival benefit in patients with cardiovascular disease [10, 27, 30].

In the general population, regular exercise has been shown to reduce the risk of myocardial infarction [25] and is accepted as an important intervention to reduce the risk of second heart attacks [81]. It is also an important therapy to delay mortality and improve quality of life in patients with congestive heart failure [44]. Exercise regimens have also demonstrated success in improving fatigue (or quality of life) in populations with diseases other than cancer including chronic heart disease [29, 68].

The improvements from exercise regimens in cardiac function and fatigue in other disease populations therefore supports evaluating exercise as a way to improve both in cancer populations and in particular those at risk for cardiac toxicity from radiotherapy to the chest.

10.4.2
Exercise Interventions: Safety and Efficacy in Cancer Survivors

Preliminary data suggest that exercise may be an effective therapeutic intervention to reduce CRF and improving cardiorespiratory function among survivors of HL and BC. For the purpose of this review and according to the National Cancer Institute, "an individual is considered a cancer survivor from the time of diagnosis, through the balance of his or her life." This definition includes cancer patients receiving treatment as well as those who have completed their therapy among the cohort considered cancer survivors.

It is important to define and differentiate between the terms physical activity and exercise because they are often used interchangeably and inappropriately. Physical activity is defined as any skeletal muscle movement that causes an increase in energy expenditure above a resting basal metabolic rate and encompasses a wide variety of lifestyle and occupational activities [8]. Exercise is defined as physical activity performed in an organized manner (e.g., a specific frequency, intensity, duration, and mode) with the intent of improving health-related outcomes, including cardiovascular fitness, muscular strength, body composition, depression, anxiety, sleep, cognition, and fatigue [8]. In this chapter, the term exercise or physical exercise is used to describe any physical activity intervention designed and delivered with the aim of improving CRF or cardiovascular function.

Physical exercise is a behavioral intervention with the potential promise of mitigating the acute CRF experienced by cancer patients during treatment, the persistent CRF they experience after treatments are complete, and the cardiorespiratory impairment associated with treatments such as radiation therapy [62, 64, 65]. MUSTIAN and colleagues [67], JACOBSEN and colleagues [45], GALVAO and NEWTON [26], KNOLS and colleagues [47], STEVINSON and colleagues [82], SCHMIDTZ and colleagues [78], and MCNEELY and colleagues [54] recently summarized the evidence from randomized controlled clinical trials regarding the benefits from physical exercise interventions implemented with adult cancer survivors during and after treatment. The outcomes that were examined included CRF, emotional distress (e.g., depression, anxiety), quality of life, aerobic capacity, muscular strength, flexibility, body composition, functional capacity, and immunological parameters. In total, 15 of these studies assessed CRF and/or cardiorespiratory function as a primary or secondary outcome among Hodgkin's and/or BC survivors and employed a randomized, controlled clinical trial experimental design. The current article restricts discussion to these 15 randomized controlled clinical trials. See Table 10.4 for a complete summary of these studies.

Of these studies, 12 included BC patients/survivors in the sample, while only three studies included HL patients/survivors. Unfortunately, the randomized clinical trials that included HL patients/survivors evaluated them in a mixed cancer population, and subgroups were not large enough to examine HL patients/survivors independently regarding the influence of exercise on CRF and cardiovascular function. OLDERVOLL and colleagues [70] examined the influence of an aerobic exercise intervention among a non-randomized sample of HL survivors and found that fatigue, physical functioning and maximal aerobic capacity were significantly improved by a home based aerobic exercise program of 20 weeks. These results did not differ based on whether the survivor reported chronic and severe fatigue at baseline or no fatigue at all. Unfortunately, this pilot study by OLDERVOLL and colleagues was a one-arm study, with no randomization and included a small sample of 15 survivors without chronic fatigue, and nine survivors with chronic fatigue in the exercise intervention. Additionally, cardiac and/or pulmonary function were not evaluated [70].

The results of these 15 studies provide preliminary evidence suggesting that exercise is safe and well-tolerated by cancer survivors with a wide range of diagnoses. The safety evidence is primarily generated by a priori evaluation of adverse events stemming from the exercise intervention. The tolerability evidence is primarily developed by a priori assessment of adherence and compliance with the prescribed exercise intervention. These studies also suggest the results are similar for patients throughout the cancer care continuum; during and after surgery, chemotherapy, radiation therapy, hormone therapy, and even salvage therapy. One study also suggests that low-intensity and seated exercise is safe and well-tolerated by women with metastatic BC. This growing body of research suggests that exercise interventions involving moderately intense (55%–75% of heart rate maximum) aerobic exercise (e.g., walking and cycling) ranging from 10–90 min in duration, 3–7 days/week are

Table 10.4. Exercise, cancer-related fatigue and cardiorespiratory function among cancer survivors

Reference	Sample	Treatment	Type of exercise	Results[a]
[56]	Breast cancer patients w/stages I and II diagnoses *n*=14	Chemotherapy	Home-based walking 4–5×/week for 10–45 min @ self-paced % HR maximum with support therapy for 4–6 months	↓ Fatigue ↑ **Walking ability in exercisers compared to controls**
[57]	Breast cancer patients w/stages I and II diagnoses *n*=50	Radiation therapy	Home-based walking 4–5×/week for 20–30 min @ self-paced % heart rate maximum for 6 weeks	↓ Fatigue ↑ Walking ability in exercisers compared to controls
[24]	Mixed solid tumor or lymphoma survivors *n*=62	Post high-dose chemotherapy and autologous peripheral blood stem cell transplant	Supervised bed ergometer cycling daily for 15 min @ 50% heart rate reserve during hospitalization (~ 2 days/week)	↓ Fatigue in exercisers ↑ Fatigue ↓ Vigor in controls
[58]	Breast cancer patients w/stages I –III diagnoses *n*=52	Chemotherapy and radiation therapy	Home-based walking 5×/week for 30 min @ self-paced % heart rate maximum for 6 months	↑ **Functional capacity** ↓ **Fatigue in high vs. low exercisers**
[79]	Breast cancer stages I–II *n*=123	Chemotherapy, radiation therapy and hormone therapy	Self-directed exercise (5×/week for 26 weeks), supervised exercise (3×/week for 26 weeks plus 2 days of home exercise) and usual care (no exercise program but advise on general wellness and exercise)	↑ **Aerobic capacity among the participants in both the self-directed and supervised exercise groups compared to the usual care participants**
[13]	Breast and colon cancer survivors *n*=21	Post surgery, chemotherapy and/or radiation therapy	Low-intensity aerobic exercise (25%–35% heart rate reserve), moderate-intensity aerobic exercise (40%–50% heart rate reserve) and usual care (no exercise) 3×/week for 10 weeks	↑ **Aerobic capacity** ↓ **Fatigue in the two exercise groups compared to the usual care group;** no significant differences between the two different exercise intensity conditions
[21]	Post-menopausal breast cancer survivors *n*=53	Post-surgery, chemotherapy and/or radiation therapy with no hormone therapy	Individually tailored and supervised upright cycle ergometer training 3×/week for 15 weeks versus no-exercise control	↑ **Peak oxygen consumption, peak power output, oxygen consumption at the ventilatory equivalent for oxygen, carbon dioxide and power output at the ventilatory equivalent for oxygen among exercisers compared to controls**
[20]	Cancer survivors *n*=108	Post-surgery, chemotherapy and/or radiation therapy	Group psychotherapy plus exercise versus group psychotherapy alone for 10 weeks	↓ **Fatigue** ↑ Aerobic capacity **among group psychotherapy plus exercise compared to psychotherapy alone**
[72]	Breast cancer *n*=24	Post-treatment within 5 years	Home-based walking at a moderate intensity (55%–65% maximum heart rate) 2–5×/week for 10–30 min for 12 weeks	↓ **Fatigue in exercisers compared to controls**

Table 10.4. Continued

Reference	Sample	Treatment	Type of exercise	Results[a]
[23]	Women and men with mixed solid tumors $n=72$	Post-surgery for a solid tumor, post-chemotherapy and post-radiation No current treatment	Supervised stationary cycling 5×/week for 30 min @ 80% MHR using interval training at 50 RPM	↓ **Fatigue** ↓ Dyspnea among exercisers
[35]	Metastatic breast cancer $n=38$	Chemotherapy	Home-based seated exercise program 3×/week using a videotape	↓ **Fatigue in exercisers compared to controls** ↓ **Physical function in exercisers compared to controls**
[84]	Mixed cancers (lymphomas, breast, gynecologic, testicular) $n=111$	Post-chemotherapy	Supervised home-based flexibility training combined with two exercise sessions per week for 30 min minimum for 14 weeks (mode of activity was patient choice) at a slightly strenuous intensity (13–15 on rating of perceived exertion scale; anchored from 6–20) compared to controls who received no exercise intervention but were told to continue with the normal amount of physical activity they would usually do	↑ **Aerobic capacity among the exercisers compared to the non-exercisers** with no significant differences between groups in fatigue
[14]	Breast cancer $n=22$	Chemotherapy or radiation therapy	Supervised mixed aerobic and resistance exercise 2×/week for 10–20 min at 60%–75% of maximum heart rate for 12 weeks	↓ **Fatigue in exercisers compared to controls**
[59]	Breast cancer stages 0–III $n=119$	Chemotherapy or radiation therapy	Home-based walking for 15–30 min 5–6×/week at 50%–70% maximum heart rate for 6 weeks for radiation patients and 3–6 months for chemotherapy patients versus usual care controls	↓ **Fatigue in fully compliant exercisers compared to controls**
[66]	Breast cancer $n=21$	Post-treatment 2–24 months	Supervised tai chi chuan for 60 min at moderate intensity 3×/week for 12 weeks	↑ **Walking ability in exercisers compared to controls**

[a] Results in bold print indicate a $p \leq .05$.

consistently effective at either reducing or halting the progression of CRF and improving cardiorespiratory function in Hodgkin's and BC patients during and after treatment. CAMPBELL and colleagues [14] were the only group to use both aerobic and anaerobic exercise (resistance exercise). Although the overall results were positive, the study sample was small and, at this time, it is not possible to differentiate the effects of aerobic and anaerobic exercise in this study. Therefore, the evidence supporting the safety and efficacy of anaerobic exercise for improving CRF or cardiovascular function is nonexistent among HL and BC survivors.

Recent meta-analyses by SCHMITZ and colleagues [78], and JACOBSEN and colleagues [45] suggests that the evidence for exercise as an effective therapy for managing CRF is consistently positive. The effect sizes (ES) are small [e.g., weighted mean ES = 0.13, 95% confidence interval (CI): –0.06 to 0.33 during treatment; weighted mean ES = 0.16, 95% CI: –0.23 to 0.54 post treatment]. This indicates the need for developing more targeted and effective exercise interventions.

Although the extant exercise and cancer control literature provides consistent support for the efficacy of exercise interventions in managing CRF during and after treatment, the investigations must be considered to be preliminary. The studies have small sample sizes. The studies as a body of research lack consistency in the type and amounts of exercise utilized. These limitations make it impossible to apply the results and effectively develop standards of care regarding tailored exercise prescriptions to safely meet the needs of these survivors. Additionally, the measures used to assess CRF and cardiovascular function as well as the type of control groups used are inconsistent. This makes interpreting findings and drawing conclusions across studies difficult. Appropriate statistical and follow-up analyses were not always used (e.g., intent-to-treat analyses in randomized controlled trials) which makes comparisons based on regimen and methods of exercise intervention difficult to ascertain.

Despite these limitations, this growing body of research provides consistent preliminary support for the safety of exercise interventions for HL and BC survivors across the entire cancer care continuum. This growing body of literature also suggests that early intervention with exercise during radiation may effectively prevent or reduce acute, chronic and late occurring CRF as well as improve cardiorespiratory function and prevent or delay the onset of cardiovascular disease as a consequence of radiation therapy to the chest among Hodgkin's and BC survivors. However, caution is warranted when considering an exercise prescription among this population of cancer survivors because there are many cardiovascular complications and a comprehensive subclinical assessment of cardiovascular status in long-term cancer survivors with different manifestations has not been performed. Patients should be carefully monitored by physicians and exercise physiologists since some are at risk for heart-rate-related hemodynamic instability, conduction problems, ischemia, and other complications.

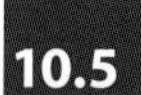

10.5
Conclusion

In conclusion, radiation therapy to the chest is associated with premature heart disease among Hodgkin's and BC survivors. Heart disease is associated with reduced quality life years and increased mortality. Exercise is a non-invasive and non-pharmacological intervention that shows promise in preventing or delaying the onset of premature heart disease in survivors of HL or BC. Systematic and thorough evaluation of CRF in this population might identify patients with covert or apparently compensated cardiac disease which is causative for this condition. Most significantly, it may identify the survivors who will benefit the most from early implementation of therapeutic exercise interventions targeting the reduction of CRF and improvement of cardiorespiratory function. Ultimately, exercise might prevent or delay the onset of heart disease after radiation therapy in this vulnerable population.

References

1. Adams MJ, Constine L, Lipshultz SE (2001a) Cardiology. Mosby International Ltd, London
2. Adams MJ, Constine L, Lipshultz SE (2001b) Radiation. In: Crawford MH, DiMarco JP (eds) Radiation. Mosby International Ltd, London, pp 1–8
3. Adams MJ et al (2003a) Radiation-associated cardiovascular disease. Crit Rev Oncol Hematol 45:55–75
4. Adams MJ et al (2003b) Radiation-associated cardiovascular disease: manifestations and management. Semin Radiat Oncol 13:346–356
5. Adams MJ et al (2004) Cardiovascular status in long-term survivors of Hodgkin's disease treated with chest radiotherapy. J Clin Oncol 22:3139–3148
6. Aleman BM et al (2007) Late cardiotoxicity after treatment for Hodgkin lymphoma. Blood 109:1878–1886
7. Aleman BM et al (2003) Long-term cause-specific mortality of patients treated for Hodgkin's disease. J Clin Oncol 21:3431–3439
8. American College of Sports Medicine (2006) ACSM's Guidelines for exercise testing and prescription. Lippincott, Williams, & Wilkins, Baltimore
9. Barton-Burke M (2006) Cancer-related fatigue and sleep disturbances. Further research on the prevalence of these two symptoms in long-term cancer survivors can inform education, policy, and clinical practice. Am J Nurs 106:72–77
10. Belardinelli R et al (1999) Randomized, controlled trial of long-term moderate exercise training in chronic heart failure: effects on functional capacity, quality of life, and clinical outcome. Circulation 99:1173–1182

11. Borger JH et al (2007) Cardiotoxic effects of tangential breast irradiation in early breast cancer patients: the role of irradiated heart volume. Int J Radiat Oncol Biol Phys 69:1131–1138

12. Brosius FC et al (1981) Radiation heart disease: Analysis of 16 young (aged 15–33 years) necropsy patients who received over 3,500 rads to the heart. Am J Med 70:519–530

13. Burnham TR et al. (2002) Effects of exercise on physiological and psychological variables in cancer survivors. Med Sci Sports Exerc 34:1863–1867

14. Campbell A et al. (2005) A pilot study of a supervised group exercise program as a rehabilitation treatment for women with breast cancer receiving adjuvant treatment. Eur J Oncol Nurs 9:56–63

15. Carlson RG et al. (1991) Radiation-associated valvular disease. Chest 99:538–545

16. Carroll JK et al. (2007) Pharmacologic treatment of cancer-related fatigue. Oncologist 12[Suppl 1]:43–51

17. Cassileth BR et al. (1985) Chemotherapeutic toxicity – the relationship between patients' pretreatment expectations and posttreatment results. Am J Clin Oncol 8:419–425

18. Clarke M et al. (2005) Effects of radiotherapy and of differences in the extent of surgery for early breast cancer on local recurrence and 15-year survival: an overview of the randomised trials. Lancet 366:2087–2106

19. Constine LS (1999) Late effects of cancer treatment. In: Halperin E, Constine L, TArbell N, Kun LE (eds) Pediatric radiation oncology. Lippincott, Williams and Wilkins, New York, pp 457–537

20. Courneya KS et al (2003a) The group psychotherapy and home-based physical exercise (group-hope) trial in cancer survivors: physical fitness and quality of life outcomes. Psycho-Oncology 12:357–374

21. Courneya KS et al (2003b) Randomized controlled trial of exercise training in postmenopausal breast cancer survivors: cardiopulmonary and quality of life outcomes. J Clin Oncol 21:1660–1668

22. Darby SC et al (2005) Long-term mortality from heart disease and lung cancer after radiotherapy for early breast cancer: prospective cohort study of about 300,000 women in US SEER cancer registries. Lancet Oncology 6:557–565

23. Dimeo F et al. (2004) Effect of aerobic exercise and relaxation training on fatigue and physical performance of cancer patients after surgery. A randomised controlled trial. Support Care Cancer 12:774–779

24. Dimeo FC et al. (1999) Effects of physical activity on the fatigue and psychologic status of cancer patients during chemotherapy. Cancer 85:2273–2277

25. Expert Panel on Detection, Evaluation, and Treatment of High Blood Cholesterol in Adults (2001) Executive Summary of The Third Report of The National Cholesterol Education Program (NCEP) Expert Panel on Detection, Evaluation, And Treatment of High Blood Cholesterol In Adults (Adult Treatment Panel III). JAMA 285:2486–2497

26. Galvao DA, Newton RU (2005) Review of exercise intervention studies in cancer patients. J Clin Oncol 23:899–909

27. Giannuzzi P et al (2003) Antiremodeling effect of long-term exercise training in patients with stable chronic heart failure: results of the Exercise in Left Ventricular Dysfunction and Chronic Heart Failure (ELVD-CHF) Trial. Circulation 108:554–559

28. Giordano SH et al (2005) Risk of cardiac death after adjuvant radiotherapy for breast cancer. J Natl Cancer Inst 97:419–424

29. Hager A et al (2005) Comparison of health related quality of life with cardiopulmonary exercise testing in adolescents and adults with congenital heart disease. Heart 91:517–520

30. Hambrecht R et al (2000) Effects of exercise training on left ventricular function and peripheral resistance in patients with chronic heart failure: a randomized trial. JAMA 283:3095–3101

31. Hancock SL et al (1993) Cardiac disease following treatment of Hodgkin's disease in children and adolescents. J Clin Oncol 11:1208–1215

32. Hancock S (1998) Cardiac toxicity after cancer therapy. National Cancer Institute. Bethesda MD, Conference Proceeding, 1[1], 3

33. Hancock S, Hoppe R (1996) Long-term complications of treatment and causes of mortality after Hodgkin's disease. Semin Radiat Oncol 6:225–242

34. Hardenbergh PH et al (2001) Cardiac perfusion changes in patients treated for breast cancer with radiation therapy and doxorubicin: preliminary results. Int J Radiat Oncol Biol Phys 49:1023–1028

35. Headley JA et al (2004) The effect of seated exercise on fatigue and quality of life in women with advanced breast cancer. Oncol Nurs Forum 31:977–983

36. Hickok JT, Mustian KM, Morrow GR, Roscoe JA, Fitch TR, Atkins JN (2005a) Differential effects of serotonin receptor antagonists on nausea (N) and vomiting (V) associated with moderately emetogenic chemotherapy. Support Care Cancer 13[6]:482 (abstract)

37. Hickok JT et al (2005b) Frequency, severity, clinical course, and correlates of fatigue in 372 patients during 5 weeks of radiotherapy for cancer. Cancer 104:1772–1778

38. Hicks GL, Jr., Hicks GLJ (1992) Coronary artery operation in radiation-associated atherosclerosis: long-term follow-up. Ann Thorac Surg 53:670–674

39. Hjermstad MJ et al (2005) Fatigue in long-term Hodgkin's Disease survivors: a follow-up study. J ClinOncol 23:6587–6595

40. Hjermstad MJ et al (2006) Quality of life in long-term Hodgkin's disease survivors with chronic fatigue. Eur J Cancer 42:327–333

41. Hofman M et al (2004) Cancer patients' expectations of experiencing treatment-related side effects: a University of Rochester Cancer Center–Community Clinical Oncology Program study of 938 patients from community practices. Cancer 101:851–857

42. Hofman M et al (2007) Cancer-related fatigue: the scale of the problem. Oncologist 12:4–10

43. Hooning MJ et al (2007) Long-term risk of cardiovascular disease in 10-year survivors of breast cancer. J Natl Cancer Inst 99:365–375

44. Hunt S et al (2008) ACC/AHA 2005 guideline update for the diagnosis and management of chronic heart failure in the adult – Summary article: a report of the American College of Cardiology/American Heart Association Task Force on Practice Guidelines (Writing Committee to Update the 2001 Guidelines for the Evaluation and Management of Heart Failure): developed in collaboration with the American College of Chest Physicians and the International Society for Lung and Heart Transplanta-

tion: endorsed by the Heart Rhythm Society. Circulation 112:1825–1852

45. Jacobsen PB et al (2007) Systematic review and meta-analysis of psychological and activity-based interventions for cancer-related fatigue. [Review] [70 refs]. Health Psychol 26:660–667

46. Jean-Pierre P et al (2007) Assessment of cancer-related fatigue: implications for clinical diagnosis and treatment. Oncologist 12:11–21

47. Knols R et al (2005) Physical exercise in cancer patients during and after medical treatment: a systematic review of randomized and controlled clinical trials. J Clin Oncol 23:3830–3842

48. Kunkler I (2005) Re: Locoregional radiation therapy in patients with high-risk breast cancer receiving adjuvant chemotherapy: 20-year results of the British Columbia randomized trial. J Natl Cancer Inst 97:1162–1163

49. Lee CK, Aeppli D, Nierengarten ME (2000) The need for long-term surveillance for patients treated with curative radiotherapy for Hodgkin's disease: University of Minnesota experience. Int J Radiat Oncol Biol Phys 48:169–179

50. Lipshultz SE et al (1993) Cardiovascular abnormalities in long-term survivors of childhood malignancy. J Clin Oncol 11: 1199–1203.

51. Loge JH et al (1999) Hodgkin's disease survivors more fatigued than the general population. J Clin Oncol 17:253–261

52. Marks LB et al. (2005) The incidence and functional consequences of RT-associated cardiac perfusion defects. Int J Radiat Oncol Biol Phys. 63(1): 214–223

53. Mauch PM et al (1995) Long-term survival in Hodgkin's disease relative impact of mortality, second tumors, infection, and cardiovascular disease. Cancer J Sci Am 1:33–42

54. McNeely ML et al (2006) Effects of exercise on breast cancer patients and survivors: a systematic review and meta-analysis. CMAJ CMAJ 175:34–41

55. Mock V (2004) Evidence-based treatment for cancer-related fatigue. J Natl Cancer Inst Monograph 32:112–118

56. Mock V et al (1994) A nursing rehabilitation program for women with breast cancer receiving adjuvant chemotherapy. Oncol Nurs Forum 21:899–907

57. Mock V et al (1997) Effects of exercise on fatigue, physical functioning, and emotional distress during radiation therapy for breast cancer. Oncol Nurs Forum 24:991–1000

58. Mock V et al (2001) Fatigue and quality of life outcomes of exercise during cancer treatment. Cancer Practice 9:119–127

59. Mock V, Frangakis C, Davidson NE et al (2005) Exercise manages fatigue during breast cancer treatment: a randomized controlled trial. Psychooncology 14:464–477

60. Mols F et al (2006) Better quality of life among 10–15 year survivors of Hodgkin's lymphoma compared to 5–9 year survivors: a population-based study. Eur J Cancer 42:2794–2801

61. Morrow G (2007) Cancer-related fatigue: causes, consequences, and management. Oncologist 12:1–3

62. Mustian KM et al (2006a) Exercise and side effects among 749 patients during and after treatment for cancer: a University of Rochester Cancer Center Community Clinical Oncology Program Study. Support Care Cancer 14:732–741

63. Mustian KM, Hofman M, Morrow GR, Griggs JJ, Jean-Pierre P, Kohli S, Roscoe JA, Simondet J, Bushunow P (2006b) Cancer-related fatigue and shortness of breath among cancer survivors: a prospective URCC CCOP study. NCI Cancer Survivorship Conference (abstract)

64. Mustian KM et al (2002) Exercise: complementary therapy for breast cancer rehabilitation. Women & Therapy 25:105–118

65. Mustian KM et al (2004) Tai Chi Chuan, health-related quality of life and self-esteem: a randomized trial with breast cancer survivors. Support Care Cancer 12:871–876

66. Mustian KM et al (2006c) A pilot study to assess the influence of tai chi chuan on functional capacity among breast cancer survivors. J Support Oncol 4:139–145

67. Mustian KM et al (2007) Integrative nonpharmacologic behavioral interventions for the management of cancer-related fatigue. Oncologist 12:52–67

68. Myers J et al (2006) Association of functional and health status measures in heart failure. J Card Fail 12:439–445

69. Ng AK et al (2005) A comparison between long-term survivors of Hodgkin's disease and their siblings on fatigue level and factors predicting for increased fatigue. Ann Oncol 16:1949–1955

70. Oldervoll LM et al (2003) Exercise reduces fatigue in chronic fatigued Hodgkins disease survivors – results from a pilot study. Eur J Cancer 39:57–63

71. Paszat LF et al (1998) Mortality from myocardial infarction after adjuvant radiotherapy for breast cancer in the surveillance, epidemiology, and end-results cancer registries.[see comment][erratum appears in J Clin Oncol 1999 17:740]. J Clin Oncol 16:2625–2631

72. Pinto BM et al (2003) Psychological and fitness changes associated with exercise participation among women with breast cancer. Psycho-Oncology 12:118–126

73. Pohjola-Sintonen S et al (1987) Late cardiac effects of mediastinal radiotherapy in patients with Hodgkin's disease. Cancer 60:31–37

74. Polikar R et al (1993) The thyroid and the heart. Circulation 87:1435–1441

75. Prue G et al (2006) Cancer-related fatigue: a critical appraisal. [Review] [84 refs]. Eur J Cancer 42:846–863

76. Ragaz J et al (2005) Locoregional radiation therapy in patients with high-risk breast cancer receiving adjuvant chemotherapy: 20-year results of the British Columbia randomized trial. J Natl Cancer Inst 97:116–126

77. Ryan JL et al (2007) Mechanisms of cancer-related fatigue. Oncologist 12:22–34

78. Schmitz KH et al (2005) Controlled physical activity trials in cancer survivors: a systematic review and meta-analysis. Cancer Epidemiol Biomarkers Prev 14:1588–1595

79. Segal R et al (2001) Structured exercise improves physical functioning in women with stages I and II breast cancer: results of a randomized controlled trial. J Clin Oncol 19:657–665

80. Slama MS, Le Guludec D, Sebag C et al (1991) Complete atrioventricular block following mediastinal irradiation: a report of six cases. Pacing Clin Electrophysiol 14:1112–1118

81. Smith SC Jr, Allen J, Blair SN et al (2006) AHA/ACC guidelines for secondary prevention for patients with coronary

and other atherosclerotic vascular disease: 2006 update: endorsed by the National Heart, Lung, and Blood Institute.[erratum appears in Circulation 2006, 113:e847]. Circulation 113:2363–2372

82. Stevinson C, Lawlor DA, Fox KR (2004) Exercise interventions for cancer patients: systematic review of controlled trials. Cancer Causes Control 15:1035–1056

83. Stewart JR, Fajardo LF, Gillette SM, Constine LS (1995) Radiation injury to the heart. Int J Radiat Oncol Biol Phys 31:1205–1211

84. Thorsen L, Skovlund E, Strømme SB et al (2005) Effectiveness of physical activity on cardiorespiratory fitness and health-related quality of life in young and middle-aged cancer patients shortly after chemotherapy. J Clin Oncol 23:2378–2388

85. Van Renterghem D, Hamers J, De Schryver A et al (1985) Chylothorax after mantle field irradiation for Hodgkin's disease. Respiration 48:188–189

86. Veinot JP, Edwards WD (1996) Pathology of radiation-induced heart disease: a surgical and autopsy study of 27 cases. Hum Pathol 27:766–773

87. Yu X, Prosnitz RR, Zhou S et al (2003) Symptomatic cardiac events following radiation therapy for left-sided breast cancer: possible association with radiation therapy-induced changes in regional perfusion. Clin Breast Cancer 4:193–197

11

Biodetection and Biointervention:
Cytokine Pathways as a Rationale for Anticytokine Interventions Post-Radiation

MITCHELL S. ANSCHER, PAUL R. GRAVES, ROSS MIKKELSEN, and ZELJKO VUJASKOVIC

CONTENTS

M. S. ANSCHER, MD
Department of Radiation Oncology, Virginia Commonwealth University Medical Center, 401 College Street, P.O. Box 980058, Richmond, VA 23298-0058, USA
P. R. GRAVES, PhD
Department of Radiation Oncology, Virginia Commonwealth University Medical Center, 401 College Street, P.O. Box 980058, Richmond, VA 23298-0058, USA
R. MIKKELSEN, PhD
Department of Radiation Oncology, Virginia Commonwealth University Medical Center, 401 College Street, P.O. Box 980058, Richmond, VA 23298-0058, USA
Z. VUJASKOVIC, MD, PhD
Department of Radiation Oncology, Duke University Medical Center, P.O. Box 3085 DUMC, Durham, NC 27710, USA

11.1
Introduction

Normal tissue tolerance limits the dose of radiation that can be used to treat most malignancies [78]. Despite the fact that many cancers present as large masses that require high doses of radiation to control, physicians are forced to limit the dose and volume irradiated in order to prevent the development of potentially serious, life threatening or fatal complications. Consequently, cure rates for some of these malignancies, such as lung cancers or malignant brain tumors, are distressingly low. Recent advances in our understanding of the molecular events underlying the pathogenesis of radiation-induced normal tissue injury has opened up the possibility of biologically-based interventions to prevent, mitigate or treat these complications. This work has also stimulated efforts to develop strategies to stratify patients according to risk of injury as a means to individualize therapy and improve the therapeutic ratio.

11.2
Molecular Mechanisms of Radiation Injury

It has been known for decades that the biologic response to ionizing radiation begins immediately after the first exposure with the generation of reactive oxygen/reactive nitrogen species (ROS/RNS) [73, 77, 90]. More recently, researchers have described how these immediate biochemical events rapidly trigger a series of genetic and molecular phenomena leading to clinically and histologically recognizable injury [11, 22, 25, 47, 53, 55, 62, 66–69, 96, 108]. This response to radiation is dynamic and involves a number of mediators of inflammation and fibrosis produced by macrophages, epithelial cells, and fibroblasts. These events appear to be sustained for months to years beyond the completion of therapy [40]; however, the mechanisms responsible for maintaining the injured phenotype, until recently, have remained unknown [74, 108].

The molecular processes responsible for radiation induced normal tissue injury have been, perhaps, most extensively studied in the lung (Fig. 11.1). As previously stated, the initial tissue damage from radiation is generated by direct action of ROS on DNA. This interaction causes tissue injury including endothelial cell damage with an increase in permeability, edema and fibrin accumulation in the extracellular matrix. Endothelial cell damage plays an important role in this process, and recent evidence suggests that the capillary endothelial cell may be the first cellular element to be damaged by RT [85]. This is followed by an inflammatory response with macrophage accumulation and activation. Macrophages, a rich source of proinflammatory and

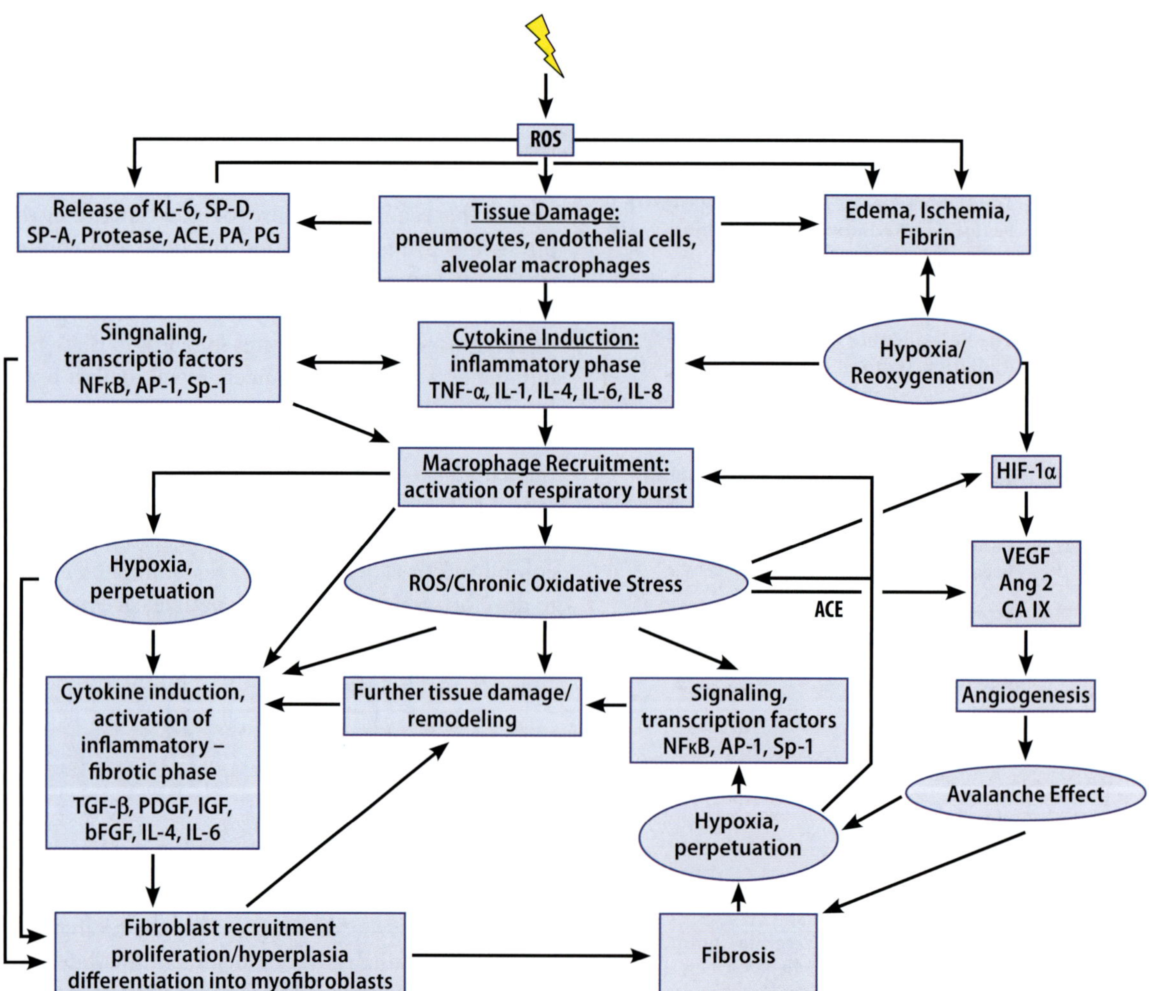

Fig. 11.1. Simplified model of processes involved in the pathogenesis of radiation-induced lung injury. As noted in the diagram, each event has the potential to influence several other processes. Exposure to ionizing radiation initiates a cascade of cytokines and growth factors. Proinflammatory cytokines promote an influx of macrophages and inflammatory cells, which are stimulated to produce ROS, proinflammatory and profibrotic cytokines. ROS serve as redox regulators of transcription factors, which further stimulate induction and activation of cytokines and growth factors. In addition, vascular changes, as well as an increase in oxygen consumption by activated macrophages, contribute to the development and perpetuation of hypoxia and chronic oxidative stress, leading to the non-healing tissue response of chronic radiation injury. *ACE*, angiotensin converting enzyme; *PA*, plasminogen activator; *PG*, prostaglandins; *Ang2*, angiotensin II; *CAIX*, carbonic anhydrase IX; *HIF*, hypoxia inducible factor; *PDGF*, platelet derived growth factor; *IGF*, insulin-like growth factors; *bFGF*, basic fibroblast growth factor. (Reproduced with permission from [37])

profibrotic cytokines, along with other inflammatory cells are recruited to an area of injury or evolving inflammation. The majority of macrophages in lung are derived from circulating monocytes that enter the lung in response to inflammation. Both vascular changes as well as an increase in oxygen consumption (due to macrophage activation) contribute to the development of hypoxia [38]. Hypoxia further stimulates production of ROS, proinflammatory, profibrogenic and proangiogenic cytokines. This perpetuates tissue damage leading to fibrosis via TGFβ1 production and stimulates angiogenesis via vascular endothelial growth factor (VEGF) production. In an attempt to respond to the proliferative stimulus of VEGF, endothelial cells die due to previously accumulated radiation damage. Hypoxia therefore continuously perpetuates a non-healing tissue response leading consequently to chronic radiation injury [6, 108].

Many of these molecular mediators of normal tissue injury are proteins, which can be measured both in tissue and blood. The ability to quantify the expression of these proteins, in the normal and diseased state, led to attempts to use them as predictors of risk of normal tissue injury after radiation therapy [4, 5, 26, 30, 44, 83, 106]. Until recently, each protein had to be quantified individually using methods such as antibody-based enzyme-linked immunosorbent assays (ELISA) or bioluminescence assays, which are laborious and time consuming [72]. Advances in bioassay technology now permit researchers to quantify multiple proteins simultaneously from the same sample in a rapid and reproducible manner [64]. This technology will greatly enhance the ability to construct protein expression profiles for individual patients and determine whether these patterns of protein expression can improve our ability to predict risk of injury from radiation therapy [51]. Along these lines, blood and tissue banks stocked with samples from patients irradiated for various malignancies will become invaluable resources for normal tissue injury research.

11.3

The Importance of Transforming Growth Factor β in Radiation-Induced Injury

The most widely studied of the potential mediators of normal tissue injury after radiation therapy is transforming growth factor-β1 (TGFβ1). TGFβ has multiple functions that are important in the development of excess fibrous tissue, one of the hallmarks of late radiation injury. TGFβ is chemoattractant for fibroblasts and also promotes differentiation of immature fibroblasts into myofibroblasts, which leads to increased production of collagen and extracellular matrix [92, 93]. TGFβ also decreases production of matrix-specific proteases and increases production of protease inhibitors, resulting in decrease collagen degradation, with a net result of increased fibrous tissue formation [45, 75]. In addition to being autocrine stimulated, TGFβ expression is also stimulated by hypoxia, which further promotes collagen formation [50, 79].

Recent evidence, indeed, confirms that TGFβ1 is important in the pathogenesis of radiation induced normal tissue injury. Rubin et al. [95] reported that alveolar macrophages obtained from bronchial lavage specimens from irradiated rabbits demonstrated increased production and release of TGFβ1 as compared to macrophages from normal lungs. These authors suggested that the fibroblast proliferation and extracellular matrix production found after irradiation are controlled by growth factors that are released from parenchymal cells following radiation exposure. Anscher et al. [3] demonstrated that TGFβ1 expression increased in a dose-dependent manner in the liver of rats following irradiation and that this increase in TGFβ1 expression correlated with the extent of connective tissue production. Barcellos-Hoff [12, 13] has shown that free radicals produced following exposure to ionizing radiation can directly activate TGFβ1. Thus, radiation therapy can both increase local expression and activation of TGFβ1, resulting in increased fibrosis formation in irradiated tissues. As further evidence to support the role of TGFβ in radiation injury, mice lacking Smad 3 (part of the TGFβ signal transduction pathway) have been shown to be resistant to radiation-induced fibrosis [36], suggesting that targeting the TGFβ pathway might be a useful strategy to prevent radiation injury (see below).

Moreover, the local activation of TGFβ1 in tissues may be an important component in sustaining the process of abnormal wound healing long after the exposure to radiation has ended. For example, active TGFβ1 both recruits and activates macrophages to secrete inflammatory and fibrogenic cytokines, including TGFβ1 itself [9, 91]. This autoinduction of TGFβ1 is important in maintaining levels of TGFβ1 in wound healing. Following radiation, however, this process contributes to overproduction of collagen and inhibition of epithelial cell proliferation, increased local oxygen consumption by activated macrophages, and decrease oxygen delivery due to microvasculature injury creating an hypoxic environment [74] which further perpetuates normal tissue injury. In addition, sustained overproduction of TGFβ may contribute not only to chronic fibrosis, but also reduce the effectiveness of cancer therapies [20], and possibly contribute to the development of radiation-induced malignancy (see below).

11.4
Using Plasma TGFβ Levels to Predict Injury Risk

Plasma TGFβ1 levels recently has been used to try and identify patients at risk for the development of normal tissue injury after exposure to chemotherapy and/or radiotherapy. In patients who develop radiation induced lung injury, Fu et al. [40] found sustained elevations in plasma TGFβ1 level for as long as 2 years after treatment. In contrast, patients who did not develop symptomatic lung injury did not exhibit sustained elevations in circulating plasma TGFβ1. In animal experiments, long term overexpression and activation of TGFβ1 has been demonstrated in tissue as well [62, 109, 110]. Thus, elevations in plasma TGFβ1 months after radiation exposure appear to reflect the presence of significantly dysregulated wound healing in the irradiated tissues. In contrast, the absence of sustained elevations of circulating TGFβ1 levels appear to reflect a more normal wound healing process. Thus, sustained elevations of plasma TGFβ1 following radiation exposure may be a useful means to identify patients at risk for late radiation-induced injury, including radiation-induced malignancy. Other investigators, however, have not found plasma TGFβ to be a reliable identifier of patients at increased risk for normal tissue injury after cancer therapy [15, 30, 83]. These discrepancies may be due to a number of factors, including differences in techniques used to measure TGFβ, differences in patient populations under study, and the fact that these series contain relatively small numbers of patients with treatment-related injury, thus the power to detect a difference between groups is not large [2].

11.5
The Role of Other Cytokines in Radiation-Induced Injury

A growing body of evidence points toward a complex web of protein interactions as being important in the pathogenesis of radiation injury (see Table 11.1 and Fig. 11.1). For example, Huang et al. [57] have found that IL-7, a cytokine that enhances T cell function and IFN-γ production, inhibits both TGFβ production and signaling, and protects against the development of bleomycin-induced pulmonary fibrosis, a model very similar to radiation injury. Fedorocko et al. [35] showed that radiation exposure could increase cytokine production both directly (IL-6, TNF-α) and indirectly (GM-CSF), either by locally acting paracrine or endocrine effects or as a result of systemic effects of early proinflammatory mediators such as IL-1 or TNF-α. There is no doubt that protein production is a dynamic process, which will change as a result of cancer treatment. Hong et al. [56] have documented temporal and spatial changes in the expression of proinflammatory cytokines (TNF-α, IL-1α and IL-1β) following thoracic irradiation in mice. Given the impact that radiation has on the expression of these, and other, proteins in tissue, and that these changes in tissue protein expression might be reflected in changes in plasma protein levels, it is reasonable to postulate that it may be possible to quantify an individual patient's inflammatory status by measuring candidate protein levels in the blood.

11.6
Using Other Markers to Predict Radiation-Induced Injury

In addition to TGFβ, several other proteins have been studied in humans to evaluate their potential as biomarkers for radiation-induced injury. Most of this work has been carried out in the lung. Of these, the most promising include interleukins (IL) 1α, IL-6, IL-8, IL-10, Krebs von den Lungen protein (KL-6, which is expressed mainly on type II pneumocytes and bronchiolar epithelial cells), soluble intracellular adhesion molecule (sICAM)-1, and surfactant proteins A and D [26, 27, 43, 44, 49, 52, 58, 71, 76, 97, 102]. Of these, KL-6 is the most extensively studied, and has been most consistently correlated with the risk of radiation-induced lung injury [37]. As with TGFβ, more prospective studies with larger patient numbers will be required to confirm its value as a predictive marker for lung injury.

11.7
Chronic Inflammation as a Mediator of Radiation Induced-Malignancy

Epidemiologic evidence has also suggested a correlation between chronic inflammation, such as that seen after exposure to radiation therapy, and the development of malignancy at the inflamed site. The underlying mechanism involves recruitment of inflammatory cells, as well as the expression of multiple mediators of inflammation, including cytokines, chemokines and enzymes. Proinflammatory cytokines, such as the interleukins and tumor necrosis factor α, cause an influx of inflammatory cells and fibroblasts into the microenvironment [63, 94]. These cells, primarily macrophages [95, 107], become stimulated to produce ROS/RNS and additional proinflammatory and profibrotic cytokines [37] (Fig. 11.1). ROS/RNS functionally regulate transcription factors that also influence expression and activation of cytokines and growth factors [77, 101, 114, 115], and ROS/RNS also are important in intracellular signaling [14, 77, 98]. Recent evidence also suggests the importance of ROS/RNS generated by macrophages and tumor cells in the processes of initiation and progression of malignancy [41, 54, 88, 113]. Thus, it is likely that many, if not all, of the proteins involved in the development of radiation-induced normal tissue inflammation and fibrosis might also be involved in the generation of radiation-induced malignancy.

In addition to creating a chronic inflammatory state, the microenvironmental stress resulting from hypoxia may also result in genomic instability [19, 23]. The ability of mammalian cells to detect and repair DNA damage has a critical impact on tumor response to ionizing radiation, but may also be important in normal tissue response. Mammalian cells have evolved a number of repair systems to deal with various types of DNA damage, and to maintain genomic integrity. The most harmful of all radiation-induced DNA damage is the double strand break (DSB). Errors in DSB repair can lead to deletions, insertions, chromosomal translocations and genomic instability that could lead to the development of malignancy [33, 103]. Specific surveillance proteins influence the balance between cell cycle arrest, DNA repair and apoptosis [17, 29]. For example, ATM is an important cellular surveillance protein, and recent evidence suggests that TGFβ is important for a fully functioning ATM response [70, 116], the loss of which might contribute to the development of malignancy. DNA damage repair mechanisms involving ATM are extremely sensitive to ROS/RNS generated in response to hypoxia/reperfusion [19, 48], and inhibition of ATM results in increased cellular levels of ROS/RNS [16, 59, 60]. Thus, chronic overproduction of ROS/RNS, as demonstrated to occur after exposure to radiation, may lead to interference with DNA damage repair, inhibition of apoptosis and regulation of oncogenes or tumor suppressor genes in a manner that may predispose people to the development of malignancy [10].

11.8
Candidate Proteins for Predicting Radiation Injury

While many proteins have been implicated in the pathogenesis of radiation-induced injury, few have been evaluated as possible predictors of predisposition to such injury. At the present time, not every protein implicated in inflammation, wound healing, fibrogenesis or radiation response can be detected in the blood, owing to the lack of availability of reliable antibodies to these proteins. Thus, it is not yet possible to screen for alterations in expression of every potential candidate protein. In addition, multiple proteins and signaling pathways are involved in these processes, and reliable antibodies are not available to target every individual protein involved in each pathway. Nevertheless, the list of proteins below represent components of all of the major mechanisms and pathways currently thought to be involved in the response of cells to radiation [99, 104]. This approach is likely to detect a profile of protein expression associated with an increased risk of radiation injury, if in fact one exists. The role of each of these candidate proteins, relevant to radiation injury, is summarized in Table 11.1.

Table 11.1. Summary of the function of candidate proteins for profiling

Protein	Function
IL-1β	Inflammation, growth factor expression
IL-5	Proinflammatory
IL-6	Proinflammatory, decrease apoptosis of activated lung fibroblasts
IL-7	Proinflammatory
IL-8	Angiogenesis, leukocyte chemotaxis, collagen synthesis
IL-10	Anti-inflammatory (decrease TNFα production, decrease upregulation of endothelial cell adhesion molecules)
IL-13	Proinflammatory
MCP-1	Inflammation, chemoattraction of monocytes
MIP-1alpha	Antiproliferative
PDGF BB	Angiogenesis, recruit smooth muscle cells
VEGF	Angiogenesis and increased vascular permeability
EGF	Epithelial cell motility, mitogenicity and differentiation
EGFR	Receptor for EGF, initial component of EGF signaling pathway
NFkappaB	Pleiotropic gene transcription responses
HIF-1	Transcription factor for genes regulating angiogenesis
TGF-alpha	Cell motility and proliferation
FGF 2	Angiogenesis and fibroblast proliferation
MMP-1	Degradation of collagen and extracellular matrix proteins
MMP-2	Matrix remodeling, growth factor release
MMP-3	Matrix remodeling, growth factor release
MMP-13	Matrix remodeling, growth factor release
SMAD 2/3	Signal transduction in the TGFß pathway
IGF-1R	Binding of IGF-1 (reepithialization and granulation tissue formation)
TNF-alpha	Growth factor expression, inflammation, matrix production and remodeling
TGFβ	Profibrotic, immunosuppression, angiogenesis, metastasis
Beta-catenin	Epithelial-mesenchymal transition
Nitric oxide synthases	Inflammation
Superoxide dismutases	Endogenous anti-inflammatory regulator

11.9
Strategies and Potential Targets for Intervention

There are 3 primary approaches to intervention in the injury process, depending upon the timing of intervention relative to radiation exposure, and whether or not injury has developed [81]. These approaches are: protection or prophylaxis, mitigation and treatment. Protection refers to treatments given before and/or during radiation. This is the most common strategy utilized in the clinic today and is illustrated by the use of the free radical scavenger amifostine in the prevention of injury following radiation to the head and neck [24]. Mitigation refers to therapies started after radiation exposure, but before overt injury is expressed, as exemplified by the use of angiotensin converting enzyme inhibitors to prevent renal injury [82]. Treatment refers to interventions begun after overt injury develops, an example of which would be the use of vitamin and pentoxifylline to treat established radiation soft tissue fibrosis [32].

As we learn more about the specific molecular pathways involved in the process of radiation injury (Figs. 11.1–11.3), more targeted therapies are being studied as approaches to the prevention of radiation injury. Given the importance of the TGFβ pathway in the pathogenesis of radiation injury, several investigators have demonstrated the efficacy of blocking TGFβ in preventing radiation injury in animals [7, 36, 87]. These agents, to date, have not been utilized in humans for this purpose. TGFβ has also been demonstrated to work through Smad independent pathways [18], and targeting one or more of these pathways may also prove to be an effective approach to prevention of radiation induced injury. For example, one of these alternative pathways involves signaling via PI3-kinase and cAbl [68], and the use of imatinib, which targets cAbl, has been shown to reduce the severity of bleomycin-induced lung injury [28]. In addition to TGFβ, other pathways have been demonstrated to be viable targets to inhibit the development of radiation-induced in-

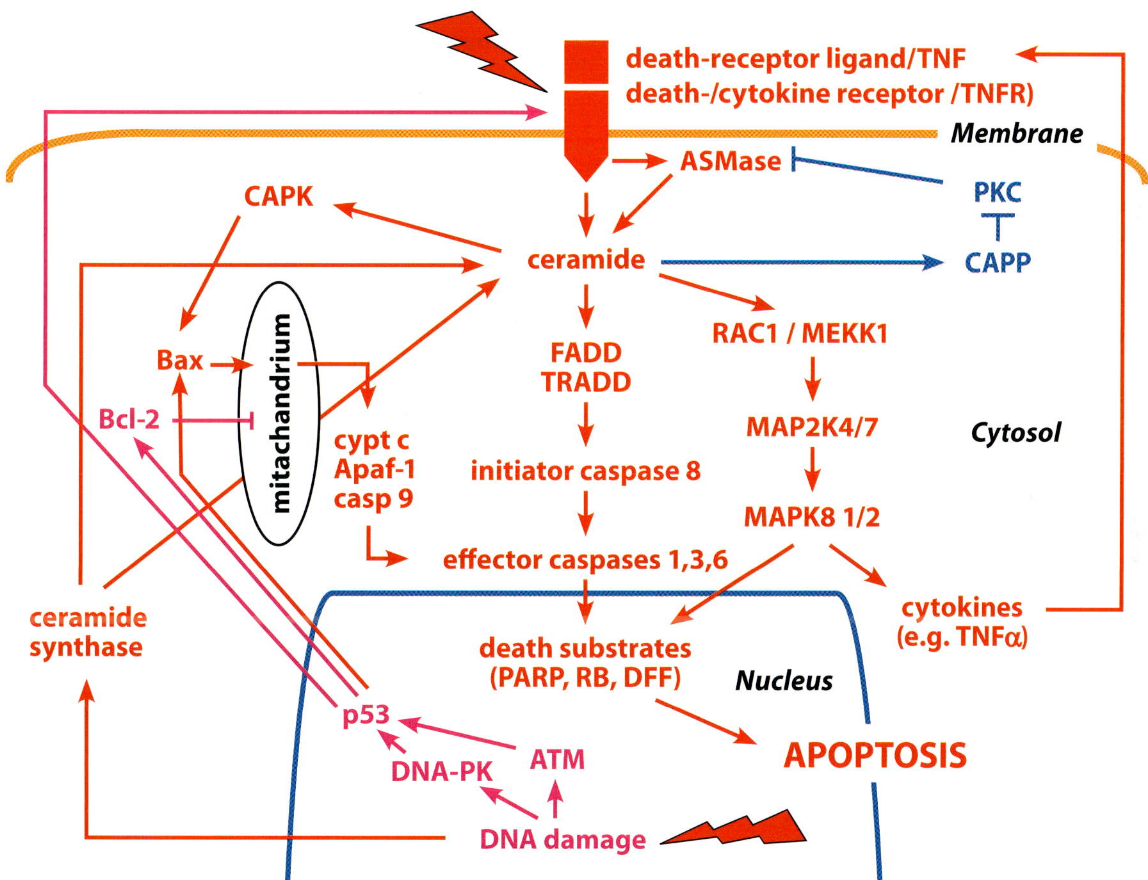

Fig. 11.2. DNA damage-independent and -dependent pathways of endothelial cell apoptosis. The primary apoptotic response to ionizing radiation in the endothelial cells is DNA damage independent and is mediated through radiation-induced activation of acid sphingomyelinase (*ASMase*) and the generation of ceramide. Ceramide mediates the activation of the MAPK8 pathway, the mitochondrial pathway or the death receptor pathway. The second source of ceramide occurs via production of DNA double-strand breaks and activation of ceramide synthase. *CAPK*, ceramide-activated protein kinase; *PKC*, protein kinase C; *TNF*, tumor necrosis factor; *BAX*, bcl-2 associated protein X; *BAD*, bcl-2 antagonist of cell death; *cyt*, cytochrome; *casp*, caspase; *PARP*, poly(adenosine-5'-diphosphate-ribose) polymerase; *RB*, retinoblastoma protein; *FADD*, Fas-associated death domain; *TRADD*, TNF-receptor associated death domain; *RAC*, receptor for activated C-kinase; *MEKK*, MAP/Erk kinase kinase; *MAPK*, mitogen activated protein kinase; *DFF*, DNA fragmentation factor; *Apaf*, apoptotic protease activating factor; *ATM*, ataxia-telangiectasis mutated. (Reproduced with permission from [93])

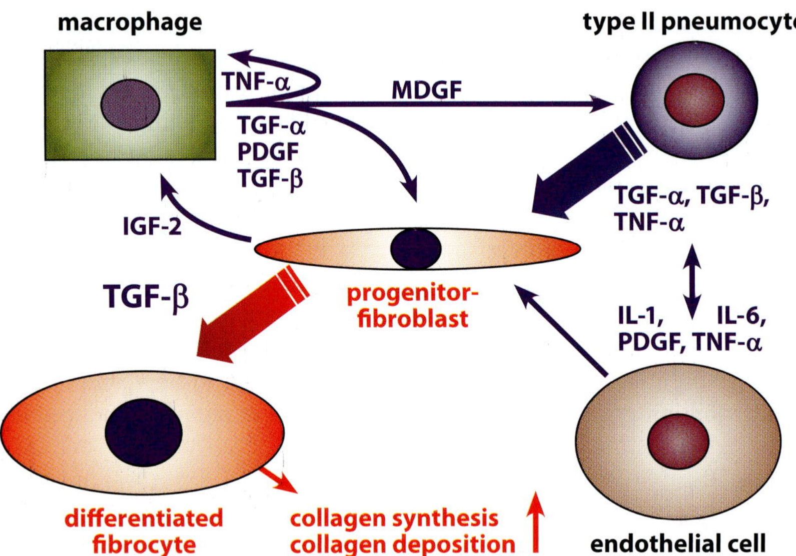

Fig. 11.3. The interaction between multiple cells, mediated via cytokines, in the process of connective tissue remodeling. *IL*, interleukin; *TGF*, transforming growth factor; *PDGF*, platelet derived growth factor; *IGF*, insulin-like growth factor; *TNF*, tumor necrosis factor; *MDGF*, macrophage derived growth factor. (Reproduced with permission from [93])

jury [1, 8, 31, 34, 46, 65, 109]. Given the redundancy and crosstalk between these multiple pathways, it is likely that strategies to prevent radiation injury may require agents that target multiple pathways simultaneously, or combinations of multiple agents with more specific targets.

An example of a class of drugs, which target multiple cellular pathways, and might prove beneficial in the struggle to prevent radiation induced normal tissue injury, are the statins. As noted above, vascular damage is an important component in the pathogenesis of radiation induced injury. Vascular damage is important in the phenotype of RT-induced rectal injury, where telangiectatic vessels are often responsible for the bleeding characteristic of this condition. The cholesterol lowering agents HMG coA reductase inhibitors (statins) have been demonstrated to reduce the risk of myocardial infarction, in part, through their vascular protective effects, which are not dependent on changes in serum cholesterol levels. In vitro, statins have been shown to protect human endothelial cells from ionizing radiation [21, 42, 84]. Multiple mechanisms appear to be involved, including attenuation of extracellular stress responses [80, 89], down-regulation of chemokines and chemokine receptors [111], and by exerting anti-inflammatory and anti-thrombotic effects [21, 86, 100, 105] on these cells. Of major interest recently has been the demonstration that statins induce the synthesis of nitric oxide synthase (NOS) in endothelial cells and may represent one mechanism for the beneficial effects of statins in chronic inflammation [61]. Elevated NOS activity is potentially a 2-edged sword and a number of other factors modulating nitric oxide activity may contribute to its beneficial, and also harmful, effect [39].

In vivo, lovastatin has been shown to protect mice from the effects of whole lung irradiation for up to 24 weeks [112]. Mice receiving lovastatin demonstrated improved survival, a decreased inflammatory response in the lung and reduced fibrosis. Thus statins may have the potential to protect against RT-induced late effects, and studies testing different statins as radioprotectors are currently underway.

Much work remains to be done, however, particularly in the areas of mitigation and treatment [109], and additional human studies will be required to identify the most effective agents and approaches to this complex problem.

References

1. Adawi A, Zhang Y, Baggs R, Rubin P, Williams J, Finkelstein J, Phipps RP (1998) Blockade of CD40-CD40 ligand interactions protects against radiation-induced pulmonary inflammation and fibrosis. Clin Immunol Immunopathol 89:222–230
2. Anscher MS, Kong FM (2005) In regard to De Jaeger et al.: significance of plasma transforming growth factor-beta levels in radiotherapy for non-small-cell lung cancer (INT J RADIAT ONCOL BIOL PHYS 2004;58:1378–1387). Int J Radiat Oncol Biol Phys 61:1276–1277

3. Anscher MS, Crocker IR, Jirtle RL (1990) Transforming growth factor-beta 1 expression in irradiated liver. Radiat Res 122:77–85

4. Anscher MS, Peters WP, Reisenbichler H, Petros WP, Jirtle RL (1993) Transforming growth factor beta as a predictor of liver and lung fibrosis after autologous bone marrow transplantation for advanced breast cancer. N Engl J Med 328:1592–1598

5. Anscher MS, Murase T, Prescott DM, Marks LB, Reisenbichler H, Bentel GC, Spencer D, Sherouse G, Jirtle RL (1994) Changes in plasma TGF beta levels during pulmonary radiotherapy as a predictor of the risk of developing radiation pneumonitis. Int J Radiat Oncol Biol Phys 30:671–676

6. Anscher MS, Chen L, Rabbani Z, Kang S, Larrier N, Huang H, Samulski TV, Dewhirst MW, Brizel DM, Folz RJ, Vujaskovic Z (2005) Recent progress in defining mechanisms and potential targets for prevention of normal tissue injury after radiation therapy. Int J Radiat Oncol Biol Phys 62:255–259

7. Anscher MS, Thrasher B, Rabbani Z, Teicher B, Vujaskovic Z (2006) Antitransforming growth factor-beta antibody 1D11 ameliorates normal tissue damage caused by high-dose radiation. Int J Radiat Oncol Biol Phys 65:876–881

8. Arango D, Ettarh RR, Holden G, Moriarty M, Brennan PC (2001) BB-10010, an analog of macrophage inflammatory protein-1alpha, protects murine small intestine against radiation. Dig Dis Sci 46:2608–2614

9. Ashcroft GS (1999) Bidirectional regulation of macrophage function by TGF-beta. Microbes Infect 1:1275–1282

10. Azad N, Rojanasakul Y, Vallyathan V (2008) Inflammation and lung cancer: roles of reactive oxygen/nitrogen species. J Toxicol Environ Health B Crit Rev 11:1–15

11. Barcellos-Hoff M (1998) How do tissues respond to damage at the cellular level? The role of cytokines in irradiated tissues. Radiat Res 150:S109–S120

12. Barcellos-Hoff MH (2003) Redox mechanisms for activation of latent TGF-β. In: 43rd Annual Meeting of the Radiation Research Society, pp 153

13. Barcellos-Hoff M, Dix T (1996) Redox-mediated activation of latent transforming growth factor-β1. Mol Endocrinol 10:1077–1083

14. Barrett DM, Black SM, Todor H, Schmidt-Ullrich RK, Dawson KS, Mikkelsen RB (2005) Inhibition of protein-tyrosine phosphatases by mild oxidative stresses is dependent on S-nitrosylation. J Biol Chem 280:14453–14461

15. Barthelemy-Brichant N, Bosquee L, Cataldo D, Corhay JL, Gustin M, Seidel L, Thiry A, Ghaye B, Nizet M, Albert A, Deneufbourg JM, Bartsch P, Nusgens B (2004) Increased IL-6 and TGF-beta1 concentrations in bronchoalveolar lavage fluid associated with thoracic radiotherapy. Int J Radiat Oncol Biol Phys 58:758–767

16. Barzilai A, Rotman G, Shiloh Y (2002) ATM deficiency and oxidative stress: a new dimension of defective response to DNA damage. DNA Repair (Amst) 1:3–25

17. Bernstein C, Bernstein H, Payne CM, Garewal H (2002) DNA repair/pro-apoptotic dual-role proteins in five major DNA repair pathways: fail-safe protection against carcinogenesis. Mutat Res 511:145–178

18. Bierie B, Moses HL (2006) Tumour microenvironment: TGFbeta: the molecular Jekyll and Hyde of cancer. Nat Rev Cancer 6:506–520

19. Bindra RS, Crosby ME, Glazer PM (2007) Regulation of DNA repair in hypoxic cancer cells. Cancer Metastasis Rev 26:249–260

20. Biswas S, Guix M, Rinehart C, Dugger TC, Chytil A, Moses HL, Freeman ML, Arteaga CL (2007) Inhibition of TGF-beta with neutralizing antibodies prevents radiation-induced acceleration of metastatic cancer progression. J Clin Invest 117:1305–1313

21. Boerma M, Burton GR, Wang J, Fink LM, McGehee RE Jr, Hauer-Jensen M (2006) Comparative expression profiling in primary and immortalized endothelial cells: changes in gene expression in response to hydroxy methylglutaryl-coenzyme A reductase inhibition. Blood Coagul Fibrinolysis 17:173–180

22. Brach MA, Hass R, Sherman ML, Gunji H, Weichselbaum R, Kufe D (1991) Ionizing radiation induces expression and binding activity of the nuclear factor kappa B. J Clin Invest 88:691–695

23. Bristow RG, Ozcelik H, Jalali F, Chan N, Vesprini D (2007) Homologous recombination and prostate cancer: a model for novel DNA repair targets and therapies. Radiother Oncol 83:220–230

24. Brizel DM, Wasserman TH, Henke M, Strnad V, Rudat V, Monnier A, Eschwege F, Zhang J, Russell L, Oster W, Sauer R (2000) Phase III randomized trial of amifostine as a radioprotector in head and neck cancer. J Clin Oncol 18:3339–3345

25. Brush J, Lipnick SL, Phillips T, Sitko J, McDonald JT, McBride WH (2007) Molecular mechanisms of late normal tissue injury. Semin Radiat Oncol 17:121–130

26. Chen Y, Rubin P, Williams J, Hernady E, Smudzin T, Okenieff P (2001) Circulating IL-6 as a predictor of radiation pneumonitis. Int J Radiat Oncol Biol Phys 49:641–648

27. Chen Y, Hyrien O, Williams J, Okunieff P, Smudzin T, Rubin P (2005) Interleukin (IL)-1A and IL-6: applications to the predictive diagnostic testing of radiation pneumonitis. Int J Radiat Oncol Biol Phys 62:260–266

28. Daniels CE, Wilkes MC, Edens M, Kottom TJ, Murphy SJ, Limper AH, Leof EB (2004) Imatinib mesylate inhibits the profibrogenic activity of TGF-beta and prevents bleomycin-mediated lung fibrosis. J Clin Invest 114:1308–1316

29. Dasika GK, Lin SC, Zhao S, Sung P, Tomkinson A, Lee EY (1999) DNA damage-induced cell cycle checkpoints and DNA strand break repair in development and tumorigenesis. Oncogene 18:7883–7899

30. De Jaeger K, Seppenwoolde Y, Kampinga HH, Boersma LJ, Belderbos JS, Lebesque JV (2004) Significance of plasma transforming growth factor-beta levels in radiotherapy for non-small-cell lung cancer. Int J Radiat Oncol Biol Phys 58:1378–1387

31. Delanian S, Baillet F, Huart J, Lefaix JL, Maulard C, Housset M (1994) Successful treatment of radiation-induced fibrosis using liposomal Cu/Zn superoxide dismutase: clinical trial. Radiother Oncol 32:12–20

32. Delanian S, Porcher R, Balla-Mekias S, Lefaix JL (2003) Randomized, placebo-controlled trial of combined pentoxifylline and tocopherol for regression of superficial radiation-induced fibrosis. J Clin Oncol 21:2545–2550

33. Elliott B, Jasin M (2002) Double-strand breaks and translocations in cancer. Cell Mol Life Sci 59:373–385

34. Epperly M, Bray J, Kraeger S, Zwacka R, Engelhardt J, Travis E, Greenberger J (1998) Prevention of late effects of irradiation lung damage by manganese superoxide dismutase gene therapy. Gene Ther 5:196–208

35. Fedorocko P, Egyed A, Vacek A (2002) Irradiation induces increased production of haemopoietic and proinflammatory cytokines in the mouse lung. Int J Radiat Biol 78:305–313

36. Flanders KC, Sullivan CD, Fujii M, Sowers A, Anzano MA, Arabshahi A, Major C, Deng C, Russo A, Mitchell JB, Roberts AB (2002) Mice lacking Smad3 are protected against cutaneous injury induced by ionizing radiation. Am J Pathol 160:1057–1068

37. Fleckenstein K, Gauter-Fleckenstein B, Jackson IL, Rabbani Z, Anscher M, Vujaskovic Z (2007) Using biological markers to predict risk of radiation injury. Semin Radiat Oncol 17:89–98

38. Fleckenstein K, Zgonjanin L, Chen L, Rabbani Z, Jackson I.L, Thrasher B, Kirkpatrick J, Foster WM, Vujaskovic Z (2007) Temporal onset of hypoxia and oxidative stress after pulmonary irradiation. Int J Radiat Oncol Biol Phys 68:196–204

39. Forstermann U (2006) Janus-faced role of endothelial NO synthase in vascular disease: uncoupling of oxygen reduction from NO synthesis and its pharmacological reversal. Biol Chem 387:1521–1533

40. Fu X, Huang H, Bentel G, Clough R, Jirtle RL, Kong F, Marks LB, Anscher MS (2001) Predicting the risk of symptomatic radiation-induced lung injury using both the physical and biologic parameters V(30) and transforming growth factor beta. Int J Radiat Oncol Biol Phys 50:899–908

41. Fukumura D, Kashiwagi S, Jain RK (2006) The role of nitric oxide in tumour progression. Nat Rev Cancer 6:521–534

42. Gaugler MH, Vereycken-Holler V, Squiban C, Vandamme M, Vozenin-Brotons MC, Benderitter M (2005) Pravastatin limits endothelial activation after irradiation and decreases the resulting inflammatory and thrombotic responses. Radiat Res 163:479–487

43. Goto K, Kodama T, Sekine I, Kakinuma R, Kubota K, Hojo F, Matsumoto T, Ohmatsu H, Ikeda H, Ando M, Nishiwaki Y (2001) Serum levels of KL-6 are useful biomarkers for severe radiation pneumonitis. Lung Cancer 34:141–148

44. Gridley DS, Bonnet RB, Bush DA, Franke C, Cheek GA, Slater JD, Slater JM (2004) Time course of serum cytokines in patients receiving proton or combined photon/proton beam radiation for resectable but medically inoperable non-small-cell lung cancer. Int J Radiat Oncol Biol Phys 60:759–766

45. Hakenjos L, Bamberg M, Rodemann HP (2000) TGF-beta1-mediated alterations of rat lung fibroblast differentiation resulting in the radiation-induced fibrotic phenotype. Int J Radiat Biol 76:503–509

46. Hallahan DE, Virudachalam S (1997) Intercellular adhesion molecule 1 knockout abrogates radiation induced pulmonary inflammation. Proc Natl Acad Sci USA 94:6432–6437

47. Hallahan DE, Geng L, Shyr Y (2002) Effects of intercellular adhesion molecule 1 (ICAM-1) null mutation on radiation-induced pulmonary fibrosis and respiratory insufficiency in mice. J Natl Cancer Inst 94:733–741

48. Hammond EM, Dorie MJ, Giaccia AJ (2003) ATR/ATM targets are phosphorylated by ATR in response to hypoxia and ATM in response to reoxygenation. J Biol Chem 278:12207–12213

49. Hara R, Itami J, Komiyama T, Katoh D, Kondo T (2004) Serum levels of KL-6 for predicting the occurrence of radiation pneumonitis after stereotactic radiotherapy for lung tumors. Chest 125:340–344

50. Haroon ZA, Amin K, Jiang X, Arcasoy MO (2003) A novel role for erythropoietin during fibrin-induced wound-healing response. Am J Pathol 163:993–1000

51. Hart J, Rabbani Z, Pizzo S, Vujaskovic Z, Anscher M (2004) Cytokine profiling to predict radiation-induced lung injury. Int J Radiat Oncol Biol Phys 60:S238

52. Hart JP, Broadwater G, Rabbani Z, Moeller BJ, Clough R, Huang D, Sempowski GA, Dewhirst M, Pizzo SV, Vujaskovic Z, Anscher MS (2005) Cytokine profiling for prediction of symptomatic radiation-induced lung injury. Int J Radiat Oncol Biol Phys 63:1448–1454

53. Hauer-Jensen M, Kong FM, Fink LM, Anscher MS (1999) Circulating thrombomodulin during radiation therapy of lung cancer. Radiat Oncol Investig 7:238–242

54. Hirst DG, Robson T (2007) Nitrosative stress in cancer therapy. Front Biosci 12:3406–3418

55. Hong JH, Chiang CS, Campbell IL, Sun JR, Withers HR, McBride WH (1995) Induction of acute phase gene expression by brain irradiation. Int J Radiat Oncol Biol Phys 33:619–626

56. Hong JH, Jung SM, Tsao TC, Wu CJ, Lee CY, Chen FH, Hsu CH, McBride WH, Chiang CS (2003) Bronchoalveolar lavage and interstitial cells have different roles in radiation-induced lung injury. Int J Radiat Biol 79:159–167

57. Huang M, Sharma S, Zhu LX, Keane MP, Luo J, Zhang L, Burdick MD, Lin YQ, Dohadwala M, Gardner B, Batra RK, Strieter RM, Dubinett SM (2002) IL-7 inhibits fibroblast TGF-beta production and signaling in pulmonary fibrosis. J Clin Invest 109:931–937

58. Ishii Y, Kitamura S (1999) Soluble intercellular adhesion molecule-1 as an early detection marker for radiation pneumonitis. Eur Respir J 13:733–738

59. Ito K, Hirao A, Arai F, Matsuoka S, Takubo K, Hamaguchi I, Nomiyama K, Hosokawa K, Sakurada K, Nakagata N, Ikeda Y, Mak TW, Suda T (2004) Regulation of oxidative stress by ATM is required for self-renewal of haematopoietic stem cells. Nature 431:997–1002

60. Ito K, Takubo K, Arai F, Satoh H, Matsuoka S, Ohmura M, Naka K, Azuma M, Miyamoto K, Hosokawa K, Ikeda Y, Mak TW, Suda T, Hirao A (2007) Regulation of reactive oxygen species by Atm is essential for proper response to DNA double-strand breaks in lymphocytes. J Immunol 178:103–110

61. Jantzen F, Konemann S, Wolff B, Barth S, Staudt A, Kroemer HK, Dahm JB, Felix SB, Landsberger M (2007) Isoprenoid depletion by statins antagonizes cytokine-induced down-regulation of endothelial nitric oxide expression and increases NO synthase activity in human umbilical vein endothelial cells. J Physiol Pharmacol 58:503–514

62. Johnston C, Piedboeuf B, Baggs R, Rubin P, Finkelstein J (1995) Differences in correlation of mRNA gene expres-

sion in mice sensitive and resistant to radiation-induced pulmonary fibrosis. Radiat Res 142:197–203

63. Johnston CJ, Williams JP, Elder A, Hernady E, Finkelstein JN (2004) Inflammatory cell recruitment following thoracic irradiation. Exp Lung Res 30:369–382

64. Jones LP, Zheng HQ, Karron RA, Peret TC, Tsou C, Anderson LJ (2002) Multiplex assay for detection of strain-specific antibodies against the two variable regions of the G protein of respiratory syncytial virus. Clin Diagn Lab Immunol 9:633–638

65. Kang S, Rabbani Z, Folz R, Golson M, Huang H, Samulski T, Dewhirst M, Anscher M, Vujaskovic Z (2002) Overexpression of extracellular superoxide dismutase protects mice from radiation induced lung injury. Int J Radiat Oncol Biol Phys 54:78

66. Kharbanda S, Saleem A, Datta R, Yuan ZM, Weichselbaum R, Kufe D (1994) Ionizing radiation induces rapid tyrosine phosphorylation of p34cdc2. Cancer Res 54:1412–1414

67. Kharbanda S, Ren R, Pandey P, Shafman TD, Feller SM, Weichselbaum RR, Kufe DW (1995) Activation of the c-Abl tyrosine kinase in the stress response to DNA-damaging agents. Nature 376:785–788

68. Kharbanda S, Bharti A, Pei D, Wang J, Pandey P, Ren R, Weichselbaum R, Walsh CT, Kufe D (1996) The stress response to ionizing radiation involoves c-Abl-dependent phosphorylation of SHPTP1. Proc Natl Acad Sci USA 93:6898–6901

69. Kharbanda S, Saleem A, Yuan Z.M, Kraeft S, Weichselbaum R, Chen LB, and Kufe D (1996) Nuclear signaling induced by ionizing radiation involves colocalization of the activated p56/p53lyn tyrosine kinase with p34cdc2. Cancer Res 56:3617–3621

70. Kirshner J, Jobling MF, Pajares MJ, Ravani SA, Glick AB, Lavin MJ, Koslov S, Shiloh Y, Barcellos-Hoff MH (2006) Inhibition of transforming growth factor-beta1 signaling attenuates ataxia telangiectasia mutated activity in response to genotoxic stress. Cancer Res 66:10861–10869

71. Kohno N, Hamada H, Fujioka S, Hiwada K, Yamakido M, Akiyama M (1992) Circulating antigen KL-6 and lactate dehydrogenase for monitoring irradiated patients with lung cancer. Chest 102:117–122

72. Kong F-M, Anscher M, Jirtle R (2003) Tumor marker protocols: plasma transforming growth factor beta, a plasma tumor marker. In: Hannausek M, Walaszek Z (eds) Methods in molecular medicine. Humana Press, Inc., pp 417–430

73. Leach JK, Van Tuyle G, Lin PS, Schmidt-Ullrich R, Mikkelsen RB (2001) Ionizing radiation-induced, mitochondria-dependent generation of reactive oxygen/nitrogen. Cancer Res 61:3894–3901

74. Li Y-Q, Ballinger J, Nordal R, Su Z-F, Wong C (2001) Hypoxia in radiation-induced blood-spinal cord barrier breakdown. Cancer Res 61:3348–3354

75. Martin M, Lefaix J-L, Delanian S (2000) TGF-β1 and radiation fibrosis: a master switch and a specific target? Int J Radiat Oncol Biol Phys 47:277–290

76. Matsuno Y, Satoh H, Ishikawa H, Kodama T, Ohtsuka M, Sekizawa K (2006) Simultaneous measurements of KL-6 and SP-D in patients undergoing thoracic radiotherapy. Med Oncol 23:75–82

77. Mikkelsen RB, Wardman P (2003) Biological chemistry of reactive oxygen and nitrogen and radiation-induced signal transduction mechanisms. Oncogene 22:5734–5754

78. Milano MT, Constine LS, Okunieff P (2007) Normal tissue tolerance dose metrics for radiation therapy of major organs. Semin Radiat Oncol 17:131–140

79. Moeller BJ, Cao Y, Vujaskovic Z, Li CY, Haroon ZA, Dewhirst MW (2004) The relationship between hypoxia and angiogenesis. Semin Radiat Oncol 14:215–221

80. Morikawa S, Takabe W, Mataki C, Kanke T, Itoh T, Wada Y, Izumi A, Saito Y, Hamakubo T, Kodama T (2002) The effect of statins on mRNA levels of genes related to inflammation, coagulation, and vascular constriction in HUVEC. Human umbilical vein endothelial cells. J Atheroscler Thromb 9:178–183

81. Moulder JE, Cohen EP (2007) Future strategies for mitigation and treatment of chronic radiation-induced normal tissue injury. Semin Radiat Oncol 17:141–148

82. Moulder JE, Fish BL, Cohen EP (2003) ACE inhibitors and AII receptor antagonists in the treatment and prevention of bone marrow transplant nephropathy. Curr Pharm Des 9:737–749

83. Novakova-Jiresova A, Van Gameren MM, Coppes RP, Kampinga HH, Groen HJ (2004) Transforming growth factor-beta plasma dynamics and post-irradiation lung injury in lung cancer patients. Radiother Oncol 71:183–189

84. Nubel T, Damrot J, Roos WP, Kaina B, Fritz G (2006) Lovastatin protects human endothelial cells from killing by ionizing radiation without impairing induction and repair of DNA double-strand breaks. Clin Cancer Res 12:933–939

85. Paris F, Fuks Z, Kang A, Capodieci P, Juan G, Ehleiter D, Haimovitz-Friedman A, Cordon-Cardo C, Kolesnick R (2001) Endothelial apoptosis as the primary lesion initiating intestinal radiation damage in mice. Science 293:293–297

86. Perez-Guerrero C, Alvarez de Sotomayor M, Jimenez L, Herrera MD, Marhuenda E (2003) Effects of simvastatin on endothelial function after chronic inhibition of nitric oxide synthase by L-NAME. J Cardiovasc Pharmacol 42:204–210

87. Rabbani ZN, Anscher MS, Zhang X, Chen L, Samulski TV, Li CY, Vujaskovic Z (2003) Soluble TGFβ type II receptor gene therapy ameliorates acute radiation-induced pulmonary injury in rats. Int J Radiat Biol Oncol Phys 57:563–572

88. Ridnour LA, Thomas DD, Donzelli S, Espey MG, Roberts DD, Wink DA, Isenberg JS (2006) The biphasic nature of nitric oxide responses in tumor biology. Antioxid Redox Signal 8:1329–1337

89. Rikitake Y, Kawashima S, Takeshita S, Yamashita T, Azumi H, Yasuhara M, Nishi H, Inoue N, Yokoyama M (2001) Anti-oxidative properties of fluvastatin, an HMG-CoA reductase inhibitor, contribute to prevention of atherosclerosis in cholesterol-fed rabbits. Atherosclerosis 154:87–96

90. Riley PA (1994) Free radicals in biology: oxidative stress and the effects of ionizing radiation. Int J Radiat Biol 65:27–33

91. Roberts AB, Piek E, Bottinger EP, Ashcroft G, Mitchell JB, Flanders KC (2001) Is Smad3 a major player in signal transduction pathways leading to fibrogenesis? Chest 120:43S–47S

92. Rodemann HP, Bamberg M (1995) Cellular basis of radiation-induced fibrosis. Radiother Oncol 35:83–90

93. Rodemann H, Blaese M (2007) Responses of normal cells to ionizing radiation. Semin Radiat Oncol 17:81–88

94. Rube CE, Uthe D, Wilfert F, Ludwig D, Yang K, Konig J, Palm J, Schuck A, Willich N, Remberger K, Rube C (2005) The bronchiolar epithelium as a prominent source of pro-inflammatory cytokines after lung irradiation. Int J Radiat Oncol Biol Phys 61:1482–1492

95. Rubin P, Finkelstein JN, Shapiro D (1992) Molecular biology mechanisms in the radiation induction of pulmonary injury syndromes: interrelationship between the alveolar macrophage and the septal fibroblast. Int J Radiat Oncol Biol Phys 24:93–101

96. Rubin P, Johnston CJ, Williams JP, McDonald S, Finkelstein JN (1995) A perpetual cascade of cytokines post irradiation leads to pulmonary fibrosis. Int J Radiat Oncol Biol Phys 33:99–109

97. Sasaki R, Soejima T, Matsumoto A, Maruta T, Yamada K, Ota Y, Kawabe T, Nishimura H, Sakai E, Ejima Y, Sugimura K (2001) Clinical significance of serum pulmonary surfactant proteins a and d for the early detection of radiation pneumonitis. Int J Radiat Oncol Biol Phys 50:301–307

98. Schmidt-Ullrich RK, Dent P, Grant S, Mikkelsen RB, Valerie K (2000) Signal transduction and cellular radiation responses. Radiat Res 153:245–257

99. Schmidt-Ullrich RK, Mikkelsen RB, Valerie K (2004) Molecular cancer and radiation biology. In: Perez CA, Brady LW, Halperin EC, Schmidt-Ullrich RK (eds) Principles and practice of radiation oncology. Lippincott Williams and Wilkins, pp 137–162

100. Shi J, Wang J, Zheng H, Ling W, Joseph J, Li D, Mehta JL, Ponnappan U, Lin P, Fink LM, Hauer-Jensen M (2003) Statins increase thrombomodulin expression and function in human endothelial cells by a nitric oxide-dependent mechanism and counteract tumor necrosis factor alpha-induced thrombomodulin downregulation. Blood Coagul Fibrinolysis 14:575–585

101. Sun Y, Oberley LW (1996) Redox regulation of transcriptional activators. Free Radic Biol Med 21:335–348

102. Takahashi H, Imai Y, Fujishima T, Shiratori M, Murakami S, Chiba H, Kon H, Kuroki Y, Abe S (2001) Diagnostic significance of surfactant proteins A and D in sera from patients with radiation pneumonitis. Eur Respir J 17:481–487

103. Thompson LH, Schild D (2002) Recombinational DNA repair and human disease. Mutat Res 509:49–78

104. Tsoutsou PG, Koukourakis MI (2006) Radiation pneumonitis and fibrosis: mechanisms underlying its pathogenesis and implications for future research. Int J Radiat Oncol Biol Phys 66:1281–1293

105. Undas A, Brozek J, Musial J (2002) Anti-inflammatory and antithrombotic effects of statins in the management of coronary artery disease. Clin Lab 48:287–296

106. Vujaskovic Z, Down JD, van Waarde MA, van Assen AJ, Szabo BG, Konings AW (1997) Plasma TGFbeta level in rats after hemithoracic irradiation. Radiother Oncol 44:41–43

107. Vujaskovic Z, Marks L, Anscher M (2000) The physical parameters and molecular events associated with radiation-induced lung toxicity. Sem Radiat Oncol 10:296–307

108. Vujaskovic Z, Anscher M, Feng Q-F, Rabbani Z, Amin K, Samulski T, Dewhirst M, Haroon Z (2001) Radiation-induced hypoxia may perpetuate late normal tissue injury. Int J Radiat Oncol Biol Phys 50:851–855

109. Vujaskovic Z, Batinic-Haberle I, Rabbani Z, Feng Q, Kang S, Spasojevic I, Samulski T, Fridovich I, Dewhirst M, Anscher M (2002) A small molecular weight catalytic metalloporphyrin antioxidant with superoxide dismutase (SOD) mimetic properties protects lungs from radiation-induced injury. Free Radic Biol Med 33:857

110. Vujaskovic Z, Feng QF, Rabbani ZN, Anscher MS, Samulski TV, Brizel DM (2002) Radioprotection of lungs by amifostine is associated with reduction in profibrogenic cytokine activity. Radiat Res 157:656–660

111. Waehre T, Damas JK, Gullestad L, Holm AM, Pedersen TR, Arnesen KE, Torsvik H, Froland SS, Semb AG, Aukrust P (2003) Hydroxymethylglutaryl coenzyme a reductase inhibitors down-regulate chemokines and chemokine receptors in patients with coronary artery disease. J Am Coll Cardiol 41:1460–1467

112. Williams JP, Hernady E, Johnston CJ, Reed CM, Fenton B, Okunieff P, Finkelstein JN (2004) Effect of administration of lovastatin on the development of late pulmonary effects after whole-lung irradiation in a murine model. Radiat Res 161:560–567

113. Wink DA, Vodovotz Y, Laval J, Laval F, Dewhirst MW, Mitchell JB (1998) The multifaceted roles of nitric oxide in cancer. Carcinogenesis 19:711–721

114. Wu X, Bishopric NH, Discher DJ, Murphy BJ, Webster KA (1996) Physical and functional sensitivity of zinc finger transcription factors to redox change. Mol Cell Biol 16:1035–1046

115. Yakovlev VA, Barani IJ, Rabender CS, Black SM, Leach JK, Graves PR, Kellogg GE, Mikkelsen RB (2007) Tyrosine nitration of IkappaBalpha: a novel mechanism for NF-kappaB activation. Biochemistry 46:11671–11683

116. Zhang S, Ekman M, Thakur N, Bu S, Davoodpour P, Grimsby S, Tagami S, Heldin CH, Landstrom M (2006) TGFbeta1-induced activation of ATM and p53 mediates apoptosis in a Smad7-dependent manner. Cell Cycle 5:2787–2795

Late Toxicity from Hypofractionated Stereotactic Body Radiation

Michael T. Milano, Jacqueline P. Williams, Louis S. Constine, and Paul Okunieff

CONTENTS

12.1 Introduction

Stereotactic body radiation therapy (SBRT) utilizes a three dimensional coordinate system to achieve more reproducible patient set-up [1, 2]. With SBRT, the margins for set-up uncertainty can be reduced, allowing greater volume sparing of the surrounding normal tissues. Since SBRT yields a reduced volume of normal tissue exposure, SBRT has been used to increase the fractional dose of radiation (hypofractionation) in an attempt to intensify the dose de-

M. T. Milano, MD, PhD
J. P. Williams, PhD
L. S. Constine, MD
P. Okunieff, MD
Department of Radiation Oncology, University of Rochester Medical Center, 601 Elmwood Avenue, Box 647, Rochester, NY 14642, USA

livery without incrementally increasing the risk of normal tissue damage. This is becoming an important approach to treating discrete tumors, and has yielded impressive local control of treated tumors without significant toxicity. The benefit of SBRT is to achieve improved local control compared to conventional radiation, via improved target localization and more intense doles delivery, without the added toxicity. Arguably, SBRT can achieve similar or even improved outcome over surgical resection. One advantage that SBRT has over a limited resection (i.e. one that does not achieve wide margins) is that the penumbra dose around the target treats microscopic disease [3].

With three-dimensional planning, detailed dose-volume information can be obtained for critical organs at risk as well as gross and microscopic targets, providing more tools for the clinician to assess the acceptability of a plan. Ideally, well characterized dose-volume constraints should be used, though certainly more clinical data is needed [4], particularly with hypofractionated regimens.

While some authors assert that SBRT implies the use of hypofractionation in extracranial sites [1, 2, 5, 6], an alternative view is that SBRT is merely a tool, employing a three-dimensional coordinate system to more accurately target radiation delivery, which may allow the safe use of hypofractionation in certainly situations. Arguably, SBRT can be used with standard fractionation schemes with cranial or extracranial tumors. One example would be the treatment of benign tumors abutting the optic chiasm and nerves, where it is well known that hypofractionation increases the risk of toxicity [7]. With standard fractionation SBRT, the risk of late toxicity can be reduced solely by virtue of better patient set-up and lowering the volume of normal tissue exposure. Therefore when choosing the dose and fractionation with SBRT, several considerations are important, primarily: (1) the predicted risks of late toxicity and

(2) the predicted efficacy of the radiation; but also: (3) patient convenience with respect to the number of treatments delivered, (4) the cost of treatment planning and delivery and (5) the number of time slots used on a given linear-accelerator.

In recent years, there has been a growing clinical experience treating patients with primary and metastatic tumors with hypofractionated SBRT. These patients certainly benefit from reduced normal tissue exposure, but the effect of a greater fraction size, albeit to a smaller volume of normal tissue, is not well understood. As clinical experience with hypofractionated SBRT matures, we will obtain much needed patient outcome data. This review will focus on the radiobiology of hypofractionation and normal tissue tolerance to hypofractionated radiation, as well as the patient outcome in select trials using hypofractionated SBRT. Generally, SBRT implies the delivery of multiple (> 1) fractions of radiation. When radiation is delivered in one fraction, it is termed stereotactic body radiosurgery (SBRS) or in the case of the treatment of cranial lesions, stereotactic radiosurgery (SRS). This review will apply to both SBRT and SBRS, but for simplicity we will only use "SBRT" in the text below (unless specifically referencing a study employing SBRS).

ple non-coplanar fields and/or arcing fields, the dose gradient is steeper than with conventional radiation, though the low dose region can encompass a larger volume and be irregularly shaped.

Intensity modulated radiation therapy (IMRT) can used to further customize the dose delivery, allowing for greater relative sparing of normal tissues. With IMRT, the radiation is modulated spatially and/or temporally with inverse planning techniques [9]. The goal of IMRT is to shape the dose distribution so as to minimize the dose to normal tissues and/or escalate the dose delivery to the target. The physician decides upon dose constraints to the target and avoidance objects, and the optimal inverse plan yields a dose-volume distribution that best achieves these pre-determined dose constraints. Generally, with IMRT, there is an increase in monitor unit delivery, which corresponds to a greater integral dose-volume distribution. There has been much concern about the possibility of IMRT resulting in a greater risk of second cancers resulting from the greater volume of low dose exposure [10–14]. Because SBRT and IMRT are separate tools (which can be used together), this will not be explored in greater detail in this review.

12.2

Technical Aspects of SBRT

SBRT requires a three-dimensional coordinate system for accurate and reproducible patient set-up. A system to detect and process this three-dimensional array is also needed. SBRT can be achieved through the use of internal fiducials or markers, external markers and/or image guidance. Systems which gate the delivery of radiation, such that radiation is only administered when the patient position falls within a predetermined set of positioning parameters, can also be used. Immobilization techniques such as relaxed patient breath-hold can allow further reduction in set-up uncertainty [8].

With SBRT, the clinician can choose the dose fraction, total dose as well as the isodose line prescribed to the periphery of the target. As a result, normal tissue adjoining the target can receive a lower dose than the target isocenter, simply by virtue of prescribing to a lower isodose line. Because the planning and delivery of SBRT often uses multi-

12.3

Radiobiology of Hypofractionated Radiation

For a given fraction of radiation, larger fraction sizes are associated with fewer surviving cells as described by the classic linear-quadratic model. In this model, the log of cell survival is affected by two components: one proportional to the dose (linear), and the other proportional to the square of the dose (quadratic) [15]. Generally, with larger fractions, the cell survival becomes more greatly impacted by the quadratic component, and thus the radiation yields incrementally greater cell kill. Classically, late responding tissues have a smaller α/β ratio. The linear component (single cell killing events, characterized by the α) and the quadratic component (cell killing from the accumulation of sublethal events, characterized by the β) are equal at lower doses (in the vicinity of 2–3 Gy), beyond which the quadratic component dominates. With early responding tissues, such as many tumors and acutely reacting normal tissue, the linear and quadratic

components are equivalent in the vicinity of 10 Gy. Thus, late-effects are more greatly impacted by fraction size than early effects. Consequently, there is a reasonable concern about late toxicity with the use of hypofractionated regimens, even when stereotactic techniques are used to reduce the volume of normal tissue exposure.

Yet another model, the multi-target model, incorporates the effects from single event killing (more shallow slope at lower doses) and multi-target killing (steeper slope at higher doses) with a threshold value in which these effects transition. It should be appreciated that the linear-quadratic and the multi-target models are simply models which describe experimental findings, and do not necessarily describe the mechanism of cell killing.

The decades-long rationale for using standard smaller fractionation (with 1.8–2 Gy fractions) with conventional radiation is to allow for dose escalation while minimizing the risk of late toxicity [5]. If new technologies allow for hypofractionated radiation delivery without the added risk of toxicity, there is great potential for improving local control [5].

With hypofractionated schemes, the linear-quadratic model appears to predict a greater tumor effect than clinically observed, due to the quadratic term over-estimating cell kill [5, 16–19]. Possible reasons for this include: (1) inadequate tumor coverage due to the tight margins used with SBRT, (2) not providing time for tumor cell reassortment and reoxygenation [15], and (3) inadequacy of the linear quadratic model with hypofractionation. Pre-clinical data suggests that the margins we use should be adequate to account for tumor motion and microscopic extent of infiltration. TIMMERMAN's group [19] from the University Texas Southwestern have suggested using a hybrid linear-quadratic model and multi-target model to better predict tumor control. Perhaps such a model would also be potentially useful to predict late effects, though as of yet, there are no data to test this. Though the linear-quadratic model does have its shortcomings, it is useful to gain insight into predicting late effects, and help in determining fractionation schemes that optimize cell kill while minimize normal tissue toxicity [20]. Researchers from Australia and Canada have performed intricate modeling of hypofractionated stereotactic radiation, and conclude that the lower absolute doses used with hypofractionated regimens, combined with the normal tissue exposure to lower isodose lines with stereotactic delivery, results in a biologically sound rationale to use such approaches [17].

While classically, radiation induced cell kill, as described by the linear-quadratic model, results from mitotic death following unrepaired DNA double strand breakage, other mechanisms can lead to cell death, particularly at higher doses. These mechanisms can be incorporated into established models [21]. Apoptosis is well characterized for lymphoma cell lines [15], and may play a role in other solid tumors at higher fractional doses. Perhaps more relevant is endothelial apoptosis, resulting in microvascular disruption and resultant death of the cells supplied by that vasculature [22]. The mechanism of apoptosis is initiated by radiation induced damage to the plasma membrane, and the resultant apoptotic pathway mediated by the ceramide pathway [23–26]. This mechanism appears to be most significant above a ~ 8–10 Gy threshold [27]. Radiation may also stimulate endothelial cells to express cell adhesion molecules, stimulating an influx of immunologic cells [28, 29]. Higher fractional doses may also result in a more potent immunologic effect, resulting from radiation induced triggering of cancer cell antigen presentation, and the resulting immunologic response [30–34], and/or the recruitment of an immunologic response resulting from cytokine or other signal release [35–37]. While it is unknown the extent to which these other mechanisms account for tumor and normal tissue response, and to what extent larger fractions may impact them, a better understanding of these mechanisms may lead to more rational design of radiation treatments with respect to fractional dose delivery, total dose delivery and dose-volume constraints.

Regardless of the mechanism accounting for radiation damage, it is accepted that eradication of the stem cells in the treated volume contribute to the observed toxicity. Arguably, hypofractionated SBRT can yields greater advantage in parallel functioning tissues, in which the functional subunits are discrete entities as opposed to serial functioning tissues, in which the functional subunits are arranged in a linear or branching fashion [1, 5, 15]. With parallel functioning tissues, SBRT reduces the number of subunits destroyed by radiation by virtue of reducing the treatment volume. Small, and perhaps even larger volumes of parallel functioning organs can tolerate supratheshold radiation dosing, because either there is enough reserve in the undamaged portion of the organ (such as lung, liver or kidney) and/or there is a capacity to regenerate (such as liver). With serial functioning tissues, there is recruitment of stem cells from neighboring tissues (though arguably much less so with tissue such as spinal cord), and thus these tissues may achieve greater radiation tolerance with more standard fractionation [5]. Certainly SBRT techniques can be employed with lower fractional doses if there is concern about an adjoining serial functioning tissue. While small volumes of serially functioning tissues, such as the spinal cord, can safely tolerate suprathreshold doses [38, 39], it is not known in humans what constitutes a safe volume, what effect the lower dose penumbra may have on toxicity from suprathreshold doses [40, 41], nor what anatomical regions of serially functioning organs can tolerate these higher doses [42].

12.4
University of Rochester Experience with Hypofractionated SBRT

The University of Rochester has been using SBRT to treat primary and metastatic lesions since 2001 using the Novalis linear accelerator with the ExacTrac positioning platform and BrainLAB planning software [8, 43–45]. Table 12.1. describes the allowed dose and dose fractionation. These dose-fractionation schedules were selected on the basis of an expected 85% tumor control probability, using the linear-quadratic model as predicted by OKUNIEFF et al. [46]. While many fractionation schemes have been employed in our patients, with the total and fractional dose depending on the tumor location and volume of disease, the preferred dose-fractionation schedule has been 50 Gy in ten daily fractions. The planning target volume is generated with a mini-

mum gross target volume expansion of 10 mm in the craniocaudal direction, and 7–10 mm in other directions, which allows for coverage of between two and three standard deviations of motion [8]. Treatment is prescribed such that the 80% isodose line covers the planning target volume. SBRT is delivered using conformal shaped arcs or multiple fixed shaped coplanar beams.

Over 160 patients were enrolled on two prospective studies investigating SBRT in the treatment of limited metastatic disease [43–45]. Though many patients experience no acute symptoms, acute grade 1–2 fatigue and grade 1 dermatitis occurred in some patients. Acute grade ≥ 3 toxicity was generally not observed. There were 57 patients who survived > 2 years, with follow-up ranging from 24–77 months in these patients. Late toxicity was not commonly seen. The thoracic and liver toxicity are outlined in the following sections. Table 12.2. describes the dose-volume constraints used in our study. These guidelines have proven to be safe, though arguably, there is the potential to exceed these constraints, since we did not test toxicity in a Phase I approach. Additionally, these were maximum allowed constraints on study, though most patients were well below these constraints. For example, although a V20 (volume of lung receiving > 20 Gy) of 40% was allowed on study, the V20 in actuality ranged from 1%–34% [45]. Table 12.2 outlines the allowed dose and dose fractionation.

12.5
Review of Select Clinical Trials Using Hypofractionated SBRT: Late Toxicity

The current literature mostly focuses on the acute and dose limiting toxicity of SBRT. The CTCAE version 3 grading system does not differentiate between early and late toxicity, and many authors (ourselves included) report overall toxicity. Arguably, more mature data is needed to more fully comprehend the risks of late toxicity with SBRT.

Extracranial SBRT is used in the treatment of many organ sites, including lung, liver, pancreas, spine, kidney, adrenal, and musculoskeletal sites [2, 18, 47, 48].Tissues such as lung and liver, with parallel functional units, are well suited for stereotactic approaches, since SBRT allows for minimizing the number of functional units exposed to suprath-

Table 12.1. Select dose fractionation schemes employed at the University of Rochester

Fractional dose (Gy)	Number of fractions	Total Dose (Gy)[a]
3	17–19	51–57
4	12–14	48–56
5	9–11	9–11
6	7–8	42–48
8	5–6	40–48

[a] All treatments were delivered on a daily (Monday through Friday) basis. The preferred schedule was 5 Gy × 10

Table 12.2. Dose-volume constraints used at the University of Rochester

Lung (in patients with chronic lung disease)	1000 ml of tumor free lung 70% of normal lung <1.7 Gy per fraction and <17 Gy total 800 cc of normal lung <1.7 Gy per fraction and <17 Gy total
Lung (in patients with healthy lungs)	1000 ml of tumor free lung 60% of normal lung <2.0 Gy per fraction and <20 Gy total
Liver (in patients with chronic liver disease)	1000 ml of tumor free lung 70% of normal liver <30 Gy
Liver (in patients with healthy liver)	1000 ml of tumor free lung 60% of normal liver <30 Gy
Kidney (in patients with two functioning kidneys)	<50% of normal kidneys to receive >16 Gy
Kidney (in patients with one functioning kidney)	<10% of functioning kidney to receive >10% of prescribed dose and >1.5 Gy per fraction
Small bowel	Total dose <50 Gy
Spinal cord	Dose to center <2 Gy per fraction and <45 Gy total Surface dose <54 Gy total
Esophagus	Attempt to keep maximum dose <4 Gy per fraction

reshold doses [1, 5, 15]. Arguably, the treatment of abdominal and pelvic tumors is inherently riskier with large fractions due to the proximity of bowel, a parallel organ.

12.5.1
Lung

The standard treatment Stage I non-small cell lung cancer remains resection. In patients with inoperable disease, or in those who refuse resection, radiation therapy is a curative option, with poorer outcome compared to resection, which is arguably a reflection of selection bias. In patients with limited lung metastases, resection is an option, particularly in the setting of isolated lung metastases. Radiofrequency ablation is another option. External radiation is the best option for those unwilling to undergo or medically unfit for more invasive procedures. Radiation can be used for tumors abutting large vessels and central structures, which are generally not safely treated with more invasive techniques.

Our group has previously reviewed the literature on the outcome and toxicity of SBRT for lung metastases [49]. Acute toxicity generally includes constitutional symptoms of fatigue and malaise, cough and mild dermatitis. Acute esophagitis is commonly seen in the treatment of central tumors [50]. Nearly all patients treated with SBRT to the lung experi-

ence acute radiographic pneumonitis, while grade ≥3 pneumonitis is uncommon. In a study from Hokkaido University in which 156 patients received SBRT for Stage I lung cancer, radiation pneumonitis requiring steroid use was not correlated with pretreatment pulmonary function tests, dose-volume metrics, total dose or fractional dose [51].

Late toxicity is reported to be relatively uncommon, with late grade ≥3 toxicity ranging from 0%–7%. Examples of reported grade ≥2 late toxicity include pneumonitis [52, 53], chronic cough [54, 55], pulmonary bleeding/hemoptysis [56, 57], pulmonary function decline [52, 57], apnea [57], pneumonia [57], pleural effusion [52, 53, 57], airway narrowing or obstruction [55, 58], tracheal necrosis [59], chest pain [52, 60], rib fracture [53, 61], and esophageal ulceration [56]. While pulmonary function decline is generally uncommon [60, 62], when its is appreciated, it is often transient or asymptomatic [63, 64]. SBRT may in fact improve the diffusion capacity in some patients [62].

The constraints to the normal lung as well as other normal structures, such as spinal cord, esophagus, liver, stomach and bowel are critical in minimizing the risk of acute and late toxicity [49]. With greater clinical experience, these constraints will become better formalized. Certainly the dose, fractionation, volume and location of the target account for much of the reported toxicity, particularly toxicity related to necrosis and hemorrhage. However, host and tumor variables, which admittedly are largely uncharacterized, are also likely to be relevant, and arguably more relevant for pulmonary symptoms. In a study from Aarhus University, late dyspneic changes were not correlated to dose-volume parameters, and no consistent temporal variations were appreciated in their analysis [65]. Chronic obstructive pulmonary disease apparently accounted for symptomatic dyspnea rather than treatment effects.

The University of Indiana has the largest published North American experience treating Stage I lung cancer with SBRT. They enrolled patients with medically inoperable Stage I non-small cell lung cancer in a prospective Phase I study of three fractions of SBRT; the dose per fraction was escalated in 2 Gy increments, starting at 8 Gy per fraction [59, 63]. The spinal cord was limited to <6 Gy per fraction. In their initial report of 37 patients, six patients received steroid treatment for acute radiation pneumonitis. The authors noted a trend towards a decline in pulmonary function in the weeks that followed SBRT, which returned to baseline by 3–6 months after SBRT. Most ($n = 25$) patients developed radiographic evidence of fibrotic lung changes [63]. With a median follow-up of 15 months, no toxicity was seen beyond 6 weeks. In a follow-up report, with more patients accrued, three of five patients treated at the 24-Gy fraction dose experienced grade 3–4 toxicity, including pneumonitis ($n = 2$) and tracheal necrosis ($n = 1$) [59]. The timing of these toxicities was not addressed. In a subsequent Phase II study, in which 70 patients received 60–66 Gy in three fractions, eight were identified as having grade 3–4 toxicity, developing 1–25 months after SBRT, included decline in pulmonary function, pneumonia, pleural effusion, apnea, and skin reaction. Six patients were reported to have grade 5 (death) toxicity at 0.6–20 months (median 12) after SBRT (arguably in a frail population, with a limited life expectancy, in which SBRT may or may not have contributed to death) [57]. Four patients died from pneumonia, one from a pericardial effusion and another from massive hemoptysis. Univariate and multivariate analyses showed that tumor location (hilar/pericentral versus peripheral, $p = 0.004$) and tumor size (GTV > 10 ml versus smaller tumors, $p = 0.017$) were strong predictors of grade 3–5 toxicity ($p = 0.004$).

The University of Rochester analyzed 49 patients who received SBRT to metastases in the thorax (either lung, hilum or mediastinum). Patients were required to have 1000 ml of tumor-free lung. For patients with chronic lung disease, 70% of the lung or 800 ml (whichever was larger), was kept under 1.7 Gy per fraction. For patients with otherwise healthy lungs, 60% of the lung was kept under 2.0 Gy per fraction. Most patients received ten fractions of 5 Gy. Grade 1, 2 and 3 toxicity (acute and late) was seen in 35%, 6% and 2%, respectively; toxicity was not well correlated with the V10 or V20 [45]. No grade 4–5 toxicity was seen. The observed grade 3 toxicity was a non-malignant pleural effusion successfully managed with pleurocentesis and sclerosis; most grade 2 toxicity was a self limited cough.

Following SBRT, characteristic radiographic changes reflect the acute and late changes in the lung parenchyma. Several authors have systematically described these radiographic changes [66–68]. The acute changes (generally occurring several months after radiation) generally demonstrate consolidation and ground glass opacities. Table 12.3 summarizes the acute changes as described in the literature. In a study from Hiroshima University, patients with the diffuse consolidation pattern as well as those with no increased density experienced a greater risk of grade ≥2 radiation pneumonitis [67]. In that same study, 80% of lesions that demonstrated acute diffuse consolidation developed into late changes of consolidation, volume loss and bronchiectasis (termed modified conventional pattern); 59% of lesions that demonstrated no acute consolidation or densities developed into late changes characterized by linear opacities with associated volume loss (termed scar-like pattern). Overall, the late changes (>6 months after SBRT) of modified conventional pattern, mass-like pattern (focal consolidation around tumor site) and scar-like pattern were seen in 62%, 17% and 21%, respectively. In a study from Kyoto University, late changes (>6 months after SBRT) were characterized as patchy consolidation (within irradiated lung, though not conforming to SBRT field) in 8%, discrete consolidation (within SBRT field, though not outlining shape of field) in 27% and solid consolidation (outlining SBRT field) in 65% [66]. The shape of the radiation changes were described as wedge (35%), round (35%) and irregular (29%) and the extent of fibrotic change was described as peripheral (48%), central (6%), both (39%) and skip lesion(s) isolated from the tumor (6%). Certainly, late pulmonary fibrosis can change in shape and extent over time. In a study from Tokyo, over the course of follow-up imaging, 6–11 months after radiation. the fibrotic changes shrunk in 44% of patients and moved (generally toward the hilum) in 38% [68]. This same group from Tokyo recently published a

Table 12.3. Acute radiographic changes after SBRT to the lung

	Diffuse changes		Patchy changes		Discrete	No change
Hiroshima University	Consolidation 9%	GGO 12%	Consolidation + GGO 15%	GGO 2%		33%
Kyoto University	Homogeneous slight ↑ in opacities 26%		Consolidation 68%		Consolidation 6%	0%

GGO, ground glass opacities

study in which late radiation fibrosis radiographically appeared as abnormal opacities, mimicking recurrent tumors [69]. The authors urged caution in the interpretation of these scans, suggesting close follow-up to monitor changes, PET scanning and/or biopsy. While all of the late changes described above reflect fibrosis, the clinical significance of these different characteristics of radiation change are not known.

12.5.2
Liver

The standard treatment for limited liver metastases or primary liver malignancies is resection. Other modalities include radiofrequency ablation and radiation. Arguably, radiation is the least invasive approach, and well suited for many patients with inoperable disease, comorbid conditions and/or several lesions.

Our group previously reviewed the literature on the outcome and toxicity of SBRT for liver tumors [49]. As with SBRT to the lung, SBRT to the liver often results in mild constitutional symptoms. Grade ≥ 3 late toxicity generally does not appear to occur.

The University of Colorado and University of Indiana enrolled 18 patients with between one and three liver metastases in a prospective Phase I study of three fractions of SBRT; the dose per fraction was escalated in 2-Gy increments, starting at 12 Gy per fraction [70]. No patients experienced grade > 2 toxicity. It was required that 700 ml of normal liver receive < 15 Gy total dose. Most patients were noted to have well circumscribed hypodense lesions corresponding to the dose distribution corresponding to ~30 Gy in 10-Gy fractions. In a follow-up analysis, including an additional 18 patients treated on a phase II study, one instance of subcutaneous tissue breakdown occurred, while no liver toxicity attributable to SBRT occurred [71].

The University of Rochester analyzed 69 patients who received SBRT to metastases in the liver, mostly treated to 50 Gy in 5-Gy fractions. The volume of liver not involved by gross tumor was required to be ≥ 1000 ml. For patients with no history of macronodular sclerosis, liver failure or hepatitis, the dose to 60% of the liver volume was required to be < 30 Gy, and, for patients with a history of hepatitis or cirrhosis, the dose to 70% of the liver volume was required to be < 30 Gy. Grade 1–2 elevation of liver function tests occurred in 28%, and no grade ≥ 3 toxicity was observed [44]. Clinically insignificant radiographic changes were seen in all patients with treated liver lesions.

In a study from Aarhus University, 44 patients with liver metastases from colorectal cancer were treated to a dose of 45 Gy in 15-Gy fractions. Dose constraints included < 30% of the liver receiving a total of > 10 Gy, and the spinal cord maximum was < 18 Gy. The dose to kidney, intestine and stomach was kept as low as possible. Acute toxicity (within 6 months) included colonic ulceration (one patient) and duodenal ulceration (two patients) and one patient developed hepatic failure. Acute grade 3–4 ulceration of the skin, pain, nausea and diarrhea were also observed. Late toxicity was not explicitly discussed [72].

Princess Margaret Hospital recently published a Phase I study, in which 41 patients with primary hepatocellular or intrahepatic biliary cancer received 24–60 Gy in six fractions, in a dose escalation study, in which patients were stratified into three different dose escalation groups based on the effective liver volume irradiated [73]. A normal tissue complication model was used to stratify patients into three separate groups of dose escalation. Generally, the mean liver dose was kept < 22 Gy and the mean kidney dose was < 12 Gy. The maximal doses (to < 0.5 ml of tissue) were as follows: 27 Gy to the spinal cord; 30 Gy to the stomach, small bowel and large bowel and 40 Gy to the heart. Roughly 25% of patients experienced acute grade 3 liver enzymes and roughly 25% experienced acute (within 3 months) progression of their Child-Pugh classification, seemingly due to disease progression. Acute transient biliary obstruction was seen in two patients. There was one late death from gastrointestinal bleeding resulting from a duodenal-tumor fistula and one patient required surgery for a bowel obstruction; both of these late toxicities were exacerbated by (and perhaps primarily attributed to) recurrent disease.

12.5.3
Pancreas

Locally advanced pancreatic cancer has an unfortunately dismal prognosis, with distant metastases and local progression almost invariably leading to death. Local control from radiation can yield palliation and prophylactic palliation of biliary obstruction, bowel obstruction and pain from splanchnic nerve invasion. SBRT may afford an advantage in terms of improved local control as well as shorter treatment duration.

In a Phase II study from Aarhus University, 22 patients with unresectable pancreatic cancer received 45 Gy in 15-Gy fractions [74]. The PTV (1-cm margins around the CTV) was covered by the 67% isodose line. Acute grade 3–4 toxicity included pain, nausea, diarrhea, severe duodenal and gastric mucositis and ulceration and perforation. Poor survival precluded a late toxicity analysis. Whether toxicity was related to disease progression or radiation could not be determined.

In the Phase I study from Stanford, 15 patients were treated with single dose, escalated from 15 to 25 Gy [75]. The 50% isodose line covered only the duodenal wall closest to the tumor. At the 25-Gy dose, the mean dose to 5% of the duodenum was 22.5 Gy and the mean dose to 50% of the duodenum was 14.5 Gy. No acute grade ≥ 3 toxicity was observed; late toxicity and symptom control were not explicitly reported, presumably due to the limited follow-up (median 5 months) and poor survival (median 11 months). The results from Stanford University conflict with those from Aarhus University in that Stanford found SBRS to be relatively tolerable. This may be a result of different dose fractionation, different treatment design and/or differences in patient population and/or disease failure. The group from Stanford attributes the differences in toxicity to their use of respiratory tracking. Stanford University enrolled 16 patients in a subsequent Phase II study in which 45 Gy of conventional radiation was followed by a single 25-Gy SBRS fraction [76]. Radiation guidelines included: 70% of the liver < 15 Gy, 70% of each kidney < 15 Gy, 95% of bowel < 45 Gy, spinal cord maximum < 30 Gy. Acute grade 3 toxicity included gastroparesis in two patients (one prior to SBRS). Late toxicity included some patients (the number not explicitly reported) who developed grade 2 duodenal ulceration 4–6 months after SBRS. In a later report, the authors document late gastrointestinal bleeding from unknown cause and duodenal obstruction in the same patient [77].

These authors from Stanford examined four patients with pancreatic cancer at autopsy, 5–7 months after SBRS, in order to characterize the histopathologic findings [77]. The primary tumors were characterized by extensive fibrosis, varying amounts of necrosis (tumor necrosis and ischemic necrosis) and widespread vascular injury (fibrinous exudate of arterial wall, necrosis and luminal occlusion). Stromal changes included fibrosis, atypical fibroblasts and fibrin deposition. Sparse residual cancer cells were seen. In the adjoining colorectal tissue in one patient, mucosal exudate with possible pseudomembrane formation and submucosal vascular damage were seen. The colonic mucosa was estimated to have received 4–11.5 Gy. Lymph nodes exposed to radiation were depleted of lymphocytes.

12.5.4
Prostate

Prostate cancer may benefit from hypofractionation due to the low α/β ratio of prostate cancer [78], though obviously there is concern about late effects given the proximity of the rectum and bladder, and the expected lengthy survival of these patients [18]. Hypofractionation can be delivered using IGRT, with ultrasound and/or CT, to improve target localization, IMRT to reduce rectal and bladder dose and/or proton therapy which can also reduce normal tissue exposure. Large fractional doses are also delivered with high dose rate brachytherapy. There is only limited published experience with SBRT, which is generally delivered with the assistance of fiducials implanted in the prostate and/or IGRT [79, 80]. Virgina Mason treated 40 prostate cancer patients with 33.5 Gy in 6.7-Gy fractions, which was expected to provide equivalent biochemical control to 78 Gy in 2-Gy fractions (assuming an α/β ratio of 1.5) [80].

The equivalent dose to the rectum (using an α/β ratio of 3) was estimated to be 65 Gy in 2-Gy fractions, which was expected to be safe given the low volume of rectum that would be exposed. SBRT was used with implanted fiducials. Late grade 1–2 toxicity (defined as >1 month post treatment) included 45% with genitourinary toxicity and 37% with gastrointestinal toxicity [79]. No late Grade 3 or higher toxicity was reported. In all, 26 patients reported potency before therapy, of which six have developed impotence.

12.5.5
Spine

Metastases to the spine can result in pain as well as neurologic symptoms, which are often well palliated with radiation. The standard approach to the treatment of spinal metastases is surgical decompression followed by radiation or radiation alone in those patients not amenable to surgery. The radiation is generally delivered in a short course (1–2 weeks) with daily fractions of 2.5–4 Gy. The prescribed dose of 20–40 Gy with these larger fraction sizes is generally accepted to be at the spinal cord tolerance (though certainly below the TD 5/5) [4], and thus further radiation of the cord is thought to be riskier, though potentially feasible [81]. Thus, in patients with previously irradiated, symptomatic spinal metastases, SBRT and SBRS can allow for a means to treat spinal tumors while minimizing the dose to the cord. While hypofractionation in this situation is counterintuitive, given the association of late toxicity with fraction size, early clinical data has shown it to be tolerable, albeit with limited patient follow-up.

Single fraction SBRS [82–89], and hypofractionated SBRT [87, 90–92] have been used to treat metastases (as well as the much rarer primary spinal tumors). SBRS has also been used as a boost treatment immediately following a course of fractionated radiation in patients who have not been previously irradiated [87]. Techniques such as IMRT can be used to help conform the dose around the spinal cord [84, 86, 89–91, 93], while IGRT and/or SBRT can be used to accurately position the patient and target [84, 85, 89–91, 93]. With SBRS and SBRT to the spine, the spinal cord dose is minimized, resulting in a maximum dose on the order of 10 Gy [82–92]. Data from 177 patients with 233 lesions treated at Henry Ford Hospital suggests that a single fractional dose of 10 Gy to <10% of the contoured spinal cord (6 mm above

and below the target) is safe, and that small volumes (<1% of the contoured cord) can safely receive higher maximal doses, perhaps up to 20 Gy. More rigid dose constraints have yet to be published.

Given the palliative nature of this treatment, long term follow-up is generally limited to the extent that late toxicity is not readily assessable. Certainly, spinal SBRS and SBRT have proven to be tolerable and have produced excellent palliation without observed neural toxicity. At least one report has suggested that the acute toxicity using these approaches is perhaps better than conventional radiation [94]. Myelopathy and radiculopathy rarely occur. Henry Ford Hospital reported 1 patient out of 177 who developed radiation related spinal cord injury, resulting in slight unilateral lower extremity weakness (4 out of 5 strength) that responded to steroids [95]. In a recent report from Memorial Sloan Kettering, in which 103 lesions in 93 patients were treated with a single dose (18–24 Gy prescribed to the PTV, with the spinal cord limited to 12–14 Gy), late toxicity included vertebral body fracture and tracheoesophageal fistula [89]. In the largest series to date from the University of Pittsburgh, in which 393 patients with 500 lesions received a single dose of SBRS (12.5–20 Gy around the periphery, with only a small volume of spinal cord exceeding 8 Gy), no patient developed a new neurologic defect [82, 83]. No late effects were reported with a follow-up of 3–53 (median 21) months.

12.6
Conclusions

SBRT uses a three-dimensional coordinate system to more accurately localize the treatment target, and therefore reduce the uncertainty in patient set-up and. Because SBRT reduces the volume of normal tissue exposed to therapeutic doses, large fractional doses can be used to achieve maximal local control of the treated tumor in certain situations. The classic radiobiology models do not appear to be adequate to predict the clinical outcome of hypofractionated radiation delivery. Mechanisms such as tumor apoptosis, endothelial apoptosis, and immunologic effect may play a more prominent role after large fractional doses.

A large body of literature supports the use of SBRT to tumors in the lung and liver, which are organ whose subunits are arranged in series. SBRT can therefore reduce the number of functional subunits destroyed by radiation. Caution must be heeded with tumors close to the esophagus, large airways and spinal cord. SBRT to liver and lung tumors appears to be safe (when adhering to published dose constraints), with minimal symptomatic acute or late toxicity.

There is a large body of literature that supports the use of SBRT/SBRS in the treatment of spine tumors, even after receiving full dose conventional fractionated radiation. Toxicity appears minimal, admittedly in a patient population with limited long-term follow-up. Other sites that have been investigated include pancreas, prostate and kidney. The proximity of these structures to bowel make SBRT potentially riskier, though single institution experience has shown promise.

The primary goal of dose escalation with SBRT is to improve tumor control. If local control rates of >90% are attained, further dose escalation may not yield further improved local control, and may not be warranted due to the risk of greater toxicity. Because toxicity is uncommon with the doses that are presently used, a large number of patients will need to be analyzed to determine optimal normal tissue dose-volume constraints. Long-term follow-up is also necessary given that late effects can occur years after radiation. Further study is needed to better assess the late toxicity of SBRT in all locations.

References

1. Kavanagh BD, McGarry RC, Timmerman RD (2006) Extracranial radiosurgery (stereotactic body radiation therapy) for oligometastases. Semin Radiat Oncol 16:77–84
2. Timmerman RD, Kavanagh BD, Cho LC et al (2007) Stereotactic body radiation therapy in multiple organ sites. J Clin Oncol 25:947–952
3. Baumert BG, Rutten I, Dehing-Oberije C et al (2006) A pathology-based substrate for target definition in radiosurgery of brain metastases. Int J Radiat Oncol Biol Phys 66:187–194
4. Milano MT, Constine LS, Okunieff P (2007) Normal tissue tolerance dose metrics for radiation therapy of major organs. Semin Radiat Oncol 17:131–140
5. Timmerman R, Bastasch M, Saha D et al (2007) Optimizing dose and fractionation for stereotactic body radiation therapy. Normal tissue and tumor control effects with large dose per fraction. Front Radiat Ther Oncol 40:352–365
6. Timmerman RD, Forster KM, Chinsoo Cho L (2005) Extracranial stereotactic radiation delivery. Semin Radiat Oncol 15:202–207
7. Harris JR, Levene MB (1976) Visual complications following irradiation for pituitary adenomas and craniopharyngiomas. Radiology 120:167–171
8. O'Dell WG, Schell MC, Reynolds D et al (2002) Dose broadening due to target position variability during fractionated breath-held radiation therapy. Med Phys 29:1430–1437
9. Intensity Modulated Radiation Therapy Collaborative Working Group (2001) Intensity-modulated radiotherapy: current status and issues of interest. Int J Radiat Oncol Biol Phys 51:880–914
10. Glatstein E (2002) Intensity-modulated radiation therapy: the inverse, the converse, and the perverse. Semin Radiat Oncol 12:272–281
11. Goffman TE, Glatstein E (2002) Intensity-modulated radiation therapy. Radiat Res 158:115–117
12. Hall EJ (2006) Intensity-modulated radiation therapy, protons, and the risk of second cancers. Int J Radiat Oncol Biol Phys 65:1–7
13. Hall EJ, Wuu CS (2003) Radiation-induced second cancers: the impact of 3D-CRT and IMRT. Int J Radiat Oncol Biol Phys 56:83–88
14. Hall EJ (2006) The inaugural Frank Ellis lecture – iatrogenic cancer: the impact of intensity-modulated radiotherapy. Clin Oncol (R Coll Radiol) 18:277–282
15. Hall EJ, Giacca AJ (2005) Radiobiology for the radiologist, 6th edn. Lippincott Williams & Wilkins, Philadelphia
16. Guerrero M, Li XA (2004) Extending the linear-quadratic model for large fraction doses pertinent to stereotactic radiotherapy. Phys Med Biol 49:4825–4835
17. Hoban PW, Jones LC, Clark BG (1999) Modeling late effects in hypofractionated stereotactic radiotherapy. Int J Radiat Oncol Biol Phys 43:199–210
18. Chang BK, Timmerman RD (2007) Stereotactic body radiation therapy: a comprehensive review. Am J Clin Oncol 30:637–644
19. Park C, Papiez L, Zhang S et al (2008) Universal survival curve and single fraction equivalent dose: useful tools in understanding potency of ablative radiotherapy. Int J Radiat Oncol Biol Phys 70:847–852
20. Jones B, Dale RG, Finst P et al (2000) Biological equivalent dose assessment of the consequences of hypofractionated radiotherapy. Int J Radiat Oncol Biol Phys 47:1379–1384
21. Ling CC, Chen CH, Fuks Z (1994) An equation for the dose response of radiation-induced apoptosis: possible incorporation with the LQ model. Radiother Oncol 33:17–22
22. Garcia-Barros M, Paris F, Cordon-Cardo C et al (2003) Tumor response to radiotherapy regulated by endothelial cell apoptosis. Science 300:1155–1159
23. Haimovitz-Friedman A, Kan CC, Ehleiter D et al (1994) Ionizing radiation acts on cellular membranes to generate ceramide and initiate apoptosis. J Exp Med 180:525–535
24. Chmura SJ, Nodzenski E, Beckett MA et al (1997) Loss of ceramide production confers resistance to radiation-induced apoptosis. Cancer Res 57:1270–1275
25. Lin X, Fuks Z, Kolesnick R (2000) Ceramide mediates radiation-induced death of endothelium. Crit Care Med 28:N87–93
26. Kolesnick R, Fuks Z (2003) Radiation and ceramide-induced apoptosis. Oncogene 22:5897–5906
27. Fuks Z, Kolesnick R (2005) Engaging the vascular component of the tumor response. Cancer Cell 8:89–91

28. Hallahan D, Kuchibhotla J, Wyble C (1996) Cell adhesion molecules mediate radiation-induced leukocyte adhesion to the vascular endothelium. Cancer Res 56:5150–5155

29. Gaugler MH, Squiban C, van der Meeren A et al (1997) Late and persistent up-regulation of intercellular adhesion molecule-1 (ICAM-1) expression by ionizing radiation in human endothelial cells in vitro. Int J Radiat Biol 72:201–209

30. Chakraborty M, Abrams SI, Camphausen K et al (2003) Irradiation of tumor cells up-regulates Fas and enhances CTL lytic activity and CTL adoptive immunotherapy. J Immunol 170:6338–6347

31. Lugade AA, Moran JP, Gerber SA et al (2005) Local radiation therapy of B16 melanoma tumors increases the generation of tumor antigen-specific effector cells that traffic to the tumor. J Immunol 174:7516–7523

32. Reits EA, Hodge JW, Herberts CA et al (2006) Radiation modulates the peptide repertoire, enhances MHC class I expression, and induces successful antitumor immunotherapy. J Exp Med 203:1259–1271

33. Demaria S, Formenti SC (2007) Sensors of ionizing radiation effects on the immunological microenvironment of cancer. Int J Radiat Biol 83:819–825

34. Zhang B, Bowerman NA, Salama JK et al (2007) Induced sensitization of tumor stroma leads to eradication of established cancer by T cells. J Exp Med 204:49–55

35. McBride WH, Chiang CS, Olson JL et al (2004) A sense of danger from radiation. Radiat Res 162:1–19

36. Chen Y, Williams J, Ding I et al (2002) Radiation pneumonitis and early circulatory cytokine markers. Semin Radiat Oncol 12:26–33

37. Neta R, Okunieff P (1996) Cytokine-induced radiation protection and sensitization. Semin Radiat Oncol 6:306–320

38. Bijl HP, van Luijk P, Coppes RP et al (2002) Dose-volume effects in the rat cervical spinal cord after proton irradiation. Int J Radiat Oncol Biol Phys 52:205–211

39. van der Kogel AJ (1993) Dose-volume effects in the spinal cord. Radiother Oncol 29:105–109

40. Bijl HP, van Luijk P, Coppes RP et al (2006) Influence of adjacent low-dose fields on tolerance to high doses of protons in rat cervical spinal cord. Int J Radiat Oncol Biol Phys 64:1204–1210

41. Bijl HP, van Luijk P, Coppes RP et al (2003) Unexpected changes of rat cervical spinal cord tolerance caused by inhomogeneous dose distributions. Int J Radiat Oncol Biol Phys 57:274–281

42. Philippens ME, Pop LA, Visser AG et al (2007) Dose-volume effects in rat thoracolumbar spinal cord: the effects of nonuniform dose distribution. Int J Radiat Oncol Biol Phys 69:204–213

43. Milano MT, Katz AW, Muhs AG et al (2008) A prospective pilot study of curative-intent stereotactic body radiation therapy in patients with 5 or fewer oligometastatic lesions. Cancer 112:650–658

44. Katz AW, Carey-Sampson M, Muhs AG et al (2007) Hypofractionated stereotactic body radiation therapy (SBRT) for limited hepatic metastases. Int J Radiat Oncol Biol Phys 67:793–798

45. Okunieff P, Petersen AL, Philip A et al (2006) Stereotactic body radiation therapy (SBRT) for lung metastases. Acta Oncol 45:808–817

46. Okunieff P, Morgan D, Niemierko A et al (1995) Radiation dose-response of human tumors. Int J Radiat Oncol Biol Phys 32:1227–1237

47. Chawla S, Okunieff P, Chen Y et al (2007) Stereotactic body radiation therapy (SBRT) for the treatment of adrenal metastases. First International Symposium on Stereotactic Body Radiation Therapy and Stereotactic Radiosurgery, Orlando, FL

48. Teh BS, Paulino AC, Lu HH et al (2007) Versatility of the Novalis system to deliver image-guided stereotactic body radiation therapy (SBRT) for various anatomical sites. Technol Cancer Res Treat 6:347–354

49. Carey Sampson M, Katz A, Constine LS (2006) Stereotactic body radiation therapy for extracranial oligometastases: does the sword have a double edge? Semin Radiat Oncol 16:67–76

50. Xia T, Li H, Sun Q et al (2006) Promising clinical outcome of stereotactic body radiation therapy for patients with inoperable Stage I/II non-small-cell lung cancer. Int J Radiat Oncol Biol Phys 66:117–125

51. Fujino M, Shirato H, Onishi H et al (2006) Characteristics of patients who developed radiation pneumonitis requiring steroid therapy after stereotactic irradiation for lung tumors. Cancer J 12:41–46

52. Onimaru R, Fujino M, Yamazaki K et al (2008) Steep dose-response relationship for stage I non-small-cell lung cancer using hypofractionated high-dose irradiation by real-time tumor-tracking radiotherapy. Int J Radiat Oncol Biol Phys 70:374–381

53. Zimmermann FB, Geinitz H, Schill S et al (2006) Stereotactic hypofractionated radiotherapy in stage I (T1-2 N0 M0) non-small-cell lung cancer (NSCLC). Acta Oncol 45:796–801

54. Blomgren H, Lax I, Goranson H (1998) Radiosurgery for tumors in the body: clinical experience using a new method. J Radiosurg 1:63–74

55. Song DY, Benedict SH, Cardinale RM et al (2005) Stereotactic body radiation therapy of lung tumors: preliminary experience using normal tissue complication probability-based dose limits. Am J Clin Oncol 28:591–596

56. Wulf J, Hadinger U, Oppitz U et al (2001) Stereotactic radiotherapy of targets in the lung and liver. Strahlenther Onkol 177:645–655

57. Timmerman R, McGarry R, Yiannoutsos C et al (2006) Excessive toxicity when treating central tumors in a phase II study of stereotactic body radiation therapy for medically inoperable early-stage lung cancer. J Clin Oncol 24:4833–4839

58. Joyner M, Salter BJ, Papanikolaou N et al (2006) Stereotactic body radiation therapy for centrally located lung lesions. Acta Oncol 45:802–807

59. McGarry RC, Papiez L, Williams M et al (2005) Stereotactic body radiation therapy of early-stage non-small-cell lung carcinoma: phase I study. Int J Radiat Oncol Biol Phys 63:1010–1015

60. Onimaru R, Shirato H, Shimizu S et al (2003) Tolerance of organs at risk in small-volume, hypofractionated, image-guided radiotherapy for primary and metastatic lung cancers. Int J Radiat Oncol Biol Phys 56:126–135

61. Nyman J, Johansson KA, Hulten U (2006) Stereotactic hypofractionated radiotherapy for stage I non-small cell lung cancer – mature results for medically inoperable patients. Lung Cancer 51:97–103

62. Ohashi T, Takeda A, Shigematsu N et al (2005) Differences in pulmonary function before vs. 1 year after hypofractionated stereotactic radiotherapy for small

peripheral lung tumors. Int J Radiat Oncol Biol Phys 62:1003–1008

63. Timmerman R, Papiez L, McGarry R et al (2003) Extracranial stereotactic radioablation: results of a phase I study in medically inoperable stage I non-small cell lung cancer. Chest 124:1946–1955

64. Fukumoto S, Shirato H, Shimzu S et al (2002) Small-volume image-guided radiotherapy using hypofractionated, coplanar, and noncoplanar multiple fields for patients with inoperable Stage I nonsmall cell lung carcinomas. Cancer 95:1546–1553

65. Paludan M, Traberg Hansen A, Petersen J et al (2006) Aggravation of dyspnea in stage I non-small cell lung cancer patients following stereotactic body radiotherapy: is there a dose-volume dependency? Acta Oncol 45:818–822

66. Aoki T, Nagata Y, Negoro Y et al (2004) Evaluation of lung injury after three-dimensional conformal stereotactic radiation therapy for solitary lung tumors: CT appearance. Radiology 230:101–108

67. Kimura T, Matsuura K, Murakami Y et al (2006) CT appearance of radiation injury of the lung and clinical symptoms after stereotactic body radiation therapy (SBRT) for lung cancers: are patients with pulmonary emphysema also candidates for SBRT for lung cancers? Int J Radiat Oncol Biol Phys 66:483–491

68. Takeda T, Takeda A, Kunieda E et al (2004) Radiation injury after hypofractionated stereotactic radiotherapy for peripheral small lung tumors: serial changes on CT. AJR Am J Roentgenol 182:1123–1128

69. Takeda A, Kunieda E, Takeda T et al (2008) Possible misinterpretation of demarcated solid patterns of radiation fibrosis on CT Scans as tumor recurrence in patients receiving hypofractionated stereotactic radiotherapy for lung cancer. Int J Radiat Oncol Biol Phys 70:1057–1065

70. Schefter TE, Kavanagh BD, Timmerman RD et al (2005) A phase I trial of stereotactic body radiation therapy (SBRT) for liver metastases. Int J Radiat Oncol Biol Phys 62:1371–1378

71. Kavanagh BD, Schefter TE, Cardenes HR et al (2006) Interim analysis of a prospective phase I/II trial of SBRT for liver metastases. Acta Oncol 45:848–855

72. Hoyer M, Roed H, Traberg Hansen A et al (2006) Phase II study on stereotactic body radiotherapy of colorectal metastases. Acta Oncol 45:823–830

73. Tse RV, Hawkins M, Lockwood G et al (2008) Phase I study of individualized stereotactic body radiotherapy for hepatocellular carcinoma and intrahepatic cholangiocarcinoma. J Clin Oncol 26:657–664

74. Hoyer M, Roed H, Sengelov L et al (2005) Phase II study on stereotactic radiotherapy of locally advanced pancreatic carcinoma. Radiother Oncol 76:48–53

75. Koong AC, Le QT, Ho A et al (2004) Phase I study of stereotactic radiosurgery in patients with locally advanced pancreatic cancer. Int J Radiat Oncol Biol Phys 58:1017–1021

76. Koong AC, Christofferson E, Le QT et al (2005) Phase II study to assess the efficacy of conventionally fractionated radiotherapy followed by a stereotactic radiosurgery boost in patients with locally advanced pancreatic cancer. Int J Radiat Oncol Biol Phys 63:320–323

77. Cupp JS, Koong AC, Fisher GA et al (2008) Tissue effects after stereotactic body radiotherapy using cyberknife for patients with abdominal malignancies. Clin Oncol (R Coll Radiol) 20:69–75

78. Fowler JF, Ritter MA, Chappell RJ et al (2003) What hypofractionated protocols should be tested for prostate cancer? Int J Radiat Oncol Biol Phys 56:1093–1104

79. Pawlicki T, Cotrutz C, King C (2007) Prostate cancer therapy with stereotactic body radiation therapy. Front Radiat Ther Oncol 40:395–406

80. Madsen BL, Hsi RA, Pham HT et al (2007) Stereotactic hypofractionated accurate radiotherapy of the prostate (SHARP), 33.5 Gy in five fractions for localized disease: first clinical trial results. Int J Radiat Oncol Biol Phys 67:1099–1105

81. Nieder C, Grosu AL, Andratschke NH et al (2006) Update of human spinal cord reirradiation tolerance based on additional data from 38 patients. Int J Radiat Oncol Biol Phys 66:1446–1449

82. Gerszten PC, Burton SA, Ozhasoglu C et al (2007) Radiosurgery for spinal metastases: clinical experience in 500 cases from a single institution. Spine 32:193–199

83. Gerszten PC, Ozhasoglu C, Burton SA et al (2004) CyberKnife frameless stereotactic radiosurgery for spinal lesions: clinical experience in 125 cases. Neurosurgery 55:89–98; discussion 98–89

84. Jin JY, Chen Q, Jin R et al (2007) Technical and clinical experience with spine radiosurgery: a new technology for management of localized spine metastases. Technol Cancer Res Treat 6:127–133

85. Ryu S, Rock J, Rosenblum M et al (2004) Patterns of failure after single-dose radiosurgery for spinal metastasis. J Neurosurg 101[Suppl 3]:402–405

86. De Salles AA, Pedroso AG, Medin P et al (2004) Spinal lesions treated with Novalis shaped beam intensity-modulated radiosurgery and stereotactic radiotherapy. J Neurosurg 101[Suppl 3]:435–440

87. Benzil DL, Saboori M, Mogilner AY et al (2004) Safety and efficacy of stereotactic radiosurgery for tumors of the spine. J Neurosurg 101[Suppl 3]:413–418

88. Hamilton AJ, Lulu BA, Fosmire H et al (1996) LINAC-based spinal stereotactic radiosurgery. Stereotact Funct Neurosurg 66:1–9

89. Yamada Y, Bilsky MH, Lovelock DM et al (2008) High-dose, single-fraction image-guided intensity-modulated radiotherapy for metastatic spinal lesions. Int J Radiat Oncol Biol Phys 71:484–490

90. Chang EL, Shiu AS, Lii MF et al (2004) Phase I clinical evaluation of near-simultaneous computed tomographic image-guided stereotactic body radiotherapy for spinal metastases. Int J Radiat Oncol Biol Phys 59:1288–1294

91. Chang EL, Shiu AS, Mendel E et al (2007) Phase I/II study of stereotactic body radiotherapy for spinal metastasis and its pattern of failure. J Neurosurg Spine 7:151–160

92. Yamada Y, Lovelock DM, Yenice KM et al (2005) Multifractionated image-guided and stereotactic intensity-modulated radiotherapy of paraspinal tumors: a preliminary report. Int J Radiat Oncol Biol Phys 62:53–61

93. Yin FF, Ryu S, Ajlouni M et al (2004) Image-guided procedures for intensity-modulated spinal radiosurgery. Technical note. J Neurosurg 101[Suppl 3]:419–424

94. Gagnon GJ, Henderson FC, Gehan EA et al (2007) Cyberknife radiosurgery for breast cancer spine metastases: a matched-pair analysis. Cancer 110:1796–1802

95. Ryu S, Jin JY, Jin R et al (2007) Partial volume tolerance of the spinal cord and complications of single-dose radiosurgery. Cancer 109:628–636

The Radiation Spectrum of Normal Tissue Toxicity and Tolerance – Multiorgan Domino Effect

PHILIP RUBIN

CONTENTS

13.1 Introduction

Conceptually, normal tissue tolerance is often viewed and defined in terms of a single specific normal tissue/organ site with the clinical illusion that during radiation treatment the adverse effects are localized and limited to those normal tissues within the radiation field. However, with the technological advances of highly computerized treatment delivery and dynamic multileaf collimation, the widespread use of intensity modulated radiation therapy (IMRT) allows for administering higher doses to defined tumor volume contours but in the process delivers more radiation to all the surrounding normal tissues in the axial segments being treated (Fig. 13.1) [1, 2].

P. RUBIN, MD
Professor and Chair Emeritus, Department of Radiation Oncology, University of Rochester School of Medicine and Dentistry, 601 Elmwood Avenue, Rochester, NY 14642, USA

Thus, there is an increasing need to recognize the spectrum of normal tissues and organs which are exposed but often obscured in color wash isodose curves. Although each critical structure has radiation tolerance limits well defined, it is important to have a more holistic view of the radiation effects in the large variety of normal tissues adjacent to the tumor, recognizing that all modalities leave the persistence of the memory of an untoward perturbation of their cellular, genetic, and molecular elements (Fig. 13.2) [3].

The four Rs of tumor radiobiology have dominated the concepts of the effectiveness of radiation cell kill and provide an understanding of cancer recurrence. The pioneering experiments of Hall, Elkind and Kallman [4–6] (Fig. 13.3) identified the processes of cell repair, reassortment, repopulation and reoxygenation. In an analogous fashion these radiobiologic concepts can be applied to the homeostatic mechanisms that apply to normal tissue preservation. That is, radiation cell kill within a normal organ or structure needs to be compensated for its continued function and to achieve a favorable therapeutic ratio. The Rs of tumor radiobiology are presented in this new context in five phases. This results in a progressive and unending biocontinuum for a lifetime (Fig. 13.4) [7].

13.2 Phase I: Release and Regeneration

The lymphocyte and macrophage are the first tissue to react due to their inherent radiosensitivity. Their lysis and rapid apoptosis releases a cytokine and chemokine cascade which is perpetuated as the radiation effects other cells in the adjacent tissues. Our group's demonstration that the initial multicel-

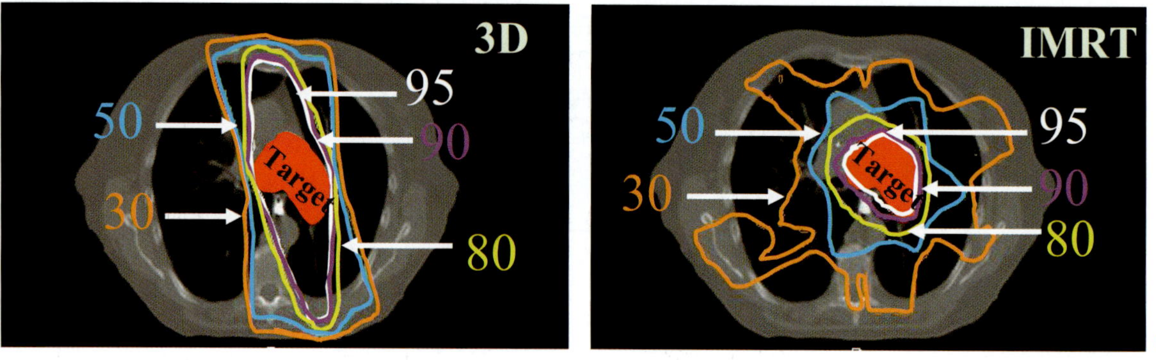

Fig. 13.1a,b. Percent relative isodose distributions for the 3DCRT plan (**a**) and IMRT-2 plan (**b**). The dose distributions show that the IMRT-2 plan is more conformal than the 3DCRT plan at the cost of slightly losing target coverage. Unlike the UTCP plan values, the UTCP$_{QALY}$ values, which incorporate clinically realistic quality of life data, suggest that the UTCP$_{QALY}$ formalism provides better differentiation between plans. (Reprinted with permission from [2])

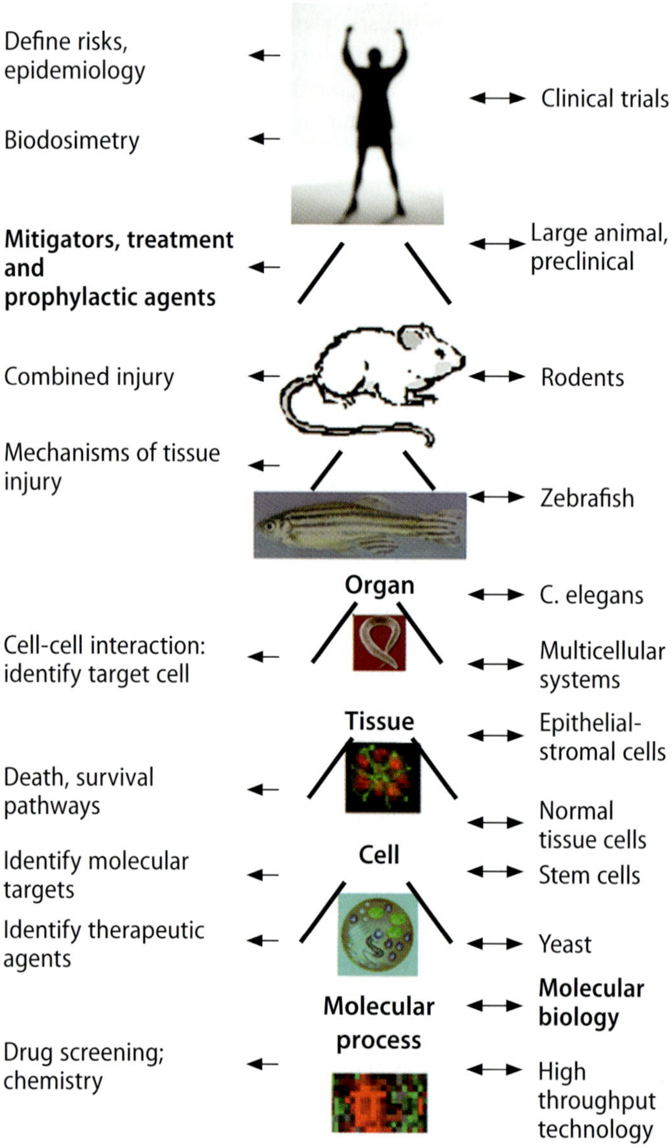

Fig. 13.2. Animal models for radiation counter-measures research. The overall goal of research is to go from underlying molecular mechanism to human application. This requires many model systems. (Adapted and reprinted with permission from [3]

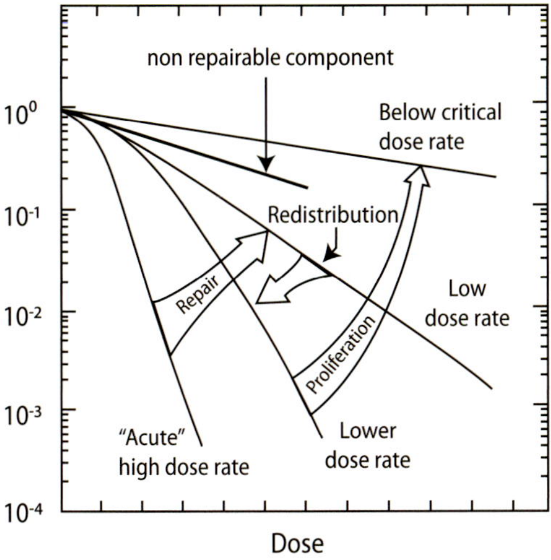

Fig. 13.3. The radiobiology of dose rate, Bedford and Hall style. (Reprinted with permission from [4])

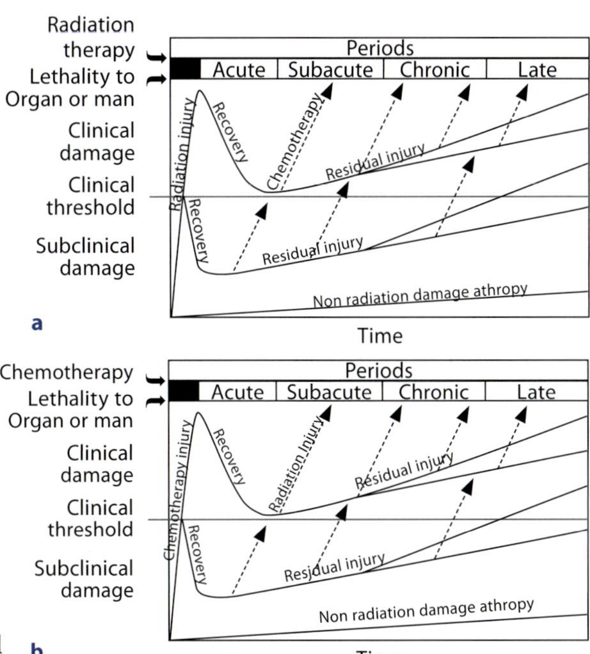

Fig. 13.4a,b. The clinicopathologic course of events following irradiation can be complicated by the addition of chemotherapy. Similarly, chemotherapy can result in parallel sets of events. **a** Classically, when radiation therapy precedes chemotherapy, the introduction of the second mode can lead to expression of subclinical damage or, when injury is present, to death. **b** The same is true if chemotherapy precedes radiation therapy. (Reprinted with permission from [7])

lular response to irradiation resulted in a perpetual cytokine cascade shifted the focus of radiobiologists from target cells to molecular messages released prior to their mitotic linked death by utilizing in vivo/in vitro set of experiments (Fig. 13.5) [8]. The first wave of early responding tissues includes the bone marrow in which alterations occur in the progenitor cells, i.e., erythroblasts, myeloblasts and thromboblasts as well as embedded lymphoid cells. This loss of bone marrow stem cells triggers the release of colony stimulating factors (CSFs) as a function of bone marrow volume as well as dose [9]. The delay in clinical expression of a falling blood count is a function of the mature blood cells' life cycle, i.e., platelets and leukocytes 2–3 weeks, red blood cells 3 months.

Since every segment of the anatomy has both lymphocytes embedded and bone marrow in its environment encased in its skeletal structure, these two systems, i.e., lymphoid and bone marrow, act as an alarm system that initiates an immediate response

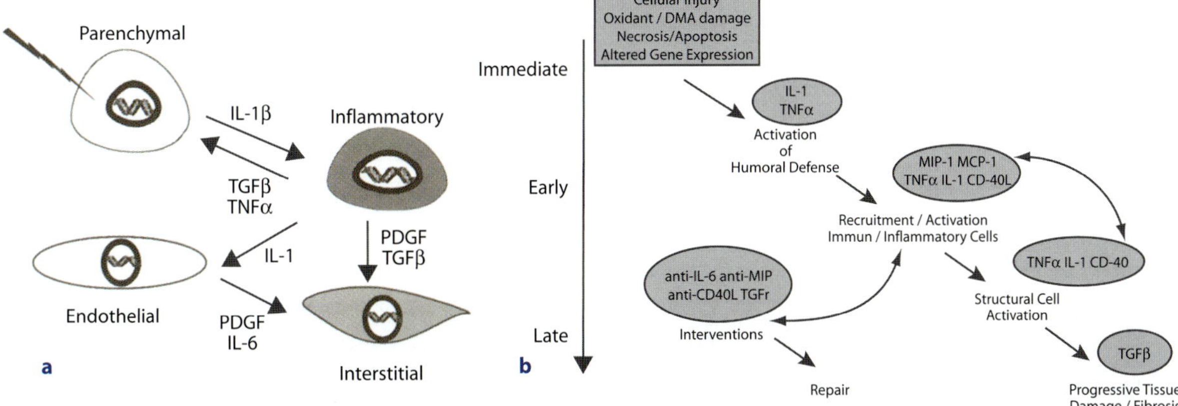

Fig. 13.5. a Suggested chain of events beginning with the initial injury to the primary target cell – the parenchymal cell – and culminating in activation of the interstitial cells (e.g., fibroblasts) to lay down extracellular matrix. **b** Hypothetical pathway indicating the chain of events from initial injury to the final late effect (e.g., fibrosis). (Reprinted with permission from [8])

mechanism so that released growth factors provoke a strong autocrine and paracrine stimulus to initiate the hematopoietic stem cell regeneration (Fig. 13.6, Table 13.1) [9, 10]. Lymphoid extranodal sites and major lymph node stations are noted for their ubiquity. The "dose volume tolerance" of the hematopoietic system was demonstrated both in the laboratory and clinic in which sterilization of defined bone marrow volumes resulted in dramatic functional compensatory alterations that persisted for years and decades [11, 12]. That is, although peripheral blood counts returned to normal, the bone marrow did not regenerate in the "irradiated local field", but resulted in either a hyperactive regeneration of shielded adjacent unexposed bone marrow or more remarkable was the ability of the bone marrow to be reactivated in the femurs, i.e., recapitulating its ontogeny [13]. These bone marrow radiation experiments demonstrated the robust systemic effects of local field treatment that once initiated continue over time for years and decades (Fig. 13.6, Table 13.2) [9].

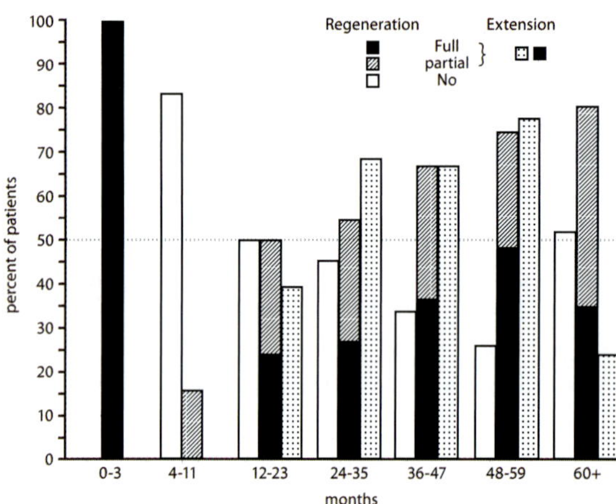

Fig. 13.6. Pattern of bone marrow regeneration and extension in Hodgkin's disease patients (after total nodal irradiation) as determined by ^{99m}Tc-S colloid. (Reprinted with permission from [9])

Phase II: Recruitment and Repopulation

The second wave of early responding tissues includes the epithelial cells of the gastrointestinal mucosal lining, from esophagus to anus, the basal germinating layer of upper aerodigestive systems and those of skin, all of which are rapidly proliferating and exist in some part in many body segments [7]. Their cell kinetic time for renewal determines the time of the expression of the inflammatory reaction, i.e., the gastrointestinal mucosa responds in a week, oral cavity, oropharynx, and esophageal mucositis starts at 2–3 weeks, dermatitis into 3–4 weeks [7]. The important observation is the inflammatory cells that provide the cytokines for epithelial cell repopulation are due to recruited unirradiated bone marrow derived white cells. That is, the acute reaction is due to the recruitment of bone marrow derived lymphocytes and macrophages interacting with dying epithelial cells. The most elegant studies are those of KRAUSE et al. [14] who demonstrated in a chimera mouse model that the pluripotent bone marrow stem cell crossed germ lines and are capable of regenerating irradiated epithelial tissues. Although controversial, numerous independent studies support the probability of a subset of bone marrow stem cells is capable of regenerating epithelial linings including esophagus and lung [15]. Most investigators have demonstrated immunochemical and histochemical markers from bone marrow stem cell chromosomes which are reconstituted in repopulated mucosal cells, i.e., female bone marrow marker in male host epithelium. This has opened the door for bioengineering irradiated normal tissue by transfusing histocompatible pluripotent hematopoietic bone marrow stem cells (HBMSC). The inherent plasticity of HBMSC allows the bone marrow stem cells' genotypes to transdifferentiate into different cell phenotypes (Fig. 13.7) [15].

Table 13.1. Table of implicated inflammatory regulators [10]

Proposed inflammatory regulators			
PDGF	TGF-β	MIP-1α, -1β, and -2	VEGF
bFGF	L-selectin	Interferon inducible protein-10 (IP-10)	Lymphotactin
MCP-1	E-selectin	Prostacyclin	Eotaxin
IL-1α	RANTES	Plasminogen activator	
IL-6	Angiotensin converting enzyme (ACE)	TNF-α	

Table 13.2. Bone marrow regeneration (BMR) patterns and compensatory mechanisms [9]

Techniques of irradiation	Regeneration			Doses (Gy)	
	Exposed bone marrow	Unexposed bone marrow	Extension	Daily	Total
Small field	N	Local-regional ↑ BMR	N	2	> 40
Large field	N	Generalized ↑↑ BMR	N	2	> 30
Subtotal body	Supressed BMR which then recovers	Generalized ↑↑ BMR	↑↑	2	40
Total body	Active	-	N	0.05–0.1	> 1

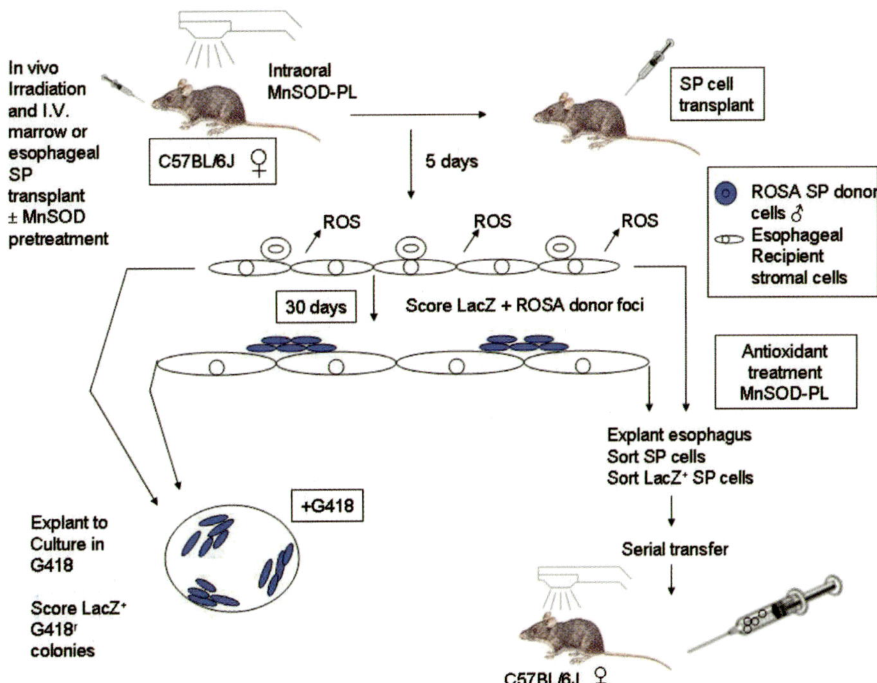

Fig. 13.7. Experimental model system to show donor marrow stem cell origin of esophageal stem cells. ROSA male donor mice have three markers (Y chromosome, G418 resistance, LAC-Z production). Recipient esophagus is irradiated 24 h after intraoral administration of MnSOD-PL, then donor marrow is given intravenously. Esophagus is removed. Cells shown to be donor origin in vivo and in vitro, and donor esophageal side population (stem cells) show self renewal by serial transfer to recipient second generation irradiated esophagus. (Reprinted with permission from [15])

13.4

Phase III: Replacement and Reoxygenation

The microvasculature and the interstitium of normal tissues are a key component of the radiation reaction. Rapidly dividing tissues in expressing their injury early interact with endothelial and fibroblast stroma which actively participate in the acute reactive phase. The importance of the capillary endothelium and stromal fibroblast is highlighted in slow responding tissues where irradiation results in the widespread damage of the microcirculation first [16]. Some of the most convincing evidence can be found in the meticulous studies by FAJARDO and STEWART (Fig. 13.8) [16] on the irradiated rabbit heart where serial histopathologic analysis demon-strated a diffuse microthrombosis of the fine capillary network in the myocardium while sparing the cardiac myocyte. The control observation was the selective effect of myocardial cell vacuolation by adriamycin in contrast to radiation injury. Disruption of the capillary bed and leakage of cells, initiates a relative hypoxia that provokes a fibrogenic response (Fig. 13.9) [17]. The aftermath of radiation often results in extensive fibrosis when parenchyma fails to regenerate and atrophies. Casarett referred to this ongoing fibrogenic process as an increase of the histohematic barrier due to a failure of the normal tissue to fully reoxygenate. Some investigators have found bone marrow derived stromal and endothelial cells contributing to fibrosis and attempts at revascularization, respectively [15].

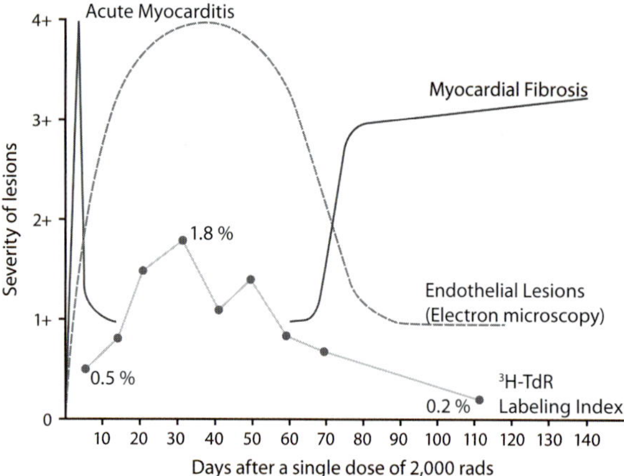

Fig. 13.8. Evolution of radiation-induced myocardial fibrosis in the rabbit heart following a single local dose of 20 Gy on day 0. The severity of the light microscopic lesions is indicated by the *solid line*, but the nature of such lesions varies: transient acute myocarditis initially and diffuse fibrosis after 70 days. The severity of the ultrastructural alterations is indicated by the *broken line*. The bottom line indicates the proportion of nuclei labeled by ³HTdR (endothelial cells). (Reprinted with permission from [16])

There are some organs that respond in a delayed fashion dramatically due to decompensation of its entire microcirculation. The most striking illustrations were the development of radiation pneumonitis during half body and total body irradiation [18, 19]. This was also evident in whole liver irradiation following whole abdominal treatment for ovarian cancer [20]. Curiously, the liver failure was attributed to venous occlusive disease of central capillary veins of hepatic lobules. The triggering mechanism was platelet adhesion probably due to release of von Willebrand factors [21]. This global versus focal effect was presented conceptually by Byfield as the "volume effect" [22]. An extensive literature has recently mushroomed on "dose volume" as the critical determinant of normal tissue tolerance and toxicity. The lung and liver have been thoroughly investigated and elaborated [23, 24] (Fig. 13.10). It is possible to attribute loss of function with volume to loss of microcirculation volume as well as loss of functional units.

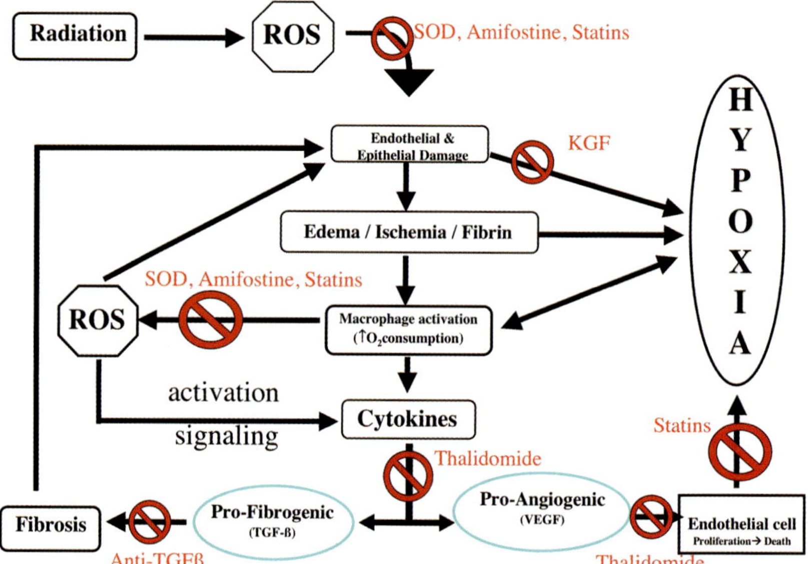

Fig. 13.9. Paradigm of hypoxia-mediated chronic lung injury. Initial tissue damage from radiation is generated by the direct action of reactive oxygen species (ROS) on DNA. This effect causes tissue injury including epithelial and endothelial cell damage, with an increase in vascular permeability, edema, and fibrin accumulation in the extracellular matrix. This tissue injury is followed by an inflammatory response including macrophage accumulation and activation. Macrophages, along with other inflammatory cells, are attracted to an area of injury or evolving inflammation. The majority of macrophages in lung are derived from circulating monocytes that enter the lung in response to inflammation. These macrophages are able to release a number of cytokines and ROS. Both vascular changes as well as an increase in oxygen consumption (due to macrophage activation) contribute to the development of hypoxia. Hypoxia further stimulates production of ROS, and profibrogenic and proangiogenic cytokines. This response to hypoxia perpetuates tissue damage leading to fibrosis via TGFß production and stimulates angiogenesis through VEGF production. While attempting to respond to the proliferative stimulus of VEGF, endothelial cells die as a result of previously accumulated radiation damage. Thus, hypoxia continuously perpetuates a non-healing tissue response leading to chronic radiation injury. This injury pathway offers numerous potential targets for therapeutic intervention. (Reprinted with permission from [17])

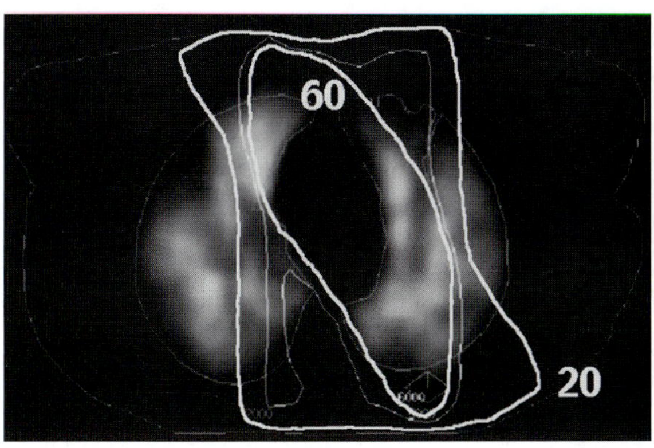

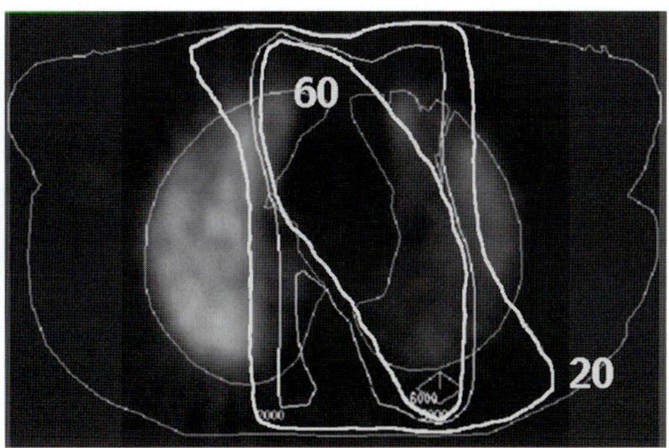

Fig. 13.10a–c. The pre- (**a**) and 6-month post-RT (**b**) transverse SPECT perfusion images from a patient irradiated for lung cancer are shown. The RT dose distribution is also shown. The post-RT perfusion defect is seen most prominently within regions of the lung receiving > 60 Gy. The dose–response curve for RT-induced reductions in regional perfusion, from this patient's SPECT scans, is shown. (Reprinted with permission from [23])

13.5
Phase IV: Reassortment and Remodeling

The late cell reassortment and remodeling phase is dominated by slow or non-renewal normal tissues that have little or no regenerative capacity. According to RUBIN and CASARETT [7], the normal tissues/organs that are dominated by parenchymal cells, which are reverting post mitotic cells have the capacity to either revert to an actively mitosing stem cell or enlarge by undergoing hypertrophy. The liver is the classic example of tissue loss being stored by reassortment and reversion of a resting cell into an actively dividing hyperplasia response to remodel the organ. Salivary glands and endocrine glands consisting of reverting post mitotic cells compensate by hyperplasia of spared volumes.

Alternatively, some normal tissues compensate by undergoing hypertrophy of the unirradiated portion of the organ system. The classic example are the kidneys when loss of one results in a compensatory hypertrophy of the other. The lung in a similar fashion compensates by hypertrophy of a lobe in response to loss of a lobe in the same lung. The hypertrophy or hyperplasia can be referred to as remodeling of an organ volume to compensate for a lost segment. The heart in an analogous fashion undergoes hypertrophy to compensate for a decrease in its ejection fraction due to myocardial cell loss either due to infarction or interstitial fibrosis (Fig. 13.11) [25, 26].

13.6
Phase V: Cell Repair and Resurgence

There are a number of normal vital parenchymal tissues that lack the mitotic potential to regenerate. These are fixed post mitotic cells. The classic example is the central nervous system, i.e., brain and spinal cord [7]. Although a temporary and transient demyelination may occur, injury to neurons are not replaced and in the spinal cord result in a permanent transection. The ganglioneurons tend to be fixed post mitotic cells and although controversy exists

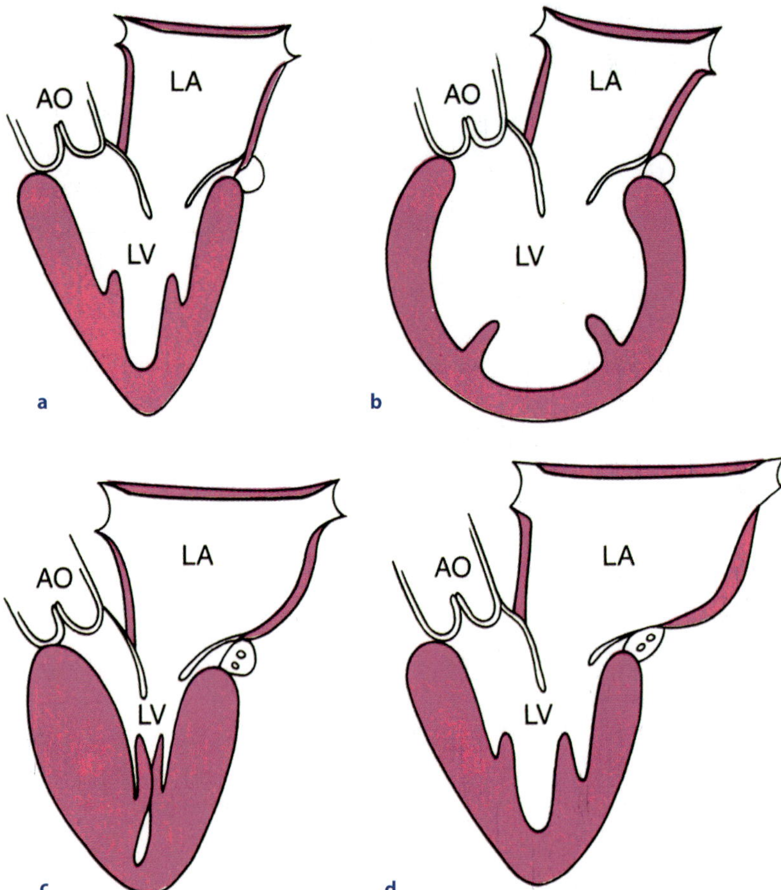

Fig. 13.11a–d. Characteristics of the normal heart and the three main types of cardiomyopathy. **a** Normal. **b** Dilated cardiomyopathy: Note the thin left ventricular (*LV*) walls and enlarged LV chamber, resulting in poor contraction of heart muscle (systolic dysfunction). **c** Hypertrophic cardiomyopathy: not related to the cardiotoxicity of cancer therapy. **d** Restrictive cardiomyopathy: note the normal to slightly thickened LV walls and slightly decreased LV chamber size. These changes are caused by fibrosis which stiffens the myocardium and results in poor chamber filling (diastolic dysfunction). (Reprinted with permission from [26])

as to the ability of periventricular stem cells to compensate, the resultant atrophy or loss of cerebral or spinal cord neurons is irreplaceable [27].

The musculoskeletal system is virtually nonreactive to large conventional radiation doses but can undergo atrophy or fail to hypertrophy with exercise as a stimulus [28]. Skeletal bone is tolerant of high doses and responds to a decrease in its vascularization by undergoing sclerosis and eventually necrosis or fracture. When a heavily irradiated long bone is fractured, the periosteal osteoblast cells fail to proliferate and are unable to form a stabilizing callous, and the bone requires pinning to seal itself [29].

Fortunately, the vital normal tissues with fixed post mitotic cells often are highly radioresistant, widely distributed and are non-responding clinically except under unusual circumstances, i.e., extremely high doses. These include the bulk of striated muscle including fascia, tendons and ligaments, peripheral and autonomic nerves, large arteries and veins. Articular cartilage and intervertebral discs allows for preservation of joint function and osteoarthritis is rarely if ever induced by radiation.

Most DNA damage is rapidly repaired [5]. However, radiation induces point mutations, gene deletions and overexpressions and in time radiation mutagenicity leads to radiation carcinogenicity and second malignant tumors (Fig. 13.12) [30–32].

13.7
Discussion

The holistic concept of the multiorgan domino effect is recapitulated by biocontinuum timelines [7]. The thorax in our illustration has been treated by IMRT and as a consequence all surrounding normal tissues have been irradiated. The Rs of radiobiology are applied to redefine reactions and interaction of the variety of normal tissues in the anatomic segments being treated.

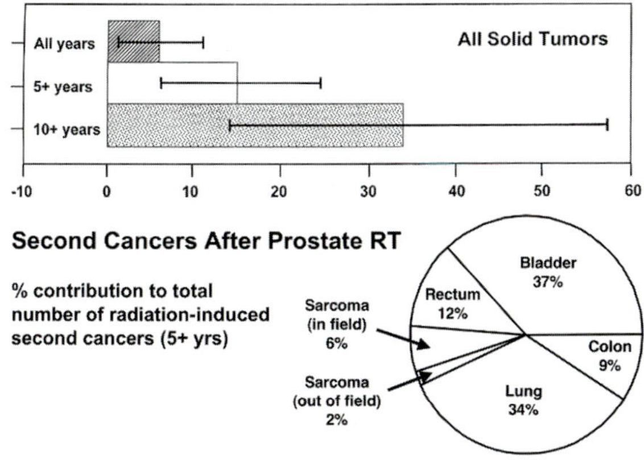

Fig. 13.12. The *upper panel* shows the percentage increase in relative risk for all solid tumors as a function of time after radiotherapy. The error bars represent 95% confidence limits. *"All years"* refer to all years post-treatment; the standard error is smaller in this case because of the larger number of patients; most did not survive to 5 or 10 years. The *lower panel* shows the distribution of the principal radiation-induced cancers, namely bladder, lung, rectum, and colon. There are also a small number of sarcomas that appear in heavily irradiated areas. (Reprinted with permission from [31])

Phase I: Release and Regeneration

The immediate lysis of lymphocytes occurs in the thymus, mediastinal lymph nodes, bronchial submucosal lymphoid tissue, and lung alveolar macrophages. The bone marrow in the sternum, thoracic vertebral bodies and ribs of their progenitor blast cells and release colony stimulating growth factors. Release of colony stimulating factors jump-starts regeneration of pluripotent hematopoietic bone marrow stem cells out of the field, i.e., cervical/lumbar vertebrae and pelvis.

Phase II: Recruitment and Repopulation

The esophageal and bronchial mucositis is followed by infiltration of bone marrow derived inflammatory cells and HBMSC that over time are recruited to repopulate the epithelial loss by transdifferentiating into epithelial cells. The infiltration of lymphocytes has been observed in unexposed ipsilateral lung segments and contralateral unirradiated lung. This abscopal "autoimmune" phenomenon attests to the systemic effects of local field irradiation (Fig. 13.13) [33]. This could be due to leakage of surfactant apoprotein, normally not present in blood, which is phagocytized by macrophages that we postulate return to the bone marrow and amplify, then home into lung bilaterally,

i.e., into the contralateral unirradiated lung, due to type II pneumocyte and stored surfactant. [34].

Phase III: Replacement and Reoxygenation

The microvasculature and the interstitium respond more rapidly in early responding mucosal tissues (esophagus) and later in slow responding organs (lung and heart). In these latter normal tissues, especially when large doses and volumes of the organ are irradiated, there are a number of pathophysiologic microvascular events that lead to hypoxia and eventually drives a replacement fibrosis and the thinning of mucosal parenchymal cells that undergo gradual atrophy. In the esophagus, loss of smooth muscle leads to strictures, in contrast to interstitial fibrosis in lung alveoli and myocardial interstitial fibrosis.

Phase IV: Reassortment and Remodeling

The cell reassortment and remodeling phase can occur both within the lung and heart due to partial loss of functional volume. Compensatory hypertrophy allows partially spared lung lobes to recover breathing vital capacity. The reverting post mitotic cardiac muscle cells are capable of some regeneration if radiation doses are moderated and/or a significant volume of the heart is spared. The whole heart hypertrophies to increase its ejection fraction.

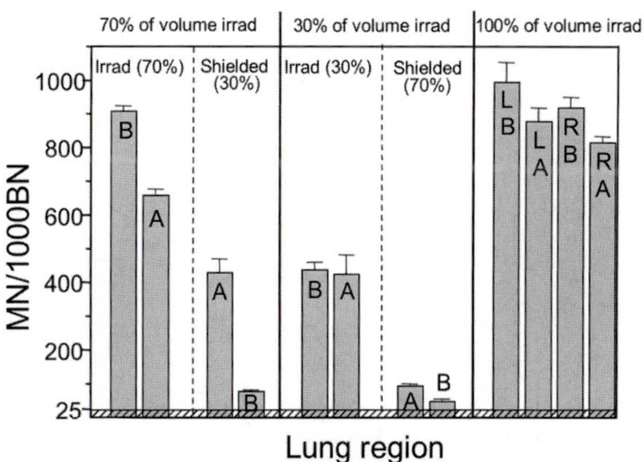

Fig. 13.13. DNA damage (micronuclei/1000 binucleate cells – MN/1000BN) observed in rat lung cells following a dose of 10 Gy given to different volumes of the lung base or lung apex. Cells from different regions of the lung were analysed (*B*, base; *A*, apex; *L*, left; *R*, right). The *bars* represent the mean (+/– SE) from groups of between four and seven rats. The *hatched region* at the bottom indicates the background level of micronuclei in non-irradiated rat lung; this does not vary for different regions of the lung. *irrad*, Irradiated. (Reprinted with permission from [33])

Phase V: Repair and Resurgence

The rapid repair of the cell's DNA was first noted in cell culture by Elkind in which the shoulder of the cell survival curve was recapitulated when radiation was fractionated over time. Most radiation induced DNA damage is rapidly repaired, but it is the occasional misrepair that can lead to the induction of point mutations, chromosomal translocations, gene fusions. This imperfect repair is initially unexpressed clinically but over time, perhaps decades later, leads to radiation induction of cancers and sarcomas. Thus, radiation can add to mutagenicity and eventually second cancers years later. This is well documented in long term Hodgkin's disease female survivors as breast cancers and more recently also lung cancer in the irradiated reactive segment of lung [35].

In summary, the multiorgan domino effect is due to a long list of Rs of normal tissue radiobiology: cell release, regeneration, recruitment, repopulation, replacement, reoxygenation, reassortment, remodeling, repair and resurgence. These new Rs provide a more holistic view of the biocontinuum of radiation as a perturbation of multiple normal tissues and organs for a lifetime. Recognizing and appreciating the systemic interactions offers new opportunities for novel interventions. The transfusion of pluripotent stem cells to regenerate parenchymal and endothelial cells is no longer the impossible dream. The new exciting advances in the bioengineering of adult skin cells by insertion of three genes into histocompatible stem cells opens the door for an improved therapeutic ratio, that is, the stabilization and reversal of the radiation biocontinuum [36].

An apocryphal study conducted with my neurobiologic research team, utilized rat embryonic grafts, implanted as a core of tissue in irradiated adult rat brain; appeared to reverse most the morphologic and functional aspects of neuronal damage. An elegant system of monitoring rat movements by interrupting laser beams documented the inevitable progression of radiation brain injury as hyperactivity in spontaneous movements standing and circling in their cages (Fig. 13.14) [37]. The fetal brain transplanted irradiated animals behaved similar to normal controls and upon sacrifice, the fetal hypothalamic graft was fully vascularized and integrated into the third ventricle of the irradiated brain which appeared free of hemorrhaging due to restoration of the blood brain barrier. There was absence of demyelination and neuronal loss in the fimbria and internal capsule in the irradiated brain suggesting migration of oligodendrolocytes, astrocytes and endothelial cells and/or release of neurotrophic cytokine factors to account for repair and regeneration of the radiation alterations (Fig. 13.15).

Upon presentation of these studies in 1989, the obvious question and dilemma was "Where would

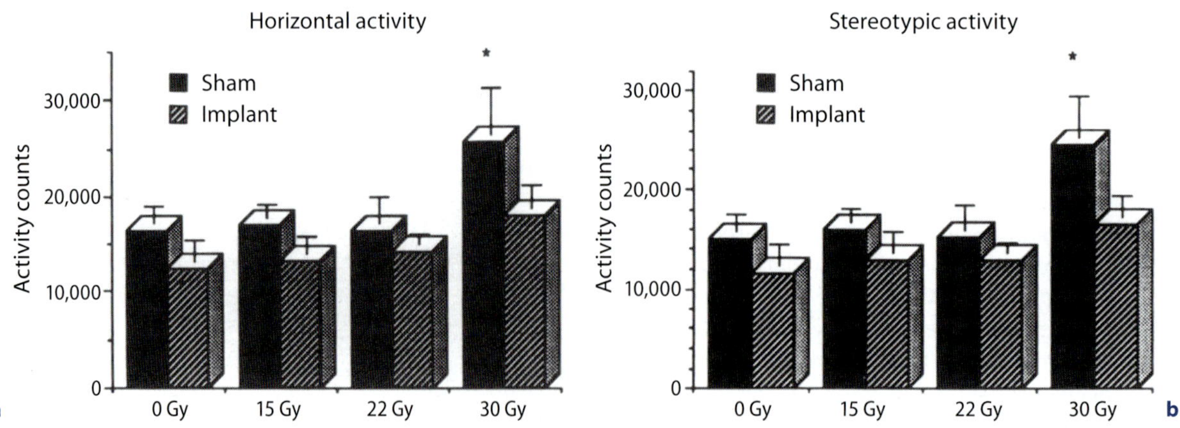

Fig. 13.14a,b. Spontaneous nocturnal locomotor activity was measured in an Omnitech Electronic automated Digiscan Analyser. Data represents total activity counts over the course of a 4-h testing period beginning at lights-off (6:00 pm). Rats in the 30-Gy sham implanted group showed significant hyperactivity in both horizontal (**a**) and stereotypic (**b**) behavioral measures as compared to non-irradiated sham implanted animals (*asterisks*, F = 2.66, $p < 0.01$; F = 2.94, $p < 0.01$, respectively). Horizontal activity represents the total number of beam intersections during the 4-h testing period, and stereotypic activity is indicative of repeated intersections of a single beam. Elevated stereotypic activity is often seen in animals with basal ganglia damage. (Reprinted with permission from [37])

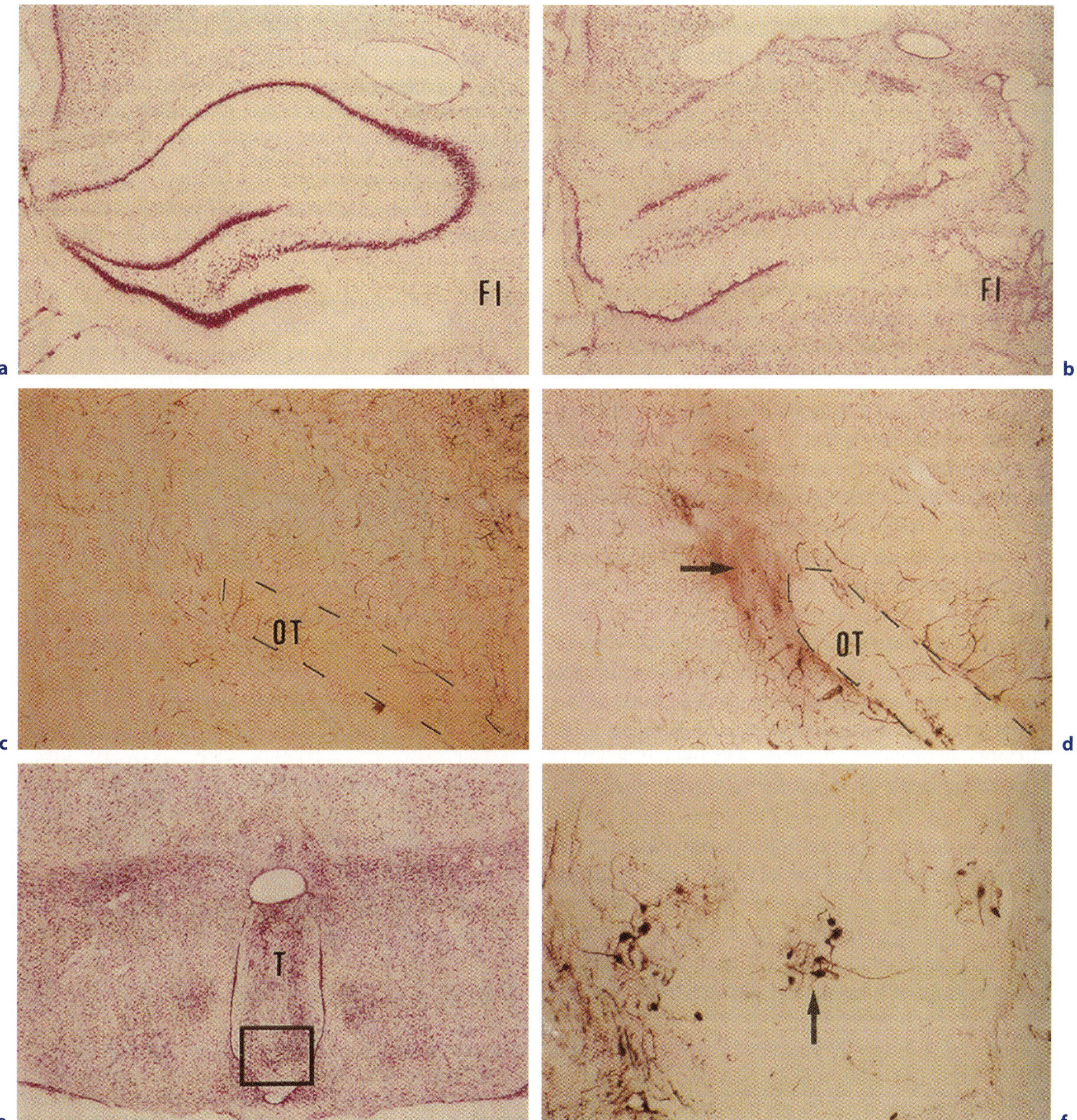

Fig. 13.15. a,b Coronal (30-μm) section through the anterior hippocampus, stained with cresyl violet. In comparison to normal controls (**a**), the 30-Gy irradiated sham animals (**b**) showed marked disruption of the cytoarchitecture of the hippocampal formation, large holes, and almost complete degeneration of the fimbria (*FI*). **c,d** The brain parenchyma around the optic tract (*OT*) of a normal (**c**) animal shows an intact blood-brain barrier while the similar region from a 30-Gy irradiated (**d**) animal shows vascular leaks (*arrow*) after radiation treatment as demonstrated by HRP-tetramethylbenzidine reaction. **e** Cresyl violet stain of a transplant (*T*) in the third ventricle of a 30-Gy irradiated rat. The grafts survived well and often filled the ventricle. **f** Enlargement of an adjacent section to the boxed region in (**e**). The grafts contain TH positive neurons (*arrow*). (Reprinted with permission from [37])

you obtain histocompatible embryos?" The current answer lies in the rapid advance in cloning, creating stem cells from somatic cells by gene insertion and hoping these designer stem cells will transdifferentiate into different cell lines and unlock the DNA double helix to recapitulate its ontogeny.

References

1. Photon Treatment Planning Collaborative Working Group (1991) State-of-the-art of external photon beam radiation treatment planning. Int J Radiat Oncol Biol Phys 21:9–23
2. Miften M, Gayou O, Parda DS et al (2008) Using quality of life information to rationally incorporate normal tissue effects into treatment plan evaluation and scoring. In: Rubin P, Constine LS, Marks LB, Okunieff P (eds) CURED I – LENT Late effects of cancer treatment on normal tissues. Springer-Verlag, Berlin Heidelberg New York, pp 83–89
3. Stone HB, Moulder JE, Coleman CN et al (2004) Models for evaluating agents intended for prophylaxis, mitigation and treatment of radiation injuries. Report of an NCI Workshop, December 3–4, 2003. Radiat Res 162:711–728
4. Hall E (2000) Radiobiology for the radiobiologist, 5th edn. Lippincott Williams & Wilkins, Philadelphia
5. Elkind MM, Sutton H (1960) Radiation response of mammalian cells grown in culture: 1. Repair of X-ray damage in surviving Chinese hamster cells. Radiat Res 13:556–593
6. Brown JM (2008) Dedication to Robert Kallman – LENT V scientific meeting. In: Rubin P, Constine LS, Marks LB, Okunieff P (eds) CURED I – LENT Late effects of cancer treatment on normal tissues. Springer-Verlag, Berlin Heidelberg New York, pp V–VI
7. Rubin P, Casarett G (1968) Clinical radiation pathology, vols. I and II. W.B. Saunders, Philadelphia
8. Rubin P, Finkelstein J, Shapiro D (1992) Molecular biology mechanisms in the radiation induction of pulmonary injury syndromes: interrelationship between the alveolar macrophage and the septal fibroblasts. Int J Radiat Oncol Biol Phys 24:93–101
9. Rubin P, Scarantino C (1978) The bone marrow organ: the critical structure in radiation-drug interaction. Int J Radiat Oncol Biol Phys 4:3–23
10. Willey CD, Hallahan DE (2008) Inflammation and cell adhesion molecules are involved in radiation-induced lung injury. In: Rubin P, Constine LS, Marks LB, Okunieff P (eds) CURED I – LENT Late effects of cancer treatment on normal tissues. Springer-Verlag, Berlin Heidelberg New York, pp 23–30
11. Croizat H, Frindel E, Tubiana M (1976) Abscopal effect of irradiation on hematopoetic stem cells of shielded bone marrow. Role of migration. Int J Radiat Biol 30:347–358
12. Croizat H, Frindel E, Tubiana M (1970) Proliferative activity of stem cells in the bone marrow of mice after single and multiple irradiations: total- or partial-body exposure. Int J Radiat Biol 18:347–358
13. Knospe W, Rayudu V, Cardello M et al (1976) Bone marrow scanning with 52 iron (52Fe). Regeneration and extension of marrow after ablative doses of radiotherapy. Cancer 37:1432–1442
14. Krause DS, Theise ND, Collector MI et al (2001) Multi-organ, multi-lineage engraftment by a single bone marrow-derived stem cell. Cell 105:369–377
15. Greenberger JS (2009) Bioengineering in the repair of irradiated normal tissue by bone marrow derived stem cell populations. In: Rubin P, Constine LS, Marks LB, Okunieff P (eds) CURED II – LENT Late effects of cancer treatment on normal tissues. Springer-Verlag, Berlin Heidelberg New York
16. Fajardo LF, Stewart JR (1973) Pathogenesis of radiation-induced myocardial fibrosis. Lab Invest 29:244–257
17. Anscher MS, Vujaskovic Z (2008) Hypoxia-mediated chronic normal tissue injury: a new paradigm and potential strategies for intervention. In: Rubin P, Constine LS, Marks LB, Okunieff P (eds) CURED I – LENT Late effects of cancer treatment on normal tissues. Springer-Verlag, Berlin Heidelberg New York, pp 61–67
18. Fryer CJH, Fitzpatrick PJ, Rider WD et al (1978) Radiation pneumonitis: experience following a large single dose of radiation. Int J Radiat Oncol Biol Phys 4:931–936
19. Keane TJ, Van Dyk J, Rider WD (1981) Idiopathic interstitial pneumonia following bone marrow transplantation: the relationship with total body irradiation. Int J Radiat Oncol Biol Phys 7:1365–1370
20. Ingold DK, Reed GB, Kaplan HS et al (1965) Radiation hepatitis. Am J Roentgenol 93:200–208
21. Sporn L, Rubin P, Marder V, Wagner D (1984) Irradiation induces release of von Willebrand protein from endothelial cells in culture. Blood 64:567–570
22. Lyman JT, Wolbarst AB (1987) Optimization of radiation therapy, III: a method of assessing complication probabilities from dose-volume histograms. Int J Radiat Oncol Biol Phys 13:103-109
23. Kocak Z, Shankar L, Sullivan DC et al (2008) The role of imaging in the study of radiation-induced normal tissue injury. In: Rubin P, Constine LS, Marks LB, Okunieff P (eds) CURED I – LENT Late effects of cancer treatment on normal tissues. Springer-Verlag, Berlin Heidelberg New York, pp 37–45
24. Lawrence TS, Robertson JM, Anscher MD et al (1995) Hepatic toxicity resulting from cancer treatment. Int J Radiat Oncol Biol Phys 31(Special Issue):1237–1248
25. Adams MJ, Lipshultz SE, Schwartz C (2003) Radiation-associated cardiovascular disease: manifestations and management. Semin Radiat Oncol 13:346–356
26. Adams MJ, Prosnitz RG, Constine LS et al (2008) Screening for cardiovascular disease in survivors of thoracic radiation. In: Rubin P, Constine LS, Marks LB, Okunieff P (eds) CURED I – LENT Late effects of cancer treatment on normal tissues. Springer-Verlag, Berlin Heidelberg New York, pp 47–59
27. Schultheiss TE, Kun LE, Ang KK et al (1995) Radiation response of the central nervous system. Int J Radiat Oncol Biol Phys 31(Special Issue):1093–1112
28. Gillette EL, Mahler PA, Powers BE et al (1995) Late radiation injury to muscle and peripheral nerves. Int J Radiat Oncol Biol Phys 31(Special Issue):1309–1318
29. Bonarigo B, Rubin P (1967) Non-union of pathologic fracture after radiation therapy. Radiol 88:889–904

30. Hall EJ, Brenner DJ (2008) Second malignancies as a consequence of radiation therapy. In: Rubin P, Constine LS, Marks LB, Okunieff P, eds. CURED I LENT Late Effects of Cancer Treatment on Normal Tissues. Berlin Heidelberg, Germany: Springer-Verlag, pp 77–81

31. Brenner DJ, Curtis RE, Hall EJ (2000) Second malignancies in prostate carcinoma patients after radiotherapy compared with surgery. Cancer 88:398–406

32. Hall EJ, Wuu CS (2003) Radiation-induced second cancers: the impact of 3D-CRT and IMRT. Int J Radiat Oncol Biol Phys 33:225–230

33. Hill RP, Khan MA, Langan AR, Yeung IWT, van Dyke J (2008) Volume effects in radiation damage to rat lung. In: Rubin P, Constine LS, Marks LB, Okunieff P (eds) CURED I - LENT Late effects of cancer treatment on normal tissues. Springer-Verlag, Berlin Heidelberg New York, pp 31–36

34. Rubin P, McDonald S, Maasilta P et al (1989) Serum markers for prediction of pulmonary radiation syndromes. Part I: Surfactant apoprotein. Int J Rad Oncol Biol Phys 17:553–558

35. Travis LB, Gospodarowicz M, Curtis RE et al (2002) Lung cancer following chemotherapy for and radiotherapy for Hodgkin's disease. J Natl Cancer Inst 94:182–192

36. Manis JP (2007) Knock out, knock in, knock down – genetically manipulated mice and the Nobel prize. New Engl J Med 357:2426–2429

37. Pearlman SH, Rubin P, White HC et al (1990) Fetal hypothalamic transplants into brain irradiated rats: graft morphometry and host behavioral responses. Int J Radiat Oncol Biol Phys 19:293–300

Risk Factors for Second Malignancies Following Stem Cell Transplant

Debra L. Friedman

CONTENTS

14.1
Introduction

Hematopoietic cell transplantation (HCT) offers potentially curative therapy for numerous malignancies, as well as immunologic, hematologic and metabolic disorders. While many patients are cured of their primary disease, a proportion develops post-transplant (secondary) malignant neoplasms (SMN) [2, 19, 29]. Individuals treated with HCT may have been exposed to pre-transplant chemotherapy or ra-

D. L. Friedman, MD
Vanderbilt-Ingram Cancer Center, 2525 West End Avenue, Sixt Floor, Nashville, TN 37203, USA

diotherapy, then to additional cytotoxic therapy as part of the preparative regimen for transplantation, and eventually, to immune suppression. All of these factors may act alone or in concert to increase the risk for SMNs. Patients may also be innately cancer susceptible and have a genetic predisposition towards multiple primary malignancies. Potential risk factors for SMN following hematopoietic stem cell transplantation are listed in Tables 14.1 and 14.2.

14.2
Risk Factors for SMN Following Autologous Versus Allogeneic Transplant

14.2.1
SMN Following Autologous HSCT

The incidence of hematologic malignancies and solid tumors following autologous transplantation varies widely across studies, with actuarial risks estimated from < 1% to 18% [14, 17, 19, 32]. Prior chemotherapy with large cumulative doses of alkylating agents as well as prior conventional radiotherapy are important risk factors for treatment-related or secondary MDS or leukemia (t-MDS, t-AML). In addition, patient age at transplant and the use of total body irradiation (TBI) in the preparative regimen, have been identified as risk factors. In some studies, patients transplanted with peripheral blood stem cells after chemotherapy priming showed a higher risk of t-MDS or t-AML than patients transplanted with cells isolated from the bone marrow without priming [35]. The incidence appears highest in patients treated for Hodgkin or non-Hodgkin lymphoma, an experience similar to that reported after conventional chemo- and radiotherapy for those diseases.

Table 14.1. General risk factors for post-transplant malignancies

Host	Disease	Treatment	Post-transplant complications	Exogenous exposures
Genetic predisposition Age at transplant Gender	Lymphoma > others	Pre-transplant therapy Total body irradiation Immunosuppressive agents Stem cell source	Graft vs. host disease Viral infections	Ultraviolet light Tobacco Alcohol Other carcinogens

Table 14.2. Post-transplant SMN specific risk factors

Type of SMN	Host	Primary disease	Treatment	Post-transplant complications
MDS/AML	Older patient age	Lymphoma	Alkylating agents Topoisomerase II inhibitors Nitrosoureas Peripheral blood stem cell source TBI Pre-transplant radiotherapy	GVHD
Hodgkin lymphoma	Unknown	Leukemia	Unknown	Acute GVHD Therapy for chronic GVHD
Skin and buccal mucosa	Male gender Older or younger patient age	Aplastic anemia	TBI	Acute or chronic GVHD
Solid tumors	Male gender Older or younger patient age Female donor	Aplastic anemia	TBI Azathioprine	Chronic GVHD

METAYER and colleagues [31] conducted a case-control study of 56 patients with t-MDS/AML and 168 matched controls within a cohort of 2,739 patients receiving autologous transplants for Hodgkin or non-Hodgkin lymphoma. In multivariate analyses, risks of t-MDS/AML significantly increased with the intensity of pre-transplantation chemotherapy with mechlorethamine or chlorambucil, compared with cyclophosphamide-based therapy. The use of TBI at doses of 12 Gy or less did not appear to increase the leukemia risk, but TBI doses of 13.2 Gy or higher increased the risk significantly. Peripheral blood stem cells were associated with a non-significantly increased risk of MDS/AML compared with bone marrow grafts [31].

In a series of 493 patients treated for NHL at The University of Texas M.D. Anderson Cancer Center, 22 patients developed tMDS or tAML. Multiple logistic regression analyses showed that TBI was independently associated with an increased risk of developing tMDS/tAML, and patients receiving TBI in combination with cyclophosphamide and etoposide were more likely to develop tMDS/tAML than patients who received TBI with cyclophosphamide or thiotepa [24].

In a series from the City of Hope National Medical Center, among 612 patients treated for lymphoma, 22 developed MDS or acute leukemia, with an estimated cumulative incidence of 8.6% ± 2.1% at 6 years. Multivariate analysis revealed stem cell priming with etoposide and pre-transplant radiotherapy to be significant risk factors [26].

Data related to 467 French patients treated with autologous transplantation for Hodgkin lymphoma was matched with 1179 conventionally treated patients listed in international databases. There were 18 secondary cancers, leading to a 5-year cumulative incidence of 8.9%. Risk factors for second cancer were age 40 years or older, the use of peripheral blood as a source of stem cells and treatment for relapsed disease. Solid tumors were more frequent in patients treated with transplantation, although the incidence of t-MDS and AML was similar in the two groups [1].

14.2.2
SMN Following Allogeneic HSCT

Risks for specific types of SMN following allogeneic HSCT range from three- to 25-fold that of the general population, with cumulative incidences reaching 3%–11% at 10–15 years [7, 8, 11, 13, 15, 16, 19, 22, 29, 41]. In particular, the risks of melanoma and non-melanoma skin cancer and cancers of the oral cavity, liver, cervix, central nervous system, thyroid, bone and connective tissue are particularly elevated [7, 8, 11, 12, 41, 27]. Risk factors include the underlying diagnosis, pre-transplant therapy, transplantation for refractory or recurrent disease, the use of TBI and immunosuppressive agents and graft versus host disease (GVHD) [7, 8, 11, 13, 15, 16, 19, 29, 41]. Host factors include younger age at diagnosis in some series [11, 41] and, for squamous cell carcinoma of the buccal cavity and skin, male gender [11, 12, 15]. A recent series by GALLAGHER and FORREST [22] found older age at transplant and female donor to be a risk factor second solid tumors. Several large studies illustrate these risks.

In a review of 3,372 patients who underwent HSCT at the University of Minnesota between 1974 and 2001, 123 cases of SMN were reported, which represented an 8.1-fold increased risk over the that of the general population. This includes a significantly elevated risk for developing t-MDS or AML [standardized incidence ratio (SIR) = 300; 95% CI, 210 to 406], non-Hodgkin lymphoma including post-transplant lymphoproliferative disorder (PTLD; SIR = 54.3; 95% CI, 39.5–41.1), Hodgkin disease (SIR = 14.8; 95% CI, 3.9–32.9), or solid tumors overall (SIR = 2.8; CI, 2.0–3.7), and specifically for melanoma, brain, and oral cavity tumors. For t-MDS or AML, the cumulative incidence reached a plateau at 1.4% (95% CI, 0.9–1.9) by 10 years post-transplant. The cumulative incidence of developing a solid tumor did not plateau and was 3.8% (95% CI, 2.2–5.4) at 20 years post-transplant [2].

Among 2,129 patients who had undergone transplantation for hematologic malignancies at the City of Hope National Medical Center between 1976 and 1998, 29 developed solid cancers, which represented a two-fold increase in risk relative to a comparable normal population. The estimated cumulative incidence (± SE) for the development of a solid cancer was 6.1% ± 1.6% at 10 years. The risk was significantly elevated for liver cancer, cancer of the oral cavity, and cervical cancer. The risk was significantly higher for survivors who were younger than 34 years of age at time of transplant. Cancers of the thyroid gland, liver, and oral cavity occurred primarily among patients who received TBI. Again, there was no plateau noted in the incidence of solid tumors [8].

The risk of SMNs was reported by CURTIS and colleagues [11] in 19,229 patients who received allogeneic (97.2%) or syngeneic transplants between 1964 and 1992 at one of 235 centers reporting to the International Bone Marrow Treatment Registry or the FHCRC. Among patients who survived 10 years or more, the risk of SMN was 8.3 times that of the general population. The cumulative incidence was 2.2% (95% CI 1.5, 3.0%) at 10 and 6.7% (95% CI 3.7, 9.6%) at 15 years. The risk was significantly elevated ($p < 0.05$) for malignant melanoma (SIR = 5.0), buccal cavity (SIR = 11.1), liver (SIR = 7.5), CNS (SIR = 7.6), thyroid (SIR = 6.6), bone (SIR = 13.4), and connective tissue cancers (SIR = 8.0). Younger age at time of transplant was associated with higher risk (p for trend < 0.001). In multivariate analyses, higher doses of TBI were associated with an increased risk. Chronic GVHD and male gender were strongly associated with an excess risk of squamous cell cancers of the buccal cavity and skin.

In a subsequent case-control study of 183 patients with subsequent solid cancers and 501 matched control patients within a cohort of 24,011 patients who underwent hematopoietic stem-cell transplantation (HSCT) at 215 centers, CURTIS and colleagues [12] found that chronic GVHD and its therapy were strongly related to the risk for squamous cell carcinoma (SCC), but not for non-squamous cell carcinoma. Major risk factors for SCC were prolonged use of chronic GVHD therapy, use of azathioprine, particularly when combined with cyclosporine and steroids and severe chronic GVHD. Additional analyses determined that prolonged immunosuppressive therapy and azathioprine use were also significant risk factors for SCC of the skin and of the oral mucosa.

Among 18,531 patients receiving allogeneic transplant between 1964 and 1992 at the same centers, the risk of Hodgkin lymphoma was also significantly increased compared with the general population, even after excluding two human immunodeficiency virus-positive patients (observed cases, $n = 6$; O/E = 4.7, 95% CI, 1.7–10.3). Mixed cellularity subtype predominated (five of eight cases, 63%). Five of six assessable cases contained Epstein-Barr virus (EBV) genome. Acute graft-versus-host disease (GVHD) or therapy for chronic GVHD were risk factors for post-transplant Hodgkin lymphoma [38].

Among 700 patients with severe aplastic anemia (AA) or Fanconi Anemia (FA), who received allogeneic HSCT at the Fred Hutchinson Cancer Research Center (FHCRC) or at Hôpital St. Louis in Paris, 23 developed malignancies at a median of 7.6 years after transplantation, with a cumulative incidence of 14% at 20 years. In univariate analysis, risk factors for solid tumors included the diagnosis of FA ($p = 0.0002$), use of azathioprine ($p < 0.0001$), radiotherapy ($p = 0.0002$), chronic GVHD ($p = 0.009$), acute GVHD ($p = 0.01$), and male gender ($p = 0.05$). In multivariate analysis, azathioprine therapy ($p < 0.0001$) and the diagnosis of FA ($p < 0.0001$) were statistically significant. Radiotherapy was statistically significant ($p = 0.004$) as a predictor only if the time-dependent variable azathioprine was not included in the analysis. Among non-FA patients, azathioprine ($p = 0.004$), age ($p = 0.03$), and radiotherapy ($p = 0.04$) were significant [15].

In an analysis of SMNs from the FHCRC, which included both allogeneic and autologous transplant, in a cohort of 5806 patients treated with transplant and who survived beyond 100 days, 381 SMNs were reported, excluding benign tumors, cancer in situ, or post-transplant lymphoproliferative disease. Using Cox proportion models, dose and fraction of TBI was analyzed, as well as the use of pre-transplant conventional radiotherapy. The analysis was adjusted for gender and age and found TBI to be a significant risk factor. As a simple yes/no factor, in adjusted analyses, the hazard of SMN among patients receiving TBI is 1.64 times (95% CI 1.3, 2.1) that of patients who did not receive TBI. Furthermore, use of TBI in a single dose increased the hazard by a factor of 2.3 (95% CI 1.6, 3.4) relative to patients receiving no TBI. Incorporation of the likelihood of pre-transplant radiation did not markedly increase the hazard ratio compared to TBI only. We also evaluated age at diagnosis. Using < 18 years as the reference group, hazard ratio for patients 18–39 years of age was 1.4 (95% CI 1.1, 1.9), and for those ≥ 40 years, 4.0 (95% CI 3.0, 5.5). The overall incidence of SMNs in our cohort was 17%, 6% and 13% at 10, 20 and 25 years, respectively. Patients with TBI exposure had a 25-year incidence of SMN of 21%, compared to 10% among patients not exposed to TBI. Risk

continues to rise with elapsed time since transplant, without an obvious plateau. Of particular interest, for patients less than 10 years of age at HSCT, those with TBI exposure had a 25-year incidence of SMN of 19%, compared to 5% among patients not exposed to TBI. For patients ≥ 10 years of age at HSCT, those with TBI exposure had a 25-year incidence of SMN of 21%, compared to 11% among patients not exposed to TBI [19].

In a subsequent analysis of 8662 transplant recipients treated at the FHCRC, who survived at least 100 days post transplant, there were 1743 autologous and 6919 allogeneic HSCT recipients. Within this cohort, there were 56 SMNs amongst the autologous recipients and 224 amongst the allogeneic recipients. Cumulative incidence of SMN at 10 years post-HSCT was 2.6% in the allogeneic and 4.2% in the autologous HCT survivors. A multivariate Cox regression model adjusted for current age, TBI, gender and length of follow-up was fit and the hazard ratio (HR) for SMN for the allogeneic transplant survivors was 0.7 [95% confidence interval (CI) 0.5, 1.0] compared to the autologous transplant survivors (reference group), suggesting that the adjusted hazard of SMN is higher for autologous SCT recipients than for allogeneic. Risk factors appeared different between the two groups. For survivors of autologous transplantation, in multivariate Cox regression models, only age > 18 years at transplant was associated with decreased risk of SMN (< 18 years HR = 1.0; 18–39 years HR = 0.04; 40+ years HR = 0.004). Use of total body irradiation (TBI) was not significantly associated with risk among the autologous HCT recipients. For allogeneic transplant survivors, increased risk of SMN was associated with TBI and the effect of TBI was stronger for younger (< 18 years at HCT: HR = 4.6; 95% CI 1.6, 13.5) than for older (≥ 18 years; HR = 1.5; 95% CI 1.0, 2.3) HCT recipients (interaction $p = 0.04$) in multivariate Cox regression models. Risk was also increased after acute graft versus host disease (HR = 1.4; 95% CI 1.0, 1.9) and with ongoing follow-up time, with HRs of 1.7 (95% CI 1.1, 2.5) at 10–14 years, 2.2 (95% CI 1.3, 3.7) at 15–19 years and 2.6 (95% CI 1.2, 5.4) at 20+ years of follow-up. Unrelated HSCT also increased risk of SMN (HR = 1.4; 95% CI 1.0, 2.0) [20].

The impact of patient-, disease-, treatment-, and toxicity-related factors on risk of basal cell carcinoma (BCC) and squamous cell carcinoma (SCC) was determined in 4,810 patients who received allogeneic HCT at the FHCRC and who survived for at least 100 days. In this cohort, 237 developed at least one skin or mucosal cancer. The 20-year cumulative incidences of BCC and SCC were 6.5% and 3.4%, respectively. Total-body irradiation was a significant risk factor for BCC, most strongly among patients younger than 18 years old at HCT. Light-skinned patients had an increased risk of BCC. Acute GVHD increased the risk of SCC, whereas chronic GVHD increased the risk of both BCC and SCC [27].

As risk for secondary breast cancer is elevated among cancer survivors treated with conventional therapy, a combined analysis at the FHCRC and the European Bone Marrow Transplant Registry evaluated the risk of breast cancer among 3337 female 5-year survivors who underwent an allogeneic hematopoietic cell transplantation. At total of 52 survivors developed breast cancer at a median of 12.5 (range: 5.7–24.8) years following HCT (SIR = 2.2). The 25-year cumulative incidence was 11.0%, higher among survivors who received total body irradiation (TBI) (17%) than those who did not receive TBI (3%). In multivariable analysis, increased risk was associated with longer time since transplantation (hazard ratio [HR] for 20+ years after transplantation = 10.8), use of TBI (HR = 4.0), and younger age at transplantation (HR = 9.5 for HCT < 18 years). Hazard for death associated with breast cancer was 2.5 (95% CI: 1.1–5.8) [21].

14.3
Genetic Risk Factors for SMNs Following Transplant

Large numbers of patients are exposed to similar treatment exposures, yet only a small proportion develop second malignancies. Therefore, there may exist genetic risk factors that interact with such exposures to increase risk of SMN.

14.3.1
Radiation Exposure and Sensitivity

There is inter-individual variation in radiation sensitivity, evidenced by different degrees of skin erythema, fibrosis, and telangiectasia following radiotherapy [44]. It is therefore likely that a number of genetic elements work in concert to determine individual response to radiotherapy. Radiation sensitivity assays on fibroblasts and lymphocytes from apparently normal individuals have established at least a three-fold range in inter-individual sensitivity. Radiosensitivity is distributed normally in the population [33, 44]. There is growing evidence that variation in the degree of radiation sensitivity is genetically determined. Family members of radiosensitive individuals are more likely to be radiosensitive than unrelated individuals [37]. There are also data to suggest that individuals who develop malignancies are radiation-sensitive [3, 6, 9, 10, 23, 34, 39]. Furthermore, there is evidence of a correlation between radiation sensitivity and susceptibility to cancer [4, 5, 18]. What remains unclear is who is at risk for cancer following radiation therapy, what proportion of patients with SMNs have increased radiation sensitivity, what genetic elements contribute to sensitivity, and how sensitivity is most effectively characterized.

14.3.2
Genetic Biomarkers for Second Malignancies Following HCT and Radiation Therapy

In identifying genetic biomarkers of susceptibility for SMN, several classes of genes can be considered. There are genes that confer high individual, low population attributable risk, such as the tumor suppressor genes RB1 or TP53, where genetic susceptibility to cancer has been described in patients with germline mutations [25, 28, 30, 43, 42, 45]. However, these do not explain most of SMN occurrence. Other genes to consider are those that may have a high population attributable risk, because of the widespread occurrence of alleles with altered function. The cancer phenotype is generated in the presence both of specific environmental influences and the specific allelic variant. Examples are genes involved in DNA repair and in provision of nucleotides. Allelic variants may alter the way in which DNA damage from radiotherapy is repaired and thus may be markers for those susceptible to SMNs [36].

14.3.3
Genetic Susceptibility to Toxicity from Combined Cancer Therapy and Environmental Carcinogens: Common Pathways of Metabolism, DNA Damage and Repair

Patients treated with HCT are exposed to cytotoxic therapy. Some of them are also exposed to known carcinogens such as components of tobacco or UV

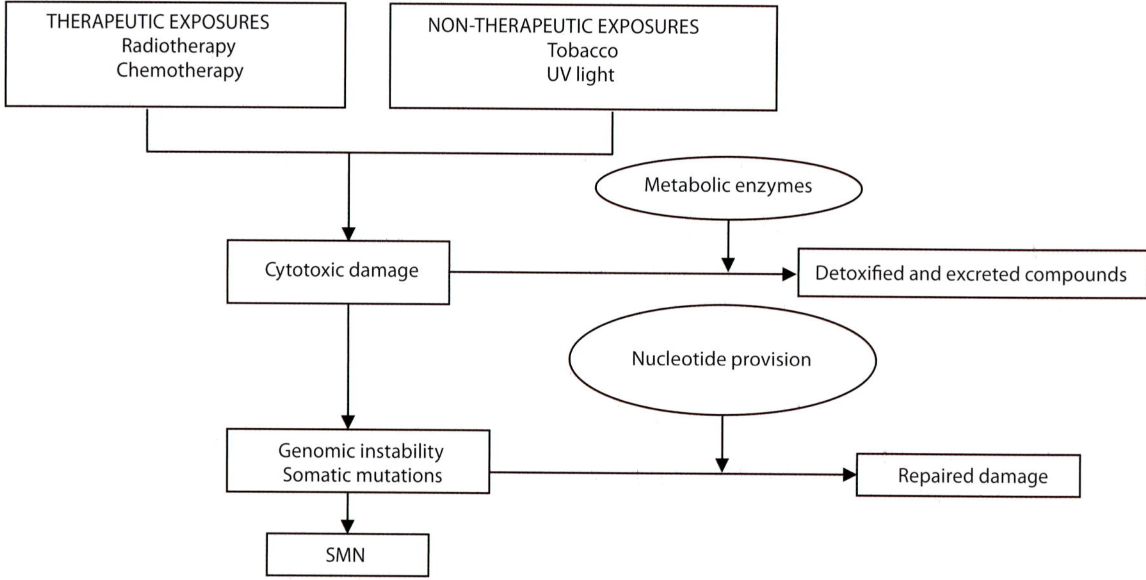

Fig. 14.1. Interaction of therapeutic and environmental exposures in SMN pathogenesis

light. This can lead to genomic instability, somatic mutations and, ultimately, malignancy. Opposing this likelihood are functional enzymes in xenobiotic metabolism, DNA repair and nucleotide provision. Specific allelic variants of these genes may result in enzymes with either increased or decreased activity, which in turn may modify the risk of SMN. This is outlined in Figure 14.1. Therefore, future research should include a simultaneous analysis of treatment, environmental and genetic risk factors, which, acting in concert may increase the risk of SMN post HCT.

14.4
Conclusions

The proportion of second cancers among all cancers in the United States has more than doubled in the past 20 years. With improving survivorship, this percentage is likely to increase. The role of genetic risk factors remains relatively unknown and is best evaluated in the context of treatment and disease-related risk factors, as well as health-related risk behaviors known to promote cancer, such as smoking, alcohol exposure, sun exposure and dietary risk factors. Identifying markers of cancer susceptibility after exposure to carcinogenic therapeutic agents can result in several important outcomes. Patients who harbor a genetic predisposition to subsequent cancers can be more closely monitored during their lifetime, and counseled regarding avoidance of potential co-carcinogens that may share similar metabolic pathways. Treatment for primary malignancies may be altered in those with identified inherited high-risk genotypes. Family members may be at a similarly increased risk of specific malignancies, when exposed to specific carcinogens and may require more targeted preventive strategies and lifetime monitoring for development of malignancy. Specific emphasis can be directed towards the interaction between environmental and therapeutic exposures and genetic susceptibility. The knowledge gained from these lines of investigation will, in part, be generalizable to the larger population of cancer survivors, treated with conventional radiotherapy and at risk for SMN, and at the very least will generate hypotheses.

References

1. Andre M, Henry-Amar M, Blaise D et al (1998) Treatment-related deaths and second cancer risk after autologous stem-cell transplantation for Hodgkin's disease. Blood 92:1933–1940
2. Baker KS, DeFor TE, Burns LJ, Ramsay NK, Neglia JP, Robison LL (2003) New malignancies after blood or mar-

row stem-cell transplantation in children and adults: incidence and risk factors. J Clin Oncol 21:1352–1358

3. Baria K, Warren C, Roberts SA, West CM, Scott D (2001) Chromosomal radiosensitivity as a marker of predisposition to common cancers. Br J Cancer 84:892–896

4. Baria K, Warren C, Eden OB, Roberts SA, West CM, Scott D (2002) Chromosomal radiosensitivity in young cancer patients: possible evidence of genetic predisposition. Int J Radiat Biol 78:341–346

5. Bennett LM (1999) Breast cancer: genetic predisposition and exposure to radiation. Molecular Carcinogenesis 26:143–149

6. Berwick M, Song Y, Jordan R, Brady MS, Orlow I (2001) Mutagen sensitivity as an indicator of soft tissue sarcoma risk. Environ Mol Mutagen 38:223–226

7. Bhatia S, Ramsay NK, Steinbuch M et al (1996) Malignant neoplasms following bone marrow transplantation. Blood 87:3633–3639

8. Bhatia S, Louie AD, Bhatia R et al (2001) Solid cancers after bone marrow transplantation. J Clin Oncol 19:464–471

9. Bondy ML, Wang LE, El-Zein R, de Andrade M, Selvan MS, Bruner JM, Levin VA, Alfred Yung WK, Adatto P, Wei Q (2001) Gamma-radiation sensitivity and risk of glioma. J Natl Cancer Inst 93:1553–1557

10. Buchholz TA, Wu X (2001) Radiation-induced chromatid breaks as a predictor of breast cancer risk. Int J Radiat Oncol Biol Phys 49:533–537

11. Curtis RE, Rowlings PA, Deeg HJ et al (1997) Solid cancers after bone marrow transplantation New Engl J Med 336:897–904

12. Curtis RE, Metayer C, Rizzo JD, Socie G, Sobocinski KA, Flowers ME, Travis WD, Travis LB, Horowitz MM, Deeg HJ (2005) Impact of chronic GVHD therapy on the development of squamous-cell cancers after hematopoietic stem-cell transplantation: an international case-control study. Blood 105:3802–3811

13. Deeg HJ, Witherspoon RP (1993) Risk factors for the development of secondary malignancies after marrow transplantation. Hematol Oncol Clin North Am 7:417–429

14. Deeg HJ, Socie G (1998) Malignancies after hematopoietic stem cell transplantation: many questions, some answers. Blood 91:1833–1844

15. Deeg HJ, Socie G, Schoch G et al (1996) Malignancies after marrow transplantation for aplastic anemia and Fanconi anemia: a joint Seattle and Paris analysis of results in 700 patients. Blood 87:386–392

16. Deeg HJ, Leisenring W, Storb R et al (1998) Long-term outcome after marrow transplantation for severe aplastic anemia. Blood 91:3637–3645

17. Deeg HJ, Schwartz JL, Friedman D, Leisenring W (2003) Secondary malignancies after hemopoietic stem cell transplantation. Turk J Med Sci 33:207–214

18. Epstein E Jr (2001) Genetic determinants of basal cell carcinoma risk. Med Pediatr Oncol 36:555–558

19. Friedman DL, Leisenring W, Schwartz JL, Deeg HJ (2004) Second malignant neoplasms following hematopoietic stem cell transplantation. Int J Hematol 79:229–234

20. Friedman DL, Leisenring W, Flowers MED, Holmberg L, Schwartz J, Deeg HJ (2004) Risk factors for second malignancies after transplantation differ between allogeneic and autologous recipients. Presented at the American Society of Hematology Annual Meeting 2004

21. Friedman DL, Rovo A, Leisenring W, Locasciulli A, Flowers MED, Tichelli A, Sanders JE, Deeg HJ, Socie G (2008) Increased risk of breast cancer among survivors of allogeneic hematopoietic cell transplantation: a report from the FHCRC and the EBMT-Late Effect Working Party. Blood 111:939–944

22. Gallagher G, Forrest DL (2007) Second solid cancers after allogeneic stem cell transplantation. Cancer 109:84–92

23. Hannan MA, Siddiqui Y, Rostom A, Al-Ahdal MN, Chaudhary MA, Kunhi M (2001) Evidence of DNA repair/processing defects in cultured skin fibroblasts from breast cancer patients. Cancer Research 61:3627–3631

24. Hosing C, Munsell M, Yazji S et al (2002) Risk of therapy-related myelodysplastic syndrome/acute leukemia following high-dose therapy and autologous bone marrow transplantation for non-Hodgkin's lymphoma. Ann Oncol 13:450–459

25. Knudson AG Jr (1971) Mutation and cancer: statistical study of retinoblastoma. Proc of the Natl Acad Sci USA 68:820–823

26. Krishnan A, Bhatia S, Slovak ML et al (2000) Predictors of therapy-related leukemia and myelodysplasia following autologous transplantation for lymphoma: an assessment of risk factors. Blood 95:1588–1593

27. LeisenringW, Friedman DL, Flowers ME, Schwartz JL, Deeg HJ (2006) Nonmelanoma skin and mucosal cancers after hematopoietic cell transplantation. J Clin Oncol 24:1119–1126

28. Li FP, Fraumeni JF Jr (1969) Rhabdomyosarcoma in children: epidemiologic study and identification of a familial cancer syndrome. J Natl Cancer Inst 43:1365–1373

29. Lowe T, Bhatia S, Somlo G (2007) Second malignancies after allogeneic hematopoietic cell transplantation. Biol Blood Marrow Transplant 13:1121–1134

30. Malkin D, Jolly KW, Barbier N, Look AT, Friend SH, Gebhardt MC, Andersen TI, Borresen AL, Li FP, Garber J (1992) Germline mutations of the p53 tumor-suppressor gene in children and young adults with second malignant neoplasms. N Engl J Med 326:1309–1315

31. Metayer C, Curtis RE, Vose J et al (2003) Myelodysplastic syndrome and acute myeloid leukemia after autotransplantation for lymphoma: a multicenter case-control study. Blood 101:2015–2023

32. Milligan DW (2000) Secondary leukaemia and myelodysplasia after autografting for lymphoma: is the transplant to blame? Leuk Lymphoma 39:223–228

33. Mossman KL (1997) Radiation protection of radiosensitive populations. Health Physics 72:519–523

34. Papworth R, Slevin N, Roberts SA, Scott D (2001) Sensitivity to radiation-induced chromosome damage may be a marker of genetic predisposition in young head and neck cancer patients. Br J Cancer 84:776–782

35. Pedersen-Bjergaard J, Andersen MK, Christiansen DH (2000) Therapy-related acute myeloid leukemia and myelodysplasia after high-dose chemotherapy and autologous stem cell transplantation. Blood 95:3273–3279

36. Potter JD (2002) At the interfaces of epidemiology, genetics, and genomics. Nat Rev Genet 2:142–147

37. Roberts SA, Spreadborough AR, Bulman B, Barber JB, Evans DG, Scott D (1999) Heritability of cellular radiosensitivity: a marker of low-penetrance predisposition genes in breast cancer. Am J Hum Genet 65:784–794

38. Rowlings PA, Curtis RE, Passweg JR et al (1999) Increased incidence of Hodgkin's disease after allogeneic bone marrow transplantation. J Clin Oncol 17:3122–3127

39. Scott D (2000) Chromosomal radiosensitivity, cancer predisposition and response to radiotherapy. Strahlenther Onkol 176:229–234

40. Seddon JM, Tarbell N, Fraumeni JF Jr, Li FP (1997) Cancer incidence after retinoblastoma. Radiation dose and sarcoma risk. JAMA 278:1262–1267

41. Socie G, Curtis RE, Deeg HJ et al (2000) New malignant diseases after allogeneic marrow transplantation for childhood acute leukemia. J Clin Oncol 18:348–357

42. Strong LC, Williams WR, Tainsky MA (1992) The Li-Fraumeni syndrome: from clinical epidemiology to molecular genetics. Am J Epidemiol 135:190–199

43. Varley JM, Evans DG, Birch JM (1997) Li-Fraumeni syndrome – a molecular and clinical review. Br J Cancer 76:1–14

44. West CM, Hendry JH (1992) Intrinsic radiosensitivity as a predictor of patient response to radiotherapy. BJR Suppl 24:146–152

45. Wong FL, Boice JD Jr, Abramson DH et al (1997) Cancer incidence after retinoblastoma. Radiation dose and sarcoma risk . JAMA 278:1262–1267

Subject Index

List of Contributors

Michael Jacob Adams, MD, MPH
Assistant Professor
Department of Community and Preventive Medicine
University of Rochester
School of Medicine and Dentistry
601 Elmwood Avenue, Box 644
USA

Email: Jacob_Adams@urmc.rochester.edu

Mitchell S. Anscher, MD
Department of Radiation Oncology
Virginia Commonwealth University Medical Center
401 College Street
P.O. Box 980058
Richmond, VA 23298-0058
USA

Email: manscher@mcvh-vcu.edu

Laurence Baker, MD
University of Michigan
Southwest Oncology Group (SWOG)
USA

Maryann Bishop-Jodoin, BS
University of Massachusetts
Quality Assurance Review Center (QARC)
USA

Walter Bosch, DSc
Washington University (ATC)
USA

James Boyett, PhD
St Jude Children's Research Hospital
Pediatric Brain Tumor Consortium (PBTC)
USA

David J. Brenner, PhD, DSc
Professor of Radiation Oncology and Public Health
Center for Radiological Research
Columbia University Medical Center
630 W. 168th Street
New York, NY 10032
USA

Email: djb3@columbia.edu

M. Giulia Cicchetti, MD
University of Massachusetts
Quality Assurance Review Center (QARC)
USA

Robert Comis, MD
Drexel University
Eastern Oncology Cooperative Group (ECOG)
USA

Louis S. Constine, MD
Professor of Radiation Oncology and Pediatrics
Vice Chair, Department of Radiation Oncology
University of Rochester Medical Center
601 Elmwood Avenue, Box 704
Rochester, NY 14642
USA

Email: Louis_constine@urmc.rochester.edu

Joseph Deasy, PhD
Washington University (ATC)
USA

Avraham Eisbruch, MD
Professor and Associate Chair for Clinical Research
Department of Radiation Oncology
University of Michigan Medical Center
Ann Arbor, MI 48109-0010
USA

Email: eisbruch@umich.edu

Thomas J. FitzGerald, MD
Chair, Department of Radiation Oncology
Quality Assurance Review Center (QARC)
University of Massachusetts Memorial Medical Center
55 Lake Avenue North
Worcester, MA 01655
USA

Email: fitzgert@ummhc.org

Debra L. Friedman, MD
Vanderbilt-Ingram Cancer Center
2525 West End Avenue, Sixth Flooor
Nashville, TN 37203
USA

Email: debra.l.friedman@vanderbilt.edu

Paul R. Graves, PhD
Department of Radiation Oncology
Virginia Commonwealth University Medical Center
401 College Street
P.O. Box 980058
Richmond, VA 23298-0058
USA

Email: prgraves@vcu.edu

Joel S. Greenberger, MD
Professor and Chairman
Department of Radiation Oncology
University of Pittsburgh School of Medicine
200 Lothrop Street
Pittsburgh, PA 15213
USA

Email: greenbergerjs@msx.upmc.edu

Carol A. Hahn, MD
Department of Radiation Oncology
Duce University Medical Center
Box 3085
Durham, NC 27710
USA

Denis E. Hallahan, MD
Department of Radiation Oncology
Vanderbilt-Ingram Cancer Center
Vanderbilt University
Nashville, TN 37232
USA

Richard Hanusik, BA
University of Massachusetts
Quality Assurance Review Center (QARC)
USA

Jessica L. Hubbs, MS
Department of Radiation Oncology
University of North Carolina at Chapel Hill
Campus Box 7512
Chapel Hill, NC 27599
USA

Geoffrey Ibbott, PhD
Radiological Physics Center (RPC)
USA

Sandy Kessel, BA
University of Massachusetts
Quality Assurance Review Center (QARC)
USA

Michael Knopp, MD
Ohio Statue University (CALGB)
USA

Andre Konski, MD, MBA, MA FACR
Director Clinical Research
Department of Radiation Oncology
Fox Chase Cancer Center
333 Cottman Avenue
Philadelphia, PA 19111
USA

Email: andre.konski@fccc.edu

Larry Kun, MD
St Jude Children's Research Hospital
Pediatric Brain Tumor Consortium (PBTC)
USA

Fran Laurie, BS
University of Massachusetts
Quality Assurance Review Center (QARC)
USA

Steven E. Lipshultz, MD
George Batchelor Professor and Chairman,
Department of Pediatrics
Professor of Epidemiology and Public Health
Professor of Medicine (Oncology)
Associate Executive Dean for Child Health
Leonard M. Miller School of Medicine
University of Miami
Chief-of-Staff, Holtz Children's Hospital of the
University of Miami-Jackson Memorial Medical Center
Director, Batchelor Children's Research Institute
Associate Director, Mailman Institute for
Child Development
Member, the Sylvester Comprehensive Cancer Center
Miami, FL 33101
USA

Bo Lu, MD, PhD
Assistant Professor
Vanderbilt University
Department of Radiation Oncology
Nashville, TN 37232
USA

Email: Bo.lu@vanderbilt.edu

Lawrence B. Marks, MD
Department of Radiation Oncology
University of North Carolina at Chapel Hill
Campus Box 7512
Chapel Hill, NC 27599
USA

Email: Lawrence.marks@duce.edu

Kathleen McCarten, MD
Hasbro Children's Hospital (QARC)
USA

JOHN MATTHEWS, PhD
Washington University (ATC)
USA

ROSS MIKKELSEN, PhD
Department of Radiation Oncology
Virginia Commonwealth University Medical Center
401 College Street
P.O. Box 980058
Richmond, VA 23298-0058
USA

Email: rmikkels@vcu.edu

MICHAEL T. MILANO, MD, PhD
Department of Radiation Oncology
University of Rochester Medical Center
601 Elmwood Avenue, Box 647
Rochester, NY 14642
USA

BHARAT MITTAL, MD
Professor and Chairman
Department of Radiation Oncology
Northwestern University Medical Center
633 Clark Street Evanston, IL 60208
USA

LUIGI MORETTI, MD
Department of Radiation Oncology
Vanderbilt-Ingram Cancer Center
Vanderbilt University
1301 22nd Avenue South, B-902 TVC
Nashville, TN 37232
USA

KAREN M. MUSTIAN, PhD
Assistant Professor
Department of Radiation Oncology
Department of Community and Preventive Medicine
Susan B. Anthony Institute for Women
and Gender Studies
Center for Future Health
University of Rochester
School of Medicine and Dentistry
601 Elmwood Avenue, Box 704
Rochester, NY 14642
USA

Email: Karen_mustian@urmc.rochester.edu

JIHO NAM, MD
Department of Radiation Oncology
University of North Carolina at Chapel Hill
Campus Box 7512
Chapel Hill, NC 27599
USA

HEIDI NELSON, MD
Mayo Clinic
American College of Surgeons Oncology Group
(ACOSOG)
USA

PAUL OKUNIEFF, MD
Department of Radiation Oncology
University of Rochester Medical Center
601 Elmwood Avenue, Box 647
Rochester, NY 14642
USA

Email: Paul_okunieff@urmc.rochester.edu

DAVID OTA, MD
Duke University (ACOSOG)
USA

MATTHEW PARLIAMENT, MD
Cross Chase Cancer Center
National Cancer Institute Canada (NCIC)
Canada

RICHARD PIETERS, MD
University of Massachusetts
Quality Assurance Review Center (QARC)
USA

JAMES PURDY, PhD
Director of Physics
Vice Chair of Radiation Oncology
University of California at Davis
Advanced Technology Consortium (ATC)
USA

UMA RAMAMURTHY, PhD
St Jude Children's Research Hospital
Pediatric Brain Tumor Consortium (PBTC)
USA

GREGORY REAMAN, MD
George Washington University Medical Center (COG)
USA

NANCY ROSEN, MD
University of Massachusetts
Quality Assurance Review Center (QARC)
USA

Barry S. Rosenstein, MD, PhD
Professor of Radiation Oncology
Departments of Radiation Oncology, Cummunity and
Preventive Medicine and Dermatology
Mount Sinai School of Medicine
Box 1236
One Gustave Levy Place
New York, NY 10029
USA
and
Department of Radiation Oncology
New York University School of Medicine
550 First Avenue
New York, NY 10016
USA

Email: barry.rosenstein@mssm.edu

Philip Rubin, MD
Professor and Chair Emeritus
Department of Radiation Oncology
University of Rochester
School of Medicine and Dentistry
601 Elmwood Avenue, Box 647
Rochester, NY 14642
USA

Email: oncophilip@earthlink.net

Joel Saltz, MD
Chair of Biomedical Informatics
Ohio State University (caBIG)
USA

Richard Schilsky, MD
University of Chicago
Cancer and Leukemia Group B (CALGB)
USA

Mitchell Schnall, MD PhD
University of Pennsylvania
American College of Radiology Imaging Network
(ACRIN)
USA

Lawrence Schwartz, MD
Memorial Sloan Kettering Cancer Center (CALGB)
USA

Ronald G. Schwartz, MD
Professor of Medicine and of Imaging Sciences
Attending in Cardiovascular Medicine,
Imaging and Prevention
Director of Nuclear Cardiology and Cardiac PET CT
University of Rochester
School of Medicine and Dentistry
601 Elmwood Avenue, Box 679
Rochester, NY 14642
USA

Email: Ronald_Schwartz@urmc.rochester.edu

Ashish Sharma, PhD
Ohio State University (caBIG)
USA

Igor Shuryak, MD
Center for Radiological Research
Columbia University Medical Center
630 W. 168th Street
New York, NY 10032
USA

Email: djb3@columbia.edu

Eliot Siegel, MD
University of Maryland (caBIG)
USA

Lois B. Travis, MD, ScD
1275 East First Avenue, #159
New York, NY 10065
USA

Email: travis1122@optonline.net

Ken Ulin, PhD
University of Massachusetts
Quality Assurance Review Center (QARC)
USA

Marcia Urie, PhD
University of Massachusetts
Quality Assurance Review Center (QARC)
USA

Stephan Voss, MD, PhD
Boston Children's Hospital
Childrens Oncology Group (COG)
USA

Zeliko Vujaskovic, MD, PhD
Department of Radiation Oncology
Duke University Medical Center,
P.O. Box 3085 DUMC
Durham, NC 27710
USA

Email: zeljko.vujakovic@duke.edu

Keith White, MD
Primary Childrens Medical Center
Salt Lake City, Utah
USA

Jackie P. Williams, PhD
Professor, Department of Radiation Oncology
University of Rochester Medical Center
601 Elmwood Avenue, Box 647
Rochester, NY 14642
USA

Eddy S. Yang, MD, PhD
Department of Radiation Oncology
Vanderbilt-Ingram Cancer Center
Vanderbilt University
Nashville, TN 37232
USA

Jeff Yorty, CMD
University of Massachusetts
Quality Assurance Review Center (QARC)
USA

Sumin Zhou, PhD
Department of Radiation Oncology
Duke University Medical Center
Box 3085
Durham, NC 27710
USA

RADIATION ONCOLOGY

Lung Cancer
Edited by C. W. Scarantino

Innovations in Radiation Oncology
Edited by H. R. Withers, L. J. Peters

**Radiation Therapy
of Head and Neck Cancer**
Edited by G. E. Laramore

**Gastrointestinal Cancer –
Radiation Therapy**
Edited by R. R. Dobelbower, Jr.

**Radiation Exposure
and Occupational Risks**
Edited by E. Scherer, C. Streffer,
K.-R. Trott

Interventional Radiation
Therapy Techniques – Brachytherapy
Edited by R. Sauer

Radiopathology of Organs and Tissues
Edited by E. Scherer, C. Streffer,
K.-R. Trott

Concomitant Continuous Infusion
Chemotherapy and Radiation
Edited by M. Rotman, C. J. Rosenthal

**Intraoperative Radiotherapy –
Clinical Experiences and Results**
Edited by F. A. Calvo, M. Santos,
L. W. Brady

**Interstitial and Intracavitary
Thermoradiotherapy**
Edited by M. H. Seegenschmiedt,
R. Sauer

Non-Disseminated Breast Cancer
Controversial Issues in Management
Edited by G. H. Fletcher, S. H. Levitt

**Current Topics in
Clinical Radiobiology of Tumors**
Edited by H.-P. Beck-Bornholdt

**Practical Approaches to
Cancer Invasion and Metastases**
*A Compendium of Radiation
Oncologists' Responses to 40 Histories*
Edited by A. R. Kagan with the
Assistance of R. J. Steckel

Radiation Therapy in Pediatric Oncology
Edited by J. R. Cassady

Radiation Therapy Physics
Edited by A. R. Smith

Late Sequelae in Oncology
Edited by J. Dunst, R. Sauer

Mediastinal Tumors. Update 1995
Edited by D. E. Wood, C. R. Thomas, Jr.

**Thermoradiotherapy
and Thermochemotherapy**
Volume 1:
Biology, Physiology, and Physics
Volume 2:
Clinical Applications
Edited by M. H. Seegenschmiedt,
P. Fessenden, C. C. Vernon

Carcinoma of the Prostate
Innovations in Management
Edited by Z. Petrovich, L. Baert,
L. W. Brady

Radiation Oncology of Gynecological Cancers
Edited by H. W. Vahrson

Carcinoma of the Bladder
Innovations in Management
Edited by Z. Petrovich, L. Baert,
L. W. Brady

**Blood Perfusion and
Microenvironment of Human Tumors**
*Implications for
Clinical Radiooncology*
Edited by M. Molls, P. Vaupel

Radiation Therapy of Benign Diseases
A Clinical Guide
2nd Revised Edition
S. E. Order, S. S. Donaldson

**Carcinoma of the Kidney and Testis,
and Rare Urologic Malignancies**
Innovations in Management
Edited by Z. Petrovich, L. Baert,
L. W. Brady

**Progress and Perspectives in the
Treatment of Lung Cancer**
Edited by P. Van Houtte,
J. Klastersky, P. Rocmans

**Combined Modality Therapy of
Central Nervous System Tumors**
Edited by Z. Petrovich, L. W. Brady,
M. L. Apuzzo, M. Bamberg

Age-Related Macular Degeneration
Current Treatment Concepts
Edited by W. E. Alberti, G. Richard,
R. H. Sagerman

**Radiotherapy of Intraocular and
Orbital Tumors**
2nd Revised Edition
Edited by R. H. Sagerman, W. E. Alberti

Modification of Radiation Response
*Cytokines, Growth Factors,
and Other Biolgical Targets*
Edited by C. Nieder, L. Milas, K. K. Ang

Radiation Oncology for Cure and Palliation
R. G. Parker, N. A. Janjan, M. T. Selch

**Clinical Target Volumes in Conformal and
Intensity Modulated Radiation Therapy**
A Clinical Guide to Cancer Treatment
Edited by V. Grégoire, P. Scalliet,
K. K. Ang

**Advances in Radiation Oncology
in Lung Cancer**
Edited by B. Jeremić

New Technologies in Radiation Oncology
Edited by W. Schlegel, T. Bortfeld,
A.-L. Grosu

**Multimodal Concepts for Integration of
Cytotoxic Drugs and Radiation Therapy**
Edited by J. M. Brown, M. P. Mehta,
C. Nieder

Technical Basis of Radiation Therapy
Practical Clinical Applications
4th Revised Edition
Edited by S. H. Levitt, J. A. Purdy,
C. A. Perez, S. Vijayakumar

**CURED I · LENT
Late Effects of Cancer Treatment
on Normal Tissues**
Edited by P. Rubin, L. S. Constine,
L. B. Marks, P. Okunieff

Radiotherapy for Non-Malignant Disorders
Contemporary Concepts and Clinical Results
Edited by M. H. Seegenschmiedt,
H.-B. Makoski, K.-R. Trott, L. W. Brady

**CURED II · LENT
Cancer Survivorship Research and Education**
Late Effects on Normal Tissues
Edited by P. Rubin, L. S. Constine,
L. B. Marks, P. Okunieff

Radiation Oncology
An Evidence-Based Approach
Edited by J. J. Lu, L. W. Brady

Primary Optic Nerve Sheath Meningioma
Edited by B. Jeremić, S. Pitz

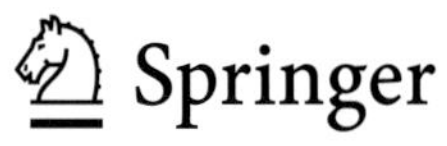

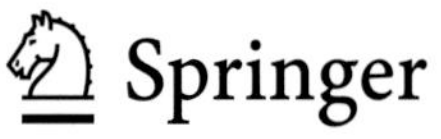

Springer